PRAISE FOR GRA.

'Engagingly written ... one of the most
nuanced portraits to date'
The Australian

'Vivid, detailed and well written'
Daily Telegraph

'A staggering accomplishment that can't be missed by
history buffs and story lovers alike'
Betterreading.com.au

'A free-flowing biography of a great Australian figure'
John Howard

'Clear and accessible ... well-crafted and
extensively documented'
Weekend Australian

'Kieza has added hugely to the depth of knowledge about
our greatest military general in a book that is timely'
Tim Fischer, *Courier-Mail*

'The author writes with the immediacy of a fine
documentary ... an easy, informative read, bringing
historic personalities to life'
Ballarat Courier

ALSO BY GRANTLEE KIEZA

Flinders

Knockout: Great Australian Boxing Stories

The Remarkable Mrs Reibey

Hudson Fysh

The Kelly Hunters

Lawson

Banks

Macquarie

Banjo

The Hornet (with Jeff Horn)

Boxing in Australia

Mrs Kelly: The Astonishing Life of Ned Kelly's Mother

Monash: The Soldier Who Shaped Australia

Sons of the Southern Cross

Bert Hinkler: The Most Daring Man in the World

The Retriever (with Keith Schafferius)

A Year to Remember (with Mark Waugh)

Stopping the Clock: Health and Fitness the George Daldry Way
(with George Daldry)

Fast and Furious: A Celebration of Cricket's Pace Bowlers

Mark My Words: The Mark Graham Story
(with Alan Clarkson and Brian Mossop)

Australian Boxing: The Illustrated History

Fenech: The Official Biography (with Peter Muszkat)

Sister Viv

GRANTLEE KIEZA

ABC
BOOKS

This book contains descriptions of wartime violence, torture and death that some readers may find distressing.

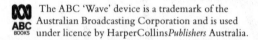 The ABC 'Wave' device is a trademark of the Australian Broadcasting Corporation and is used under licence by HarperCollins*Publishers* Australia.

HarperCollins*Publishers*
Australia • Brazil • Canada • France • Germany • Holland • India
Italy • Japan • Mexico • New Zealand • Poland • Spain • Sweden
Switzerland • United Kingdom • United States of America

HarperCollins acknowledges the Traditional Custodians
of the land upon which we live and work, and pays respect
to Elders past and present.

First published on Gadigal country in Australia in 2024
by HarperCollins*Publishers* Australia Pty Limited
ABN 36 009 913 517
harpercollins.com.au

A catalogue record for this book is available from the National Library of Australia

ISBN 978 0 7333 4329 2 (hardback)
ISBN 978 1 4607 1701 1 (ebook)

Cover design by Michelle Zaiter, HarperCollins Design Studio
Cover images: Sister Vivian Bullwinkel by Gordon Short/Fairfax Media; ocean and boat by
istockphoto.com
Author photograph by Milen Boubbov
Typeset in Bembo Std by Kelli Lonergan
Printed and bound in Australia by McPherson's Printing Group

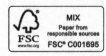

For Philippa, Alessia and Matthew Barone

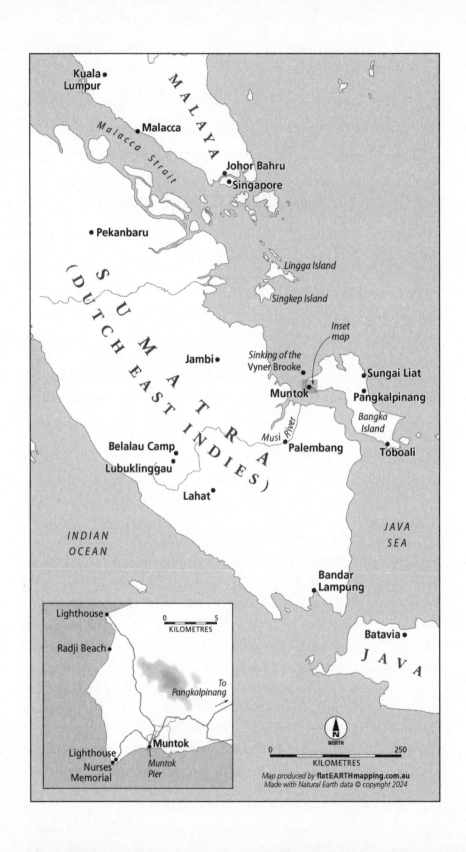

Kuala
Lumpur

MALAYA

Malacca

Malacca Strait

Johor Bahru
Singapore

Pekanbaru

SUMATRA
(DUTCH EAST INDIES)

Lingga Island

Singkep Island

Inset
map

Jambi

Sinking of the
Vyner Brooke

Muntok

Sungai Liat

Pangkalpinang

Bangka
Island

Belalau Camp

Lubuklinggau

Musi River

Palembang

Toboali

Lahat

INDIAN
OCEAN

JAVA
SEA

Bandar
Lampung

Batavia

JAVA

Lighthouse

Radji Beach

0   5
KILOMETRES

To
Pangkalpinang

Lighthouse

Nurses
Memorial

Muntok

Muntok
Pier

0   250
KILOMETRES

N
NORTH

Map produced by **flatEARTHmapping.com.au**
Made with Natural Earth data © copyright 2024

Forewords

As a vivacious 26-year-old army nursing sister, my aunt Vivian Bullwinkel miraculously survived the massacre of her colleagues on Radji Beach by Japanese troops during World War II.

Faced with unimaginable horror under the Japanese, Vivian called upon the greatest of human drives, the fight for survival. As her friends died around her, Vivian survived despite a gaping bullet wound in her body and she then lived through three and a half years of starvation, disease and cruelty in prisoner of war camps while tormented by sadistic guards.

Vivian's immense courage and tenacity were exhibited daily to preserve not only herself but also to ensure the survival of the many other nurses and civilians around her.

Every day she drew on her resilience, resourcefulness, determination and compassion to maintain her own spirits and assist others who were weaker than herself.

Caring for the sick and dying without food and medicine was a constant struggle for Vivian and all her colleagues, and she called on not just her nursing skills but also her natural cunning and immense physical and mental strength.

Often she found that laughter was the best medicine to deal with difficult situations. This was certainly a tonic that she used in dark times, not just in wartime but also in the years that followed as she became a leading figure in Australian nursing and the Australian Army.

In the years after World War II, Vivian continued to help the chronically sick and dying especially at the outbreak of and throughout the AIDS epidemic. She was instrumental in helping to raise educational standards and recognition for nurses while encouraging so many others to follow her example of great compassion and empathy.

She was an extraordinary woman and a great Australian.

I hope you enjoy reading the story of her remarkable life.

John Bullwinkel, January 2024

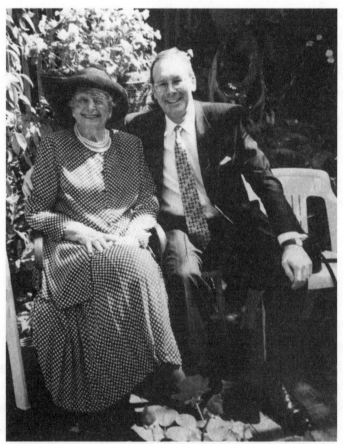

John Bullwinkel with his beloved Aunt Viv in the twilight of her remarkable life. *Vivian Bullwinkel collection*

Lieutenant Colonel Vivian Bullwinkel was an extraordinary woman; she was humble, generous and had an unbreakable fortitude. She was the sole survivor of a horrendous war crime on Bangka Island in 1942. But more than that, Vivian was dedicated to all people, a true leader – honourable and dignified. She was a true humanitarian.

The Australian War Memorial is a place that stirs the soul; it helps us reflect on love and loss, on sacrifice and gratitude, on war and peace. It was where I felt we needed to have Lt Col Vivian Bullwinkel and nurses remembered forever.

In February 2019, I met with Dr Brendan Nelson AO in his capacity as Director of the Australian War Memorial, along with retired Wing Commander and Australian War Memorial Council Member Sharon Bown FACN. That meeting kick-started our four-and-a-half-year journey – through the pandemic – that resulted in raising a statue of Lt Col Vivian Bullwinkel in bronze, the first Australian female and nurse commemorated in this way.

Recent years have reminded us that nurses work when and where others don't or won't. Yet, our military nursing colleagues take it one step further; they are loyal to the profession and country, prepared to sacrifice so much personally. They ensure that our military personnel have the care they need to defend us as well as carry out their humanitarian duties.

Lt Col Vivian Bullwinkel embodied what we stand for as nurses. She was dedicated in her career, in protecting others, in driving nursing education through university and ensuring the profession was respected. She had every right to return home from the war and live a quiet life, but Vivian went on to have a profound civilian career championing the rights of nurses, while also working as Matron of the Fairfield Infectious Diseases Hospital in Melbourne.

In August 2023, it was my honour on behalf of the Australian College of Nursing, to recognise Lt Col Vivian Bullwinkel, the 21 fallen nurses and one civilian who died on Bangka Island, along with the 65 nurses who boarded the doomed *Vyner Brooke* on 12 February 1942, as they evacuated Singapore. Vivian's story is embedded in the historical fabric of our society and has shaped how the nurses of Australia define themselves. All Australians deserve to honour her alongside the nursing profession.

The statue will inspire and educate future generations, and it has been a privilege to have played a part to ensure all nurses are remembered in Australian history. Thank you to Grantlee Kieza for writing such a vivid recollection of Vivian's life.

Adjunct Professor Kylie Ward RN, MMgt, FACN, FCHSM (HON), Wharton Fellow, FAICD
CEO of Australian College of Nursing
CEO of Australian College of Nursing Foundation
Board Chair Australian Nursing & Midwifery
Accreditation Council (ANMAC)

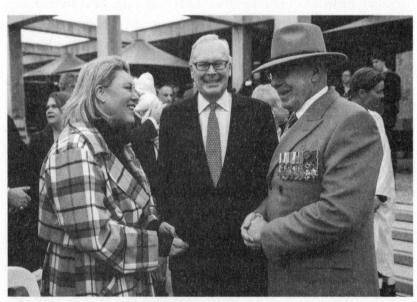

Adjunct Professor Kylie Ward, with John Bullwinkel (centre) and Governor-General David Hurley at the unveiling of the Vivian Bullwinkel statue at the Australian War Memorial in August 2023. *Australian College of Nursing*

Prologue

THE SHOCKING ROAR OF GUNFIRE sent a blast of adrenaline and fear through Vivian Bullwinkel. As flocks of birds burst from their jungle hiding places, the young woman's gaze darted towards where, beyond a headland about a hundred metres away, Japanese soldiers[1] had marched two groups of prisoners, about 25 of them, many of them badly wounded British soldiers and sailors. Viv's face devolved into a mask of shock and dread.

In the two months since Japanese fighter planes had obliterated the pride of America's naval strength in their lightning attack on Pearl Harbor, Japan had unleashed hell as its armed forces surged south in their conquest of Malaya, their sophisticated, heavily armed fighter planes and bombers opening the way for their small, rapid tanks and well-trained, ruthless fighting men to destroy anything and anyone in their path.

A few days earlier, Viv had survived the Japanese annihilation of Australian, British and Indian troops in Singapore. In the fear and chaos of that attack, she and other Australian nurses, along with civilians and wounded soldiers and sailors, had made their escape south on a small, overloaded cargo ship,[2] but the vessel had soon been assailed by Japanese aerial bombardment. After a harrowing, life-and-death battle with the sea, some of the evacuees had washed up here, on Bangka Island's Radji Beach off the coast of Sumatra in the Dutch East Indies.

3

Now, just after 10 a.m. on 16 February 1942, under the cruel gaze of Japanese captors, Viv, twenty-one of her nursing comrades, and an elderly British woman whose husband was dying, were assembled on the beach, too terrified to move. Their captors were a brutal detachment of Japan's 229th regiment, who only a few weeks earlier had raped and murdered their way through the hospital that had been St Stephen's College in Hong Kong, leaving a trail of mutilated corpses on Christmas Day.[3]

Viv wasn't certain what the Japanese soldiers had done to the men after they'd marched them away. She wasn't sure that they'd killed them all, but she knew it was wishful thinking to believe the blasts coming from beyond the headland were warning shots. Some of those men were her dear friends.

Huddled together, the Australian nurses told each other to be brave no matter what. But their hearts sank when the Japanese soldiers returned from the headland without any of their prisoners.

As they walked in single file behind their captain, Orita Masaru, a small intense young officer with a neatly cut uniform and a sword by his side, the soldiers were laughing.[4] When they reached the captive women, they began to wipe blood from their bayonets with rags.[5]

Viv's mind raced. *No prisoners … no prisoners … they're not taking prisoners.*[6] She and the other nurses had heard rumours that the Japanese killed all their captives. Now Viv was mortified to realise that the rumours were true. The fact that this grim reality had hit her on a pristine, sunny beach surrounded by an azure sea and swaying palm trees was incomprehensible.

How could something so evil be happening in such a beautiful place?

Viv was a brave, tough girl who had grown up in the hardscrabble world of Broken Hill and had spent years giving comfort to the sick and the dying, a young woman who had mended broken bones and shattered hearts as a nurse in a mining centre, and then on the frontline of a fiendish war. Now, after spending so many years saving lives, she and her comrades knew for sure that their own lives were about to end thousands of miles from the warm embrace of home. Many badly wounded men and women were lying on stretchers nearby. What would the Japanese do with them?

Viv watched, frozen, as Japanese soldiers set up a machine gun beneath picture-perfect palm trees fringing the beach.

Then they ordered Viv and the others to walk towards the water.

Chapter 1

BULLWINKEL (nee Shegog). – On the 18th December,
at Kapunda, to Mr. and Mrs. G. A. Bullwinkel – a daughter.[1]

THUS VIVIAN BULLWINKEL arrived kicking and screaming joyous sounds of new life into a world gone mad with killing.

It was seven days before Christmas, 1915, and Vivian's birth was a godsend to her first-time parents Eva[2] and George Bullwinkel.[3] The baby girl's first cries came at the same time as thousands of Australian soldiers were at war on the far side of the world.

Although the fighting in what had already been dubbed 'The Great War' had not come close to Vivian's birthplace – a small South Australian farm town called Kapunda, about an hour north of Adelaide on the locomotive – its aftershocks had. Local clergymen had already started making the sad pilgrimage to some of the Bullwinkels' neighbours to break the news that a son or brother, husband or father had died on a foreign field.

Eva was twenty-seven when she brought Vivian into the world. From a well-established South Australian family, she was the daughter of William Shegog,[4] a veteran policeman who was born in Londonderry, the second largest city in what is now Northern Ireland. William had come to Australia in 1857 as an infant when his family migrated to the Victorian goldfields. A relative, James Shegog, had been a rough-riding sergeant-major in the Charge of the Heavy Brigade in the Crimea in 1854, an attack on Russian forces that took place just prior to the celebrated Charge of the Light Brigade.[5] William had been schooled in the central Victorian gold town of Maryborough before working as a farmer in the area.[6] At the age of twenty-five he had moved to Adelaide to join the mounted police, his life for the next four decades. At his first posting in Port Augusta, he married a local girl named Emily Robinson.[7] Eva, their second child, was born there three years later.

Shegog was a good rough rider, one of the best horsemen in the force and a proven performer when it came to taming wild horses and even wilder criminals.[8] He set an example of service to the community, accepting assignments in small and often far-flung South Australian towns.[9] Wherever he went, his young family followed.

The man who would become Vivian Bullwinkel's grandfather came to national attention in 1899 after the 70-metre-long Scottish ship *Loch Sloy* was smashed to pieces on the Brothers Rocks just off Kangaroo Island in the early hours of 24 April 1899.

Of the thirty-four passengers and crew on board, only four men managed to reach the shore after making it through the raging surf as they dodged pieces of the ship's shattered masts that were flying about like missiles. Once on land the four went in search of help.[10] Three men were rescued, utterly spent, shoeless and almost mad with hunger and thirst after two weeks in the elements, but there was no sign of the fourth survivor, David Kilpatrick, an injured 25-year-old cook from Glasgow.

William was sent with Aboriginal trackers to look for the missing man around the Rocky River on the west end of Kangaroo Island. A few days later they found what was left of Kilpatrick and buried him, along with many of the dead from the *Loch Sloy*, whose bloated bodies had washed up on shore.

WILLIAM'S DAUGHTER EVA had gone to a variety of schools as her father took up remote postings. The colonies of the Australian continent became a federated nation in 1901 and began raising a combined military force for mutual defence, with both Russia and Japan perceived as threats.

However, on the subject of recruiting women for the armed forces, Eva's brother Bill,[11] then fifteen, wrote a letter to the editor of the Adelaide newspaper *The Chronicle* from his father's posting in Yongala in 1901 to declare that women had no place in a war zone.[12] Not everyone agreed, and the Australian Army Nursing Service was formed the next year.

Eva had grown into a tall teenager with a huge smile, and was an accomplished pianist, performing at school events and functions for the Anglican church and country sporting associations. She was a handy cricketer too, captaining women's sides in park games.

At the age of twenty-six she made a partnership for life with a gregarious Englishman named George Bullwinkel, who was nine years older. George was the second son of a liquor merchant from Essex, John Bullwinkel, and the grandson of Johann Bullwinkel, who was born in Hanover, Germany, in 1819 and had started the family business in wine and spirits after moving to London aged eighteen and becoming the publican of the Kings Arms in Whitechapel.

George Bullwinkel was also on the move at eighteen, arriving in Australia to work as a jackaroo and bookkeeper on the vast sheep property Mutooroo Station on the border of South Australia and New South Wales. It was a vastly different world from the narrow lanes of London, but George fell in love with the never-ending plains by day, and at night the wondrous glory of the everlasting stars. He travelled vast distances on horseback and formed lifelong friendships.[13]

George had spent thirteen years at Mutooroo before making his way about 100 kilometres to the north-east where the flourishing mines of Broken Hill on the edge of outback New South Wales[14] had drawn workers and investment from around the world. Broken Hill had become one of the richest cities on the globe, its Line of Lode – a treasure chest of silver, lead and zinc – earning the desert town the nickname of 'Silver City'. By the time George arrived, Broken Hill had steam trams running down its main streets and seventy pubs, more per capita than any other place in Australia. It also had one of the most heavily unionised workforces in the British Empire.[15]

George found a job as a clerk and timekeeper at Amalgamated Zinc, or De Bavay's, as the company was better known after its founder Auguste de Bavay,[16] a Belgian who, after being tasked with improving the lager output at Melbourne's Foster's brewery, took his knowledge of chemistry to Broken Hill. George dabbled in mining investments in a small way, too, but none made him rich. He spent much of his spare time involved in Freemason activities and, after being elected chairman, organising soccer matches for the Norths Club.[17]

George met William Shegog's son Bill, who was working as an auctioneer in Broken Hill. Bill introduced George to his sister Eva and the couple became engaged.

George and Eva were married on 16 April 1914 at Adelaide's gothic-style St Paul's Church.[18] It was a day of scattered showers over Adelaide but storm clouds were gathering over the entire globe, with an unprecedented arms race in Europe. Warfare was being industrialised like never before, with rapid and dramatic improvements to weapons. In August 1914, just four months after George and Eva's wedding, Australia was drawn into a world war.

The couple were living in Broken Hill at the end of October 1914 when the first great wave of Australian soldiers headed into battle to support their King and the British Empire. The First Australian Imperial Force and the New Zealand Expeditionary Force – together known as the Australian and New Zealand Army Corps or ANZAC – left King George Sound off Albany, Western Australia, in a convoy of thirty-eight troopships. The convoy stretched for 12 kilometres, with the Japanese cruiser *Ibuki* one of four warships enlisted to give the transports safe escort. Japan, seeing a chance to expand its influence in China, had formed an alliance with the United Kingdom, France and their old enemy, Russia. The Australians felt safe now that the Japanese were on their side.

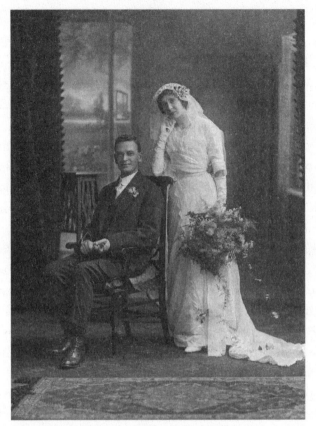

Vivian's parents, George and Eva Bullwinkel, on their
wedding day in Adelaide in 1914. *Vivian Bullwinkel collection*

THE WAR HAD COME TO BROKEN HILL on the first day
of 1915. At 10 a.m., a long and crowded train made up of open
ore wagons carrying more than 1200 New Year's Day picnickers
pulled away from the Broken Hill platform heading for a holiday
gathering beside a shady creek in Silverton, 25 kilometres away.

Ten minutes into the journey the train slowed because of sand
across the tracks and the passengers saw a small two-wheeled
cart on which was painted 'Lakovsky's Delicious ITALIAN ICE
CREAM. A Food fit for Children and Invalids'.[19]

The cart belonged to Badsha Mahomed Gool, a 39-year-old
from the mountainous Tirah region close to what is now the
border between Pakistan and Afghanistan. Gool had come to
Australia as a cameleer and worked in a silver mine until the

outbreak of war but was laid off after contracts with German smelters were cancelled. He had become a popular figure in Broken Hill, dispensing lollies and ice cream for threepence a scoop. With Gool beside the railway track on New Year's Day 1915 was his friend Mullah Abdullah, a sixty-year-old imam, most likely from the same region.

The two men each had an antiquated rifle, a home-made Ottoman flag, and a burning, fire-eyed zeal to answer the call of Mehmed V, sultan of the Ottoman Empire, who on 11 November 1914 had signed a treaty with Germany and declared a holy war against Great Britain and her allies.

Gool and Abdullah opened fire on the train. Alma Cowie, a seventeen-year-old dairyman's daughter, had half her head blown off. Two men, William Shaw and Alf Millard were also killed, before the train driver lurched the vehicle away as quickly as he could. Another man, Jim Craig, also died in what was termed 'The Battle of Broken Hill', after he was hit by a stray bullet while cutting wood in his yard.[20]

The pair of terrorists were surrounded by a posse from town and gunned down. The following night, police fought hard to stop attacks on Broken Hill's Muslim community, but a furious mob burned down the local German Club.[21] Broken Hill was placed under what was essentially martial law.[22] Peace was eventually restored, and as auditor of Broken Hill's British Association Football – or soccer competition – George Bullwinkel absorbed himself in trying to keep some semblance of normal life in his community. He urged everyone who could to 'don the jersey and short knickers, and play the game'.[23]

The previous football season had been the biggest and most successful that soccer fans had experienced in Broken Hill. A team representing the city had visited Adelaide to play the South Australian side, and there was a local country-of-origin match for players representing England against Scotland.[24]

A YEAR AFTER THEIR WEDDING, Eva became pregnant. George continued with his work at De Bavay's but the local soccer competition petered out as most of Broken Hill's star players volunteered for active duty.[25]

News began to reach home about the first major campaign of the war to involve troops who were becoming known as 'Anzacs'. On 25 April 1915, at what would be called Anzac Cove, 16,000 Australian and New Zealand troops stormed a stony beach to start a campaign to capture the Gallipoli Peninsula in Türkiye – part of the Ottoman Empire – and ensure safe supply routes to Russia through the waterway known as the Dardanelles. More than 600 Australians died on the first day of fighting, most of them torn apart by Turks defending their homeland from the rugged cliffs over the landing places.

Over the next few months as Eva's pregnancy progressed, attacks and counterattacks continued over those maddeningly twisted ravines at Gallipoli. More than 8700 Australians died fighting at places such as Sari Bair, Krithia, Lone Pine and the Nek. The dead were buried in hastily dug graves while the wounded were ferried out under machine-gun and artillery fire to hospital ships off the coast or to primitive hospitals on Lemnos, where dedicated Australian nurses worked around the clock.

As Eva's delivery approached, the Gallipoli campaign had become mired in a grim stalemate, and Allied commanders had started to discuss an evacuation of the peninsula. They wanted to avoid thousands more casualties at Gallipoli and instead redeploy the troops to the killing fields of the Western Front in Europe.

A ruse would be needed to minimise casualties in such difficult terrain with little cover. So it was that the Anzac soldiers adopted an escape plan in which they would bluff their way out of Gallipoli in stages, leaving on barges under the cover of darkness.

The evacuation started after sunset on 13 December and within three days the Anzac garrison had been reduced from 41,000 to 26,000.

Eva had decided to have her baby in Kapunda because her father was stationed there and her mother, Emily, would provide the comfort and support that only a mother could. As Eva was just hours away from going into labour, General William Birdwood, the Englishman in command of all Australian forces, went along the whole kilometre and a half of Gallipoli territory held by the troops under Melbourne engineer John Monash, shaking hands with all the officers.

If the Turks suspected the Anzac ranks were being thinned out on the peninsula they would attack with overwhelming force. So the Anzacs moved about at night and in deadly silence, shooting back at the Turks throughout their withdrawal. They even created a device for firing rifles automatically to make it appear the Anzacs were still maintaining their positions.

On 18 December, the night that Eva Bullwinkel gave birth to Vivian, the Anzacs had begun the final stages of their exit from Gallipoli.

The next day, as Eva held baby Viv close and wondered what sort of life her darling might have, the Turks bombarded the Gallipoli beaches as usual. Under the cover of darkness that night, however, the last Anzacs on the peninsula gradually made their way to the boats.

At 1.55 a.m. on 20 December 1915, Monash's last man had left that barren, deadly place. 'Thus dramatically with the bullets whistling harmlessly overhead,' Monash wrote later, 'we drew off in the light of the full moon, mercifully screened by a thin mist – and so ended the story of the Anzacs on Gallipoli.'[26]

Little Vivian Bullwinkel was now two days old. Soon news was circulating around Kapunda that thousands of Australians had somehow escaped certain death on a foreign field.

The campaign had resulted in at least 130,000 deaths but some called the survival of the last Anzacs there a miracle.[27]

Chapter 2

VIVIAN BULLWINKEL'S PARENTS were presented with her Certificate of Holy Baptism on 15 October 1916.[1] She took her first tottering baby steps in Broken Hill during a time of immense agitation and distress. As she spoke her first words, the Great War was becoming a series of long, gruelling, bloody campaigns of attrition in France, Flanders, Egypt and Palestine. Millions were being devoured in combat and the pandemics that began to spread as a result of the conflict. Broken Hill was typical of so many cities and towns in Australia, with large numbers of young local men and boys volunteering to lubricate the insatiable machinery of war. Eventually more than 3000 men and boys from Broken Hill volunteered to fight. The Bullwinkels knew many of the 365 who were eventually killed in the conflict.[2]

George was working in an essential service, and with a new baby he was not leaving home. His beloved soccer competition had been discontinued for the duration of the war, but he and Viv's uncle Bill Shegog spent some of their spare time at meetings of the Broken Hill YMCA Stamp Club, where George was the secretary and treasurer and custodian of the city's most prized collection of stamps from around the world.[3] George also became a life member of the Broken Hill Masonic Club,[4] and presided over meetings of Broken Hill's gatherings of the Ancient Order of Foresters,[5] a British friendly society, and of his local Buffalo lodge, another club designed to foster conviviality among local men. He was not so much old school as ancient in his thinking, and as a defender of masonic values he developed an abiding grudge against all things Catholic. At the time Broken Hill was roughly half Catholic, mostly of Irish descent, and half Protestant, mostly of British ancestry. George believed in religious separation. The Catholics had their ways and the Protestants theirs and the two should not mix, he said.[6]

Finally, after the most destructive four years mankind had yet recorded, World War I ended with an armistice signed aboard a railway carriage in a French forest on 11 November 1918. Viv was not quite three years old but she could not help but be caught up in the joy that peace, temporary as it might be, had arrived. As the world breathed a sigh of relief, a veil of tension was lifted from everyone around her. Before long Viv was a happy little girl at Broken Hill's Morgan Street Kindergarten.

The fighting between 1914 and 1918 had killed about ten million soldiers and an equal number of civilians, around four times the entire population of Australia in total. Another twenty million people had been seriously wounded or maimed, and as many as fifty million people had died from the Spanish flu pandemic that raged across the globe in the war's aftermath.

The Treaty of Versailles, signed in June 1919, forced the Germans to accept responsibility for all the aggression that led to the war and for all the deaths and damage it caused. It stripped Germany of its colonies and about 13 per cent of its European territories. The nation was forced to pay huge reparations to the Allied powers, and the German military was disarmed. Almost immediately, resentment began to ferment. A League of Nations was formed as a global police force designed to prevent further wars.

VIV'S GRANDFATHER, another ardent Freemason, was now Sergeant Shegog. He had been transferred from Kapunda to Renmark on the banks of the Murray River,[7] and then back to Port Augusta. In 1919 he was made a sub-inspector in charge of South Australia's Far Northern Division.[8] The following year he retired from the force, taking his police pension, a gold medal

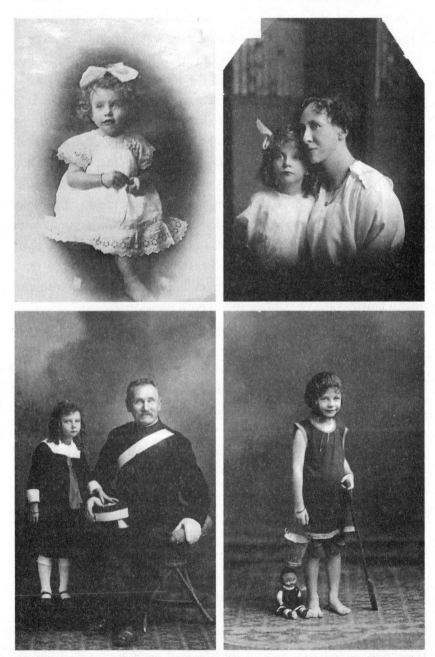

Clockwise from top left: Vivian aged 17 months; at age 6 with her mother Eva; ready for a day at the beach with her favourite doll; at age 7 with her grandfather William Shegog in Adelaide. *Vivian Bullwinkel collection*

'suitably inscribed' and a shaving kit as gifts from a grateful department.[9] He and Viv's grandmother Emily moved to Prospect, an inner-city Adelaide suburb, and Viv and her mother became frequent visitors, taking the train from Broken Hill. For a little girl the rattle and hum of the locomotive heading out of Broken Hill across the desert landscape of South Australia's arid north before reaching the grand city of churches on the Torrens was the thrill of her young life.

Broken Hill remained a hotbed of strife. Mining was still a dangerous job undertaken mostly with hand tools and horse- and mule-drawn carts working underground. With the end of the war and the return of a workforce that had already undergone years of trauma, dissent at the Broken Hill mines escalated in a fight for better conditions. In May 1919, strike action was taken over long hours and unsafe work practices. The industrial action forced many families into hardship and even starvation.[10]

Viv's mother was pregnant again near the end of the 'Great Strike' and Viv's grey-eyed baby brother, John William,[11] named in honour of both his grandfathers and often called 'Jack' in childhood, was born in Broken Hill in April 1920. Although the workers were fighting for better conditions, achieving success was a long process and long periods of industrial action saw the Silver City starting to sag at the knees. Thousands were queueing for food rations. John Bullwinkel joined Viv at a time when *The Bulletin* magazine reported:

> What was once a prosperous city is now something spiritless, existing only like a man with an incurable disease. The greatest mass of machinery south of the line is idle, the unionists' savings bank accounts are all gone, and in many cases their homes are gone too.[12]

The Great Strike lasted until November 1920, and although it eventually won the miners a workers' compensation scheme and a 35-hour week, there was still hardship all around. With a new baby to look after, George and Eva decided little Viv would probably fare better at school in Adelaide and living with her grandparents for a time. So when Viv was six, after a brief time at Broken Hill North Primary, they sent her to William and Emily. Viv had relatives nearby as well and would attend the Prospect Primary School just down the road from the Shegog home in Airlie Avenue for much of the next five years, returning to Broken Hill only for the holidays.[13] Viv's grandfather had mellowed from fearless rough rider into a quiet and kindly man with a drooping moustache. He taught Viv to play chess and told her stories of how he survived tough times in the bush, once having to ride more than 200 kilometres through the night from Port Augusta east to the Teetulpa Goldfields.[14] It was staggering how you could push your body to do things that seemed impossible when your life was on the line, he said. Viv's grandmother Emily once took her to see Australia play England in a Test cricket match and at another time, when Viv was ten they watched Pavlova dance at Adelaide's Theatre Royal. Viv told her grandmother that she wanted to be a world famous ballet dancer too.

In 1924, when he was sixty-eight, William bought a new Chevrolet motor car[15] and took Viv for regular runs in it, though he told her that driving the gleaming machine was still not as exciting as his days as a rough rider. At the same time, Viv's father, George, was starting to run on empty in Broken Hill. In 1925 he lost his job at De Bavay's along with eighty-seven other men when the plant closed.[16] He called on all his Freemason connections and found a job as a store clerk at Broken Hill's South Mine. Money remained tight in the household, though. George's old-school prejudices against Catholics were stirred up and he came to see his new role as a Justice of the Peace as important in enforcing what he saw as the Protestant values of the British Empire.

VIV WAS GROWING INTO A TALL girl with a wide smile, shining blue eyes and a mass of curls in her mane of light-brown hair. Not long before her tenth birthday, John Monash, now Lieutenant-General Sir John Monash and a man who admitted he thoroughly despised the whole 'business of war … the awful horror of it, the waste, the destruction',[17] arrived in Broken Hill to perform a melancholy duty. It was one he had performed many times. After the Armistice, Monash had returned to his engineering business and was now in charge of Victoria's State Electricity Commission, having built the town of Yallourn and its power station in Victoria's Gippsland to generate coal-fired electricity and light up much of south-eastern Australia. He was often called away from that work to unveil monuments to Australia's fallen in towns and cities across Australia. Sometimes the sadness overwhelmed him.

Despite inclement weather, a crowd of more than 4000 turned up in the rain on Sunday, 11 October 1925 on the corner of Argent and Sulphide streets to see Monash unveil a memorial to which was attached four bronze tablets with the names of the 365 volunteers from the surrounding area who had not returned from the Great War.[18]

One lady, well advanced in age and blinded by sobbing, was led to the monument by a girl on either side. She looked hard at the names on the plaque in front of her but could not read them through her veil of tears. The girls pointed to the position where the wreath should be placed to be directly under the name. A sobbing father also laid a wreath for his only son.

A boy and girl placed bunches of flowers for a father they could hardly have known. Young women were there, too, mourning sweethearts buried in foreign soil.[19]

The hearts of the whole audience, Monash said, went out in sympathy to those in the crowd who had lost loved ones, but the monument was also a tribute, he said, 'to the great tradition created by the Australian Imperial Forces, the tradition of service, sacrifice, and comradeship ...'[20]

VIV RETURNED TO BROKEN HILL in 1927 to prepare for her high school education, while her brother Jack, a bright boy in the fourth grade at the Broken Hill primary school, was regularly topping his class and showing great promise as a third baseman in baseball.

Viv was a good, if not outstanding, student at the Broken Hill and Districts High School, finishing the year 1929 eighth in her class and coming third in business studies. Her favourite subject was French but only because the teacher was a handsome young man. Hard times remained in Broken Hill, though, and after the Black Tuesday sharemarket crash on New York's Wall Street in October, the market continued to decline for the following three years.

Income from Australian exports nosedived and local industry ground to a halt.[21] Amid all this economic gloom, George Bullwinkel's mood was brightened by his stamp collection, his secret handshakes and other rituals of the Freemasons, and the camaraderie among the conservative voices of the friendly societies. But as he puffed on his pipe amid blue clouds of smoke in his armchair by the fire at the modest Bullwinkel home at 305 Oxide Street, he was often a tightly wound and sombre man.

Viv's home was a small brick building built in the Federation style with a bullnose verandah and an iron roof. As was the case in most Australian homes of the time, George was the sole breadwinner; wives were consigned to the occupation 'home duties' in the regular census collections. Despite the influence of George as head of the little household, Viv took after her mother, with a brighter, more optimistic personality and a great love for sports.[22] Eva had become something of an ace at the local tennis tournaments in Broken Hill and Viv, now a teenager, would eventually win blues at school for basketball, tennis and vigoro.[23] Despite her athleticism and the heat of Broken Hill, though, she did not learn to swim.

Her grandparents William and Emily Shegog died within a year of each other, and Viv's Adelaide holidays ended. She spent much of her free time playing sport instead. George encouraged those sporting ambitions but only to a point. In 1931, when Viv was fifteen and her basketball skills towered above those of the other girls at school, her headmaster, Malcolm Mackinnon, called her into his office to tell her the exciting news that she had been selected as captain of the school's Burke House. Mackinnon had recently arrived at Broken Hill after stints as headmaster at Lismore and Grafton,[24] and he was impressed by the teenager's hard work at her studies and her speed and skill on the basketball court.

Viv broke into a huge smile. She thanked the headmaster profusely, but he told her to wait. There was more. The coach at St Joseph's, the local convent school, had invited Broken Hill's basketball protégé to play for their side, the best in the local competition, that season.[25]

Viv was so excited she ran to tell her best friend, the small and dark-eyed Zelda Treloar,[26] the daughter of a metallurgist. Then she raced down Argent Street to her home on Oxide, eager to tell her parents. Eva was genuinely excited about Viv becoming a house captain but warned her to be prepared for a lukewarm response from her father when it came to playing for a Catholic team.

Times were tough, unemployment in Australia was about to reach 32 per cent and many conservatives like George were blaming the country's financial woes on James Scullin, the first Catholic and first Irish-Australian to serve as prime minister of Australia. Waiting in the wings to become the second Catholic prime minister was Joe Lyons. The political situation could not have seemed worse for George and his friends at the Masonic Club. A boy had shocked the community by hoisting the 'red rag of communism' on the Broken Hill High School flagpole as a lark. Headmaster Mackinnon had been forced to deny any links to communism and the boy had been 'severely dealt with',[27] but the conservative way of life that George and his pals enjoyed appeared to be threatened from all directions.

The world was a troubled place. In *The Barrier Miner* at the end of 1931 George read how Japan, Australia's ally in the Great War, had reacted to the economic freeze of the Depression by storming into what is now northern China to seize what it could from Manchuria amid waves of burning, looting, rape and mass executions. Japan had limited natural resources and a rapidly growing population, and its military leaders saw China as a treasure chest of raw materials, farm land and a population that could be eliminated.

The response from the west had been tepid. Japan had faced diplomatic isolation but the League of Nations was proving to be useless in enforcing world peace. Japan withdrew from the League but did not go quietly. The scenes of carnage left in China – burning cities, fleeing refugees and weeping, wounded children whose homes had been bombed – horrified the rest of the world, but nothing was done to slow the Japanese onslaught. The central government in Tokyo seemed to have no control over the army and before long the rapid victory on the Asian mainland whipped up war fever in Japan. The military became the dominant force in the nation's politics, and soon the Japanese Army was attacking Shanghai. When Prime Minister Inukai Tsuyoshi tried to rein in his generals he was assassinated,[28] and the military effectively took control of the Japanese government.

EVA HAD WARNED VIV that George might be less than impressed by her selection to play basketball for a Catholic team, but Viv was ready for him. He arrived home from his job at the mine store, a middle-aged man who looked older under the weight of money stress and a political and economic climate that was a constant worry. Viv told her father about her joy at being made the captain of Burke House. George congratulated her, but his smile became a frown when she began to relate details about the offer from the convent school.

'I'm afraid that's impossible,' he said impassively, with no room for negotiation.[29]

Viv had been braced for the reaction, but she still thought there might be some wriggle room. 'But why?' she protested. 'What possible reason could there be for not allowing me to play for the district's top team?'[30]

There were several, George said, expressionless. He explained that he was a senior Freemason and his brothers at the lodge would be aghast if his daughter played for a Catholic team. 'Saint Joseph's is a Roman Catholic high school, Vivian, run by the

Sisters of Mercy. We happen to be a Protestant family and the two do not mix.'[31] That's the way it was, he said, and the way it would always be.

Viv looked to Eva for some motherly support but Eva went on preparing dinner without comment.

Viv was crestfallen but her father told her to buck up. He leaned back in his armchair and blew out another plume of blue smoke from his pipe.

He told his downcast daughter to stop worrying about all this basketball nonsense and think more about what she would do when she left school. A third of Australia was out of work and jobs were hard to find.

Viv lifted her head, stuck out a defiant chin and marched off to her room.

In time she would forgive George. He was, after all, a good man, even if his ideas were often rooted in another, less-enlightened age. Vivian Bullwinkel hadn't yet left high school but she was already a tough and resilient young woman, with great powers of recovery.

Chapter 3

IT WAS EVA BULLWINKEL'S idea that her daughter become a nurse. Viv was well aware that money was tight at 305 Oxide Street and that she would have to find a way to support herself when she left high school. With a third of Australia's workforce now unemployed, jobs for women in Broken Hill during the Great Depression were even more limited. Viv later recalled that, at the time, the only real career opportunities for women were in nursing, teaching or as shop assistants. She promised her mother that she'd think about nursing but in truth she wasn't that keen on the idea. Working with sick or injured people might be depressing, and as for being stuck in a hospital, with all those hospital smells, and everyone in close contact ... well, she was an outdoors girl and that didn't sound like her cup of tea.

For a while Viv dreamed of making money from her sporting talent but realised that even the young Don Bradman, racing across the Australian sporting landscape like a shooting star, struggled to make money from cricket, so what chance a high school basketball player from Broken Hill at a time when female athletes, even the greatest ones on the world stage, were rarely given accolades let alone paid?

By the time Viv turned sixteen, she was still keeping her options open. Viv, or 'Bully', as most of her classmates called her, was a popular figure in a school that now numbered 500 students, with a kindly nature, a good work ethic in the classroom and determination, evident in her sporting passions. At the start of the 1932 school year, she was appointed a prefect,[1] and posed with the other prefects, including her pal Zelda Treloar and the school's new principal Walter Hammond, for a photograph that ran in *The Barrier Miner* at the end of the year.[2] Vivian and the other young ladies were dressed in the school uniform of knee-length skirt, white blouse and striped tie, uniforms that were often uncomfortable in the desert heat.

The Depression still weighed on the world, but Viv, with that huge smile and kind eyes, was already a beaming beacon of good cheer for her friends and teachers. Broken Hill High made her their school captain in 1933,[3] her last year as a student, and she again ran her opponents ragged on the tennis courts.[4] If only life was always this innocent and uncomplicated.

AS JAPAN CONTINUED ITS WAVE of terror in China, a pall was descending again over Europe. From the angst of Germany's enforced payment of war reparations and the resulting widespread poverty rose a right-wing voice that ignited a bonfire of resentment.

In the middle of 1933, not long after George had helped organise a visit to Broken Hill by the Grand Officers from the Independent Order of Odd Fellows[5] – another of the friendly societies – Viv and the rest of Broken Hill read over their toast and tea on the morning of 16 June:

> In all the important items of news from Germany of late months, one name stands out clear – that of Adolf Hitler, Chancellor of the Reich and leader of the Nazi party, which is claimed to number fifteen million in Germany alone. Until comparatively recently an obscure figure, Hitler now dominates the political horizon in Germany ... His methods may be theatrical and his speeches may have a strong smack of the street corner orator, but he seems to have captured the popular imagination in Germany, where he is almost as deeply worshipped by his followers as he is hated by his opponents ... In his own opinion he is a man with a mission,

and he intends to allow nothing to stand in the way of his carrying that mission to completion; a fanatic many people would probably call him ...[6]

Before long, Hitler instituted the Night of the Long Knives to kill his political enemies, and that was just the start of the murders. The worsening political situation added to George's many woes. He was not a well man, often complaining of shortness of breath and chest pains.

AT THE END OF 1933, Viv was farewelled from Broken Hill High with a glowing report from headmaster Walter Hammond, who, at the school's speech night, told the audience that as the girls' school captain Viv and 'her able lieutenant Zelda Treloar', the vice-captain, had assisted in improving the school spirit and the conduct of the school. He was glad of the public opportunity to thank them 'for the splendid work that they had done'.[7] At the conclusion of Hammond's speech Viv and the boys' school captain, Dick White, came forward on the stage to ask the students to rise and sing the school song. After the applause had subsided, Dick led the school in their war cry.

Viv's results for her leaving certificate were creditable if not outstanding. She received a first-class pass in geography and second-class passes in modern history, geology and dressmaking[8] – there was a heavy emphasis on needlework for the girls at Broken Hill High.

AT HOME, EVA WAS DOING HER BEST to convince Viv that nursing was a respectable profession that offered security, a steady income and the chance to help others. Viv had some ideas about becoming a sports mistress but her mother told her that not only was nursing essential to maintaining the health of Australia but it was a job that would stand her daughter in good stead for the rest of her life.[9] Viv then thought she might have a crack at being a telephonist, and she sat for an exam, receiving 39 out of 50 for handwriting, which even she must have thought was exceedingly generous for the scrawl that featured in many of her letters. She scored 94 out of 150 for spelling, and 125 out of 200 for arithmetic. She finished with a good pass of 258 out of a possible 400.[10]

Eva had already obtained application forms from the Broken Hill and Districts Hospital for Viv to train there, but despite her mother's assurances that she would make a wonderful nurse, Viv was still undecided. Then Zelda Treloar announced that she was starting as a probationary nurse; Viv decided to join her.

VIV, ZELDA AND FIVE OTHER young local women enrolled as probationers in training at the Broken Hill and Districts Hospital, a two-storey U-shaped building almost a half century old. The hospital had long wings with ornate wrought-iron lace work on the verandahs. Here Viv met the imperious 37-year-old matron, Rachel Hunter,[11] a farmer's daughter from Grenfell, New South Wales. Matron Hunter demanded the highest standards of all her staff, young and untrained as Viv and the other new recruits might be. The matron assigned Viv to the male surgical ward, and Viv recalled her first nervous visit there. She had been raised to have all the decorum and regal bearing of a well brought up Protestant woman. Just the thought of blood and bodily fluids made her queasy, and she walked quickly past the rows of sickbeds, hoping none of the patients would ask her for assistance. Just as she reached the end of the line and breathed a sigh of relief, a feeble voice called out, 'Nurse?' *Oh, no*, she thought. *What do I do now?* With butterflies dancing in her belly, she wondered for a moment whether she should pretend she was hard of hearing and walk out of the ward. But the cry became louder: '*Nurse.*' There was no escape now. Pretending that she was in complete control, Viv marched over to the bedside of a young man and, with what she thought was a degree of professional aloofness, asked him what he needed.

He told her he desperately wanted a bottle.

'A bottle of what?' she asked.

'No, I want to *use* a bottle,' he said.

'Whatever for?'

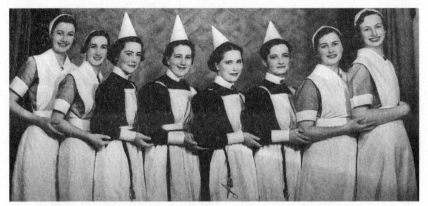

Viv (far right) with fellow nurses at the Broken Hill and District Hospital in 1935. Her great friend Zelda Treloar is third from the left. *Vivian Bullwinkel collection*

The young man was too embarrassed to explain.

Mystified, Viv went off to report the situation to her ward sister, who, roaring with laughter, handed Viv a bedpan and explained how it was to be used and how it was to be emptied and cleaned.

With her face flushed with embarrassment, Viv returned to the young man's bedside with the required equipment, doing her best to remain composed.

The male surgical ward was under the supervision of round-faced 28-year-old Irene Drummond.[12] She had been educated at Catholic schools in Adelaide and had trained as a nurse at Miss Lawrence's Private Hospital in that city. She qualified in obstetrics at Adelaide's Queen's Home before working at the Angaston Hospital, about 100 kilometres north-east of the South Australian capital. Irene had been back in Broken Hill for a year and had impressed Matron Hunter with her compassion and diligence. She was a no-nonsense professional. Irene looked Viv up and down through thick, round glasses and told her abruptly what was expected of her staff: absolute devotion to the care of their patients. Irene could be abrupt and stern, but she became Viv's mentor. It was the start of a beautiful friendship.

The young trainee worked long days and long nights in the surgical ward, helping to ease the suffering of men with broken limbs or burst appendix. Between twelve-hour shifts she would hit the books and attend lectures. Viv fitted in sleep when she could, and socialised whenever there was free time, which wasn't often. She was sometimes put on cooking duties, though whichever way she made eggs earned her only a ribbing from her fellow trainees.

In time she learned a lot about cooking and life at the Broken Hill hospital. She also learned a lot about death, seeing the final outcome for those patients beyond help, those who failed to survive operations or had been critically injured in mining and road accidents, and those who were wheeled out of the surgical ward under a sheet and dispatched to the undertaker's van when the nurses were satisfied most of the other patients were asleep.

LATE ONE EVENING, Viv was sitting alone at the nurses' station in the surgical ward, with just a small lamp to read by. There had been more strife that week at the mines, with the management of the South Mine, where her father worked, under fire from the unions for unsafe blasting during shifts.[13] A concert by the Sydney University Musical Society was playing ever so softly on the radio and there was an article on the front page of the local paper about a young waitress who had just died after being shot by her boyfriend in a murder-suicide.[14]

As Viv rose to quietly go about her rounds, she was unaware that her father was fighting for life only a few metres away in the same hospital. George had presided over a meeting of the Foresters Lodge after work at the South Mine store and was heading home to Oxide Street in a taxi when he started gasping for air. The driver, Jim Crocker, knew immediately that something was desperately wrong, and as George slumped face first in his seat, Jim floored the accelerator and raced to the hospital's front door.

Dr Vivian Ramsay Smith,[15] newly arrived from Adelaide, went to work, pumping George's chest to save him. Ramsay Smith was from a famous medical family, and if anyone could save Viv's father it was him.

Not long after George was brought into the hospital, Viv heard the soft click of footsteps in the ward. She went out into the corridor to see if a patient needed assistance and came face to face with the senior night sister.

The sister told Viv that her father had suffered a heart attack. She asked Viv to follow her into a nearby vacant room. Before the sister had finished talking Viv had become dizzy. She heard the words 'heart attack' and 'cab driver', and that Dr Ramsay Smith had done all he could.

'I'm so sorry, Vivian,' the sister said, ashen faced. 'Your father's gone.'

It seemed as though the room was spinning. Viv felt numb as her senses shut down, somehow shielding her from the pain. The sister's mouth was moving, but all Viv heard was 'best go home straight away to your mother'.

It had been nearly 30 degrees Celsius[16] in Broken Hill that evening and Viv walked out into a night that was still hot and suddenly painful. She headed home to a broken-hearted Eva.

A POST-MORTEM THE FOLLOWING day performed by the Government Medical Officer confirmed that George had died of heart failure. No inquest was necessary.[17]

George died aged fifty-five on 18 September 1934. Praise in the newspaper obituaries was fulsome. Two days after his death, a 'lodge of sorrow' was held at the Masonic Temple, just down Oxide Street from the Bullwinkels' home. As soon as it concluded George's funeral procession left his former home at 4 p.m. for Broken Hill's Church of England Cemetery.

Viv, her mother and brother were joined by more than 100 mourners. More than fifty members of the South mine staff paid their respects and thirty men marched in front of the hearse.[18]

As Viv watched her father being lowered into the red earth of the town that had embraced him, she realised that the family's fight for survival in the Great Depression had become even harder. At just eighteen, Viv would have to step up as the family breadwinner.

Eva received 877 pounds, ten shillings in death benefits from the South mine but knew that would not last long, so Viv resolved to become the best nurse she could in order to provide the best care for her patients and to support the people at home relying on her. There would be no time for boyfriends.

THE BROKEN HILL HOSPITAL was in a dilapidated condition[19] and had a shortage of doctors,[20] but it still provided Viv with a first-class training. Eva and brother John, who was just entering his teens, relied on Viv's income during these tough times. Still, at the hospital she made great friends and there were social nights to take the edge off the hard work and grim tasks.

Working in a hard, tough, mining environment was an apt preparation for a woman who would become a military nurse. Forced to show initiative and resilience, Viv forgot about ever being faint-hearted and learned to be independent. 'In those days, Broken Hill, being a mining town, we had some terrible mine accidents,' she recalled, 'and the miners were always so brave.'[21]

By the middle of 1937 the medical staff at the hospital included the 'surgeon-superintendent' Dr S.P. Barnett, the senior resident medical officer, Dr W.B. Dorsch, Drs Schlink and Meagher, and a new arrival, Adelaide-born Gavin Crabbe,[22] an experienced 35-year-old who had been working in Western Australia.[23]

It had taken almost four years of constant application, but in December that year, when she had just turned twenty-two, Viv and seven other Broken Hill nurses passed the examination by the Nurses Registration Board for acceptance into the General Branch of Broken Hill Hospital.[24] Among the graduating class were Viv's friends Zelda Treloar and Connie Sampson.[25] Another of her close friends Gwen McMahon,[26] had graduated a few months earlier.

Viv and her girlfriends celebrated their success unconcerned for the time being about the looming threat to Australia that was taking place over the horizon. Four days before Viv's exam results were made public, Japanese troops stormed into the city of Nanjing, then the capital of the Republic of China, and carried out a series of atrocities on an industrial scale. Chinese soldiers were executed in violation of the laws of war, and looting and rape took place in a frenzy that would shock the world.[27] The International Military Tribunal for the Far East, established after World War II, estimated as many as 300,000 murders were committed over a six-week period following the Japanese invasion and that there were at least 20,000 cases of rape.[28] An American missionary, Dr Ralph Phillips, later told a California State Legislative Committee that 'the Japanese took thousands of girls aged between nine and sixteen and turned them over to 58,000 soldiers for a week. Girls still alive at the end of the week were put to death in what he said was 'the most cruel and unspeakable manner'.[29]

'An 87-year-old woman was attacked 37 times in six hours,' Dr Phillips said, 'and a six-year-old girl was attacked seven times. Both died.'[30]

Soon after the fall of the city, Japanese troops marched thousands of young Chinese men to the Yangtze River, tied them up and spent an hour killing most of them with machine-gun fire. Survivors were run through with bayonets before being tossed into the water.

In one massacre at the ancient Taiping Gate, 1300 Chinese soldiers and civilians were massed together and blown up with landmines. The great mounds of corpses were doused in petrol and set on fire. Those who had survived the bombing and bayonets were burned alive. Dr Phillips said he was forced to watch while some of the Japanese troops disembowelled a Chinese soldier and then ate his heart and liver.[31]

The following year, members of the Waterside Workers' Federation of Australia at Port Kembla, outside Wollongong, New South Wales, refused to load Australian pig iron – also known as crude iron – for shipment to a Japanese arms manufacturer, in protest against the Japanese attack.[32] When Australia's Attorney-General, Robert Menzies threatened legal action, he was dubbed 'Pig Iron Bob'.

At the same time, Adolf Hitler's rapidly expanding forces annexed his homeland of Austria, marched on the Sudetenland in Czechoslovakia and unleashed 'Kristallnacht', the 'night of broken glass', when Nazi activists looted and burned as many as 7500 Jewish businesses across Germany. It was just the beginning.

VIV AND HER FRIENDS had decided to stay on at the Broken Hill Hospital for another year to study midwifery, and at the end of 1938, Viv, Gwen, Zelda and Connie all graduated with the extra qualification.[33]

As 1939 dawned, Viv decided to chase fresh opportunities. While John Bullwinkel had decided to stay in Broken Hill for a while and look for work, Eva was moving in with her sister Nell[34] in Mount Gambier, South Australia. Viv, Zelda and Connie, all doubly certified after almost five years of training at 'The Hill', took up positions at the Kia Ora Private Hospital, a series of small, low-set buildings on Gray Street in Hamilton in Victoria's Western Districts,[35] 300 kilometres west of Melbourne. The hospital had been established in the 1920s and had become a facility offering a degree of exclusivity for wealthy pastoralists and business people. There were fewer patients per nurse than there had been at 'The Hill' so Viv and her friends had more time to see the latest movies or to attend the local dances. To her delight, Viv could have a hit of tennis now and then, too.

On 12 May, Viv, now aged twenty-three, wrote to her friend Wyn James,[36] who was Zelda's cousin, to tell her how beautiful and green Hamilton was and how delighted she was to be working in the same hospital as 'Zel'.[37] Kia Ora provided the nurses with delicious morning teas and there were social gatherings that made Viv feel she was in a magical place. Maybe in Hamilton, Viv might even fall in love.

However, world events were taking a much darker turn. A few weeks after Viv wrote to Wyn, Japan invaded Mongolia.[38] In early August 1939 with fearful eyes on the German military might, Britain began experimenting with blackouts across the country to shield its people from possible enemy bombing raids. On the 18th of that month the Nazis began implementing their plans to euthanise children aged under three who showed signs of mental or physical disability. On 23 August, Germany and the Soviet Union signed the Molotov–Ribbentrop Pact to divide Eastern Europe between them. Then, on 1 September 1939, Germany invaded Poland.

Two days later, on the evening of 3 September 1939, Viv and the other nurses huddled around a wireless at the hospital along with the rest of Australia, waiting to hear an address by Robert Menzies, Australia's new prime minister. Menzies was seated in a Melbourne radio studio, rehearsing the most important speech of his life. Most of Australia already knew what was coming but millions still waited, hushed, for confirmation.

Menzies spoke in a low, slow, sombre voice. 'Fellow Australians,' he started:

> it is my melancholy duty to inform you officially that, in consequence of a persistence by Germany in her invasion of Poland, Great Britain has declared war upon her, and that, as a result, Australia is also at war. No harder task can fall to the lot of a democratic leader than to make such an announcement. Great Britain and France, with the cooperation of the British Dominions, have struggled to avoid this tragedy. They have, as I firmly believe, been patient; they have kept the door of negotiation open; they have given no cause for aggression. But in the result their efforts have failed and we are, therefore, as a great family of nations, involved in a struggle which we must at all costs win, and which we believe in our hearts we will win.[39]

Menzies knew that thousands of Australians would die, and that the nation's very survival was now on the line. Australian military capabilities had dwindled during the Depression years because of cuts to defence expenditure. Many of those listening to Menzies' speech had already lived through the ordeal of one global war and had lost loved ones in it. Now it seemed certain that this latest conflict would descend into a second world war.

Nurses from around Australia were quickly mobilised for service in the army, both from the civilian community and the Army Nursing Service Reserve. There were approximately 13,000 trained nurses in Australia, and 600 on the army reserve.[40] Viv knew that nurses would be vital to saving the lives of the young Aussie men heading to the front. She was willing to put her life on the line to help them.

Chapter 4

IN THE EARLY MONTHS of the war, nursing volunteers far exceeded requirements for the government, and by 1940 about 4000 applications had been received for overseas service. Viv, Connie and Zelda decided to continue their civilian careers and wait for their call-up.[1] But they were soon on the move again.

In early 1940, all three nurses transferred to the Guildford Private Hospital in the eastern Melbourne suburb of Camberwell, but the social life was dull and the hours exhausting. Then, Viv and Connie found jobs in the Jessie McPherson Community Hospital, the private wing at the Queen Victoria Hospital in William Street. Their new job was right in the centre of a beautiful and elegant city, a long way both geographically and aesthetically from the frontier heat of Broken Hill. Viv was enthralled with her new home and made the most of everything it offered, working hard but revelling in the social life too: nightclubs and dances, picture theatres and stage productions, horse races at Flemington and cruises on the Yarra, walks through the art gallery and steam train rides through the forests and fields of Gippsland.

Even though Japan had supported Britain and Australia in World War I, Australians had feared a Japanese invasion from the time of the Russo–Japanese battles of 1904 and 1905. Australia's defences were threadbare now, but the British government assured Menzies that Japan did not pose an immediate threat.

Twelve days after the declaration of war in September 1939, Menzies had announced the formation of the Second Australian

Imperial Force (AIF), which initially would comprise 20,000 men to fight overseas. The following month he announced that conscription would be introduced. In early 1940, Australia's 6th Division, formed during October and November 1939, left for the Middle East to aid the British as fighting was expected to soon break out there over vital shipping lanes.

War was the last thing on Viv's mind as she enjoyed a wonderful new life working at the Jessie McPherson hospital under Senior Sister Olive 'Dot' Paschke.[2] Tall and dark-haired, 35-year-old Olive had been born to parents of German background in Dimboola, Victoria, a town in the Wimmera wheat country north-west of Melbourne near the South Australian border. She was a farmer's daughter with an earnest face and a zeal for saving lives. Olive had finished her schooling as a pupil-teacher at Dimboola before riding the train through the wide, flat wheat country to Melbourne and gaining her nursing certificate at the Queen Victoria. She also gained certificates in midwifery and infectious disease nursing.[3] Back at Dimboola, Olive had been appointed matron at the Airlie Private Hospital for four years before returning to Melbourne as assistant-matron at Jessie McPherson. Like Viv, she was a warm and compassionate soul with a love for sports, particularly tennis and golf. Also like Viv, she had never learned to swim.

EUROPE WAS NOW IN FLAMES. The Germans and Russians were both ravaging Poland. Warsaw had fallen and Hitler's wicked program of mass murder, his Holocaust, had begun. German U-boat submarines had started placing mines in the Thames estuary. Britain had commenced food rationing and conscription.

As the Nazis ransacked France and reached the English Channel, 340,000 Allied troops were evacuated from the coastal city of Dunkirk near the Belgian border. Meanwhile, the Japanese parliament announced a record high budget with more than half the nation's expenditure now going on its military.

Viv's brother, John, had just turned twenty and was working as a ledger keeper at the Commonwealth Bank in Broken Hill.

He was a lean and fit six foot and one half inch (184 cm) tall, and weighed 11 stone, 2 pounds (71 kg) when, on 25 June, he visited a mobile recruiting unit in town to join the Royal Australian Air Force (RAAF) Reserve.[4] On his enlistment form he swore that he was a British subject 'of pure European descent'.[5]

The German advance through Europe continued, and in July 1940 the Nazis began their blitzkrieg of Britain, with lightning air raids against what they now saw as a besieged island.

Menzies directed that the 7th and 9th Divisions of the Second AIF be deployed overseas to support Britain and, despite long-held fears that Japan would enter the war on the side of the Germans, he also sent RAAF aircrews and a number of Royal Australian Navy (RAN) ships to fight for Britain. The 8th Division remained to defend Australia.

Viv and many of her fellow nurses wanted to support the fighting men but were awaiting an official call-up. That was until the day Connie Sampson called Viv over to a window at the hospital to witness a parade of air force men marching down William Street. They were four abreast, resplendent in their dark-blue uniforms, ever so handsome and keeping time to the beat of a military band, their jaws stuck out in defiance of anything the Germans might throw at them.

All around Viv, doctors, nurses, even patients in pyjamas craned their necks to watch and cheer.

Connie was swept up in the euphoria and patriotic fervour. 'I'm not waiting any longer,' she said.

Viv replied that there was a recruiting office for army nurses right there in William Street.[6]

The next day, the two young nurses went down to the recruiting office to volunteer. 'I just felt,' Viv said later, 'that if my friends were prepared to go and fight for their country, well, they deserved the best care that we could give them, and I believed I was able to help in providing that care.'[7]

But recruiting nurses was not the army's top priority and a month went by with no response to the applications. So on 8 August 1940, Viv and Connie applied to the air force. Fifteen days later they attended medical exams.[8] Connie was elated to be accepted but Viv, despite her sporting prowess, was rejected for having flat feet, the medical examiner telling the young nurse that flat feet would only slow her up in His Majesty's service because they caused pain with prolonged standing and running.

Viv had to cool her heels and keep her flat feet where they were for the time being, but Connie underwent X-rays on her lungs the following day and, after passing her medical with flying colours, was finally approved as a staff nurse for the RAAF on 31 August.

A week later, Constance Eva Sampson was sent to the RAAF Hospital on the Laverton Air Base, about 20 kilometres west of the Jessie McPherson Hospital. Connie and Viv said their goodbyes and embraced. Soon after, Japanese forces moved into French-controlled Indochina, and by 26 September 1940 had at their mercy the airbase and rail line outside Hanoi in what is now northern Vietnam. The following day Japan signed a pact with Germany and Italy.

Robert Menzies became increasingly worried that Japan, a militaristic nation of 73 million people with a huge army and navy, an aggressive foreign policy and a reputation for ruthlessness, would begin eyeing the small nation of seven million of which he was prime minister.[9]

SISTER OLIVE PASCHKE and some of Viv's other colleagues had also left the Jessie McPherson, signing on at the William Street Drill Hall to join the Australian Army Nursing Service (AANS) as part of the Australian Army Medical Corps.[10] To qualify for the AANS, nurses had to be aged between twenty-five and thirty-five and had to have impressive qualifications far above the basic training that all hospital nurses completed. Matrons could not be older than forty, though that number was revised up to forty-five later in the war. By January 1941 Olive had been made a matron and was posted to the 2/10th Australian General Hospital in preparation to support 6000 men of Australia's 8th Division which had been deployed to various parts of the Asia-Pacific region amid fears that the Japanese planned to continue their onslaught to Australia.

Olive was heading to Malaya, a key British colony that produced vital quantities of tin and rubber and provided a huge defensive barrier of thick jungle to defend Singapore and its naval base, the cornerstone of British power and wealth in Asia.

The Japanese Army had started planning for an invasion of Malaya in October 1940, despite assuring the world that it was the last thing on its mind. In fact, newspapers had reported:

> The [Japanese] Government spokesman (Mr Ishii) said today that he had been authorised ... to deny absolutely and flatly that Japan intended to send an army or navy force against, or to, Singapore ... Mr Ishii made direct reference to the rumours which, he said, were entirely groundless and the propaganda of warmongers.[11]

Olive had hardly arrived at her new posting in Malaya when her energy and enthusiasm prompted her nurses to christen her 'Dashing Dot' after a popular American comic strip character. January 1941 also saw Australians in their first major land battle of the war, as men of the 6th Division, under Major General Iven Mackay, along with other Allied troops, overcame Italian forces at the town of Bardia on the coast of Libya. As many as 36,000 Italians were taken captive, some of them eventually being sent to the prison camp at Cowra, a rural community 300 kilometres west of Sydney.

The day after the Italians had been routed, John Bullwinkel left his mother's home in Valmai Avenue in the Adelaide suburb of Kings Park and reported to the No. 5 Recruiting Centre for the RAAF in that city. Having volunteered for the RAAF Reserve in Broken Hill, on 6 January 1941 he told the recruiting officer he was twenty years and eight months of age and was ready to train as air crew in the RAAF with the hope of one day becoming a pilot. John listed Eva Kate Bullwinkel as his next of kin,[12] and was assigned to the RAAF's No. 4 Initial Training School at Victor Harbor.[13]

With John having signed up, and with so many of the other

nurses from the Jessie McPherson having been admitted to the forces, Viv marched into the depot of the Australian Army Medical Corps in William Street on 18 February 1941 to be weighed, measured and interrogated further about her suitability as an army nurse. She was listed as being twenty-five years and two months of age, with fair complexion, light-brown hair and blue eyes. She was 5 feet, 7½ inches tall (171 cm) and weighed 9 stone, 10 pounds (62 kg). She gave Church of England as her religious denomination.[14]

Viv swore that she had never had rheumatic fever or a weak heart, asthma, tuberculosis, venereal disease, kidney disease, malaria or dysentery. She had corns on both feet and a couple of her toes overlapped, but she had never had a fit, had never undergone an operation, was not suffering from any disease or disability, and had never been rejected for military service. Her eyesight was not 20/20 but 6/9 – well short but still good enough. She had no identifying scars but she did have a mole on her left buttock.[15]

Viv was allocated the service number VX61330 and told to be prepared for call-up.

Weeks went by and Viv began to despair over a lack of response. But finally the army wrote to say she should report to the quartermaster store at the recruiting depot in William Street to be issued her grey and scarlet uniform.

Viv's outdoor uniform was a grey Norfolk jacket and skirt, the skirt 14 inches (35 cm) from the ground; a white silk shirt with a chocolate-coloured tie; a silver brooch; brown laced shoes; brown leather gloves and a grey felt hat. The uniform for duty in the wards was a grey overall made of thick cotton called cesarine that buttoned from neck to hem, with white starched-linen collar and cuffs, a white organdie cap and a scarlet shoulder cape.[16]

Viv would be assigned the rank of lieutenant.

The army allocated twenty pounds for nursing sisters as a clothing allowance for service within the country that was paid to the nurses when they entered camp. They would be given another twenty pounds if they were assigned overseas duty. But nurses had to pay for their uniforms up front before receiving the initial money.

Despite having worked for almost a decade since leaving Broken Hill High, Viv's bank balance was low. She calculated that she would have to pay seven pounds, seven shillings for her uniform and greatcoat, and twelve shillings, eleven pence for gloves, as well as find the money for stockings, a blouse, tie and hat. She begged the issuing officer to let her put the goods on hold until the army allowance came through.

To her great surprise she scored her first victory of the war.

AFTER THE AUSTRALIAN forces had played a decisive role in the victory at Bardia, they were involved in fierce fighting in Greece in April 1941. About 3000 Australians were stranded on Crete in the wake of the Nazi invasion and most became prisoners of war of the Germans.[17] At about the same time, a Japanese spy named Takeo Yoshikawa,[18] posing as a vice-consul, was walking around the docks in Honolulu to gather information on the American fleet stationed at Pearl Harbor. Japan had just signed a neutrality pact with the Soviet Union to prevent an attack while its own forces continued to subdue much of Asia. By the middle of 1941, 14,000 Australian troops were in a force of 35,000 Allies fighting desperately as the Afrika Corps under German General Erwin Rommel besieged them in the Libyan city of Tobruk.

The 'diggers' made their homes in defensive positions underground, and German propaganda mocked the men for living like rats. Yet the 'Rats of Tobruk' would earn everlasting fame for their valour in some of the fiercest fighting of the war.

Viv learned that the nurses and troops posted to Malaya were having a far less torrid experience. In a case of unfortunate timing, the life and death struggles of the Australians in the North African desert came as the magazine *The Australian Women's Weekly* ran a series of articles about the AIF camps in Malaya.

Melbourne journalist Adele Shelton Smith was making a tour of the camps with photographer Wilfred 'Bill' Brindle. There wasn't much fighting, none at all really, and everyone seemed to be having a good time, even though the nursing staff had a week of intense emergency war training soon after they arrived in Malaya.

Banned from writing military articles, 'Tilly' Shelton Smith wrote about the daily lives of the soldiers and nurses, remarking that their living quarters were 'more comfortable than home'.[19] One of Bill Brindle's photographs showed a soldier tripping the light fantastic with a glamorous paid dance partner. Tilly wrote that the Australian soldiers and nurses were enjoying picnics under swaying palms on tropical beaches, cocktail parties beside hotel swimming pools, golf and tennis outings, lavish dinners and nightclub gatherings amid a sea of beautiful people.

On 3 May 1941, Viv flicked through the pages of the magazine to the latest dispatch: 'The people of Malaya cannot do enough for the Australian nurses. Off duty could be a whirl of gaiety were the girls not too interested in their work and in sightseeing'.

The *Women's Weekly* team paid a visit to the 2/10th Australian General Hospital in Malacca in what is now south-western Malaysia, about 250 kilometres north-west of Singapore. There, Olive Paschke told the writer: 'Some days we feel like film stars. The local residents send us huge baskets of orchids, presents of fruit, and invitations to their homes ...'[20]

The nurses were made honorary members of the prestigious local clubs.

They all looked extremely well and crisp in their grey cotton uniforms with red cotton capes. Like the men of the AIF the nurses look wonderfully fit and have become used to the heat of the tropics.

One sister said, 'Nursing makes one a realist. I used to think the glamor of the tropics was a lot of "hooey", but the colour of this country gets you ... Some of us are playing golf, and whenever transport is available a party of us goes to the swimming club. Others play tennis. We are feeling very proud because an AIF sister, partnered by one of our officers, won the club tennis tournament.'[21]

When on leave the Australian nurses could visit exotic Kuala Lumpur or travel to the delights of Singapore on air-conditioned trains.

Olive took the *Weekly*'s writer and photographer on a tour of the wards, where they met the convalescing patients.

'The wards run the full length and breadth of the building,' Shelton Smith told her readers. 'The outside walls are made entirely of glass and wood venetian shutters, allowing a maximum of ventilation. The Red Cross has equipped a recreation centre in the convalescent ward, where the men can play various table games. The Red Cross Commissioner, Basil Burdett, showed us round his store, which is packed to the ceiling with packing-cases filled with luxury tinned foods, books, sports equipment, and medical supplies.'

'Many of the boys over here are putting on weight,' a doctor said, adding that there was 'very little illness and not much work for the AIF hospital.'[22]

Viv was worried about going to Malaya, where it all seemed like a bit of a lark. She hoped she would be sent someplace where she could be more useful.

Chapter 5

ON THURSDAY, 15 MAY 1941, the day after Maurice Bavaud, a Swiss theology student, died by guillotine in Berlin after a failed attempt to assassinate Hitler, Viv was at the Jessie McPherson when she received a telephone call from an army officer, who instructed her to report to headquarters in William Street at 14:30 hours on the following Monday.

Viv would later recall that her fellow nurses treated her to a dinner and show the next night, and that they 'had quite a nice time'. Then the staff of Jessie Mac's gave her 'the loveliest writing case' as a farewell gift.[1]

The army told Viv to be prepared to board a train at 17:00 hours that night for the military training camp at Puckapunyal, just outside the town of Seymour, about 100 kilometres north of Melbourne. The grazing paddocks and farms around Seymour had been used for military training since the late nineteenth century, and Puckapunyal had been a centre for military mobilisation and training since the previous war. The camp facilities were inhospitable and confronting – timber huts with corrugated-iron roofs, unlined and windowless, which, in that bleak winter of 1941, were like ice boxes.

Viv packed an extra coat. She arrived at Puckapunyal late on the evening of 19 May to find long rows of the spartan huts, broken up here and there by ablution blocks. At the heart of the camp were separate mess rooms for the top brass, non-commissioned officers and other ranks. There was also a cinema that doubled as a conference hall and church. Troops were arriving at the camp by train every day and the small number of nurses passed almost unnoticed.

Viv was assigned to a twin room in one of the huts, which shuddered in the wind. The room contained two beds made of cyclone wire topped by a mattress stuffed with straw. There were two thin blankets, a pillow, and a dresser for clothes and personal items. She was told she would start work the next morning.

On Viv's second night at Puckapunyal she wrote a letter to her mother, using a pen from the writing case the staff at Jessie Mac's had given her. Viv told Eva that she had never slept on such a hard bed, even though she had been used to them for seven years at different hospitals. It was so cold at Puckapunyal, she said, it was as though she had been transported to the very centre of the South Pole. The quarters were of wood and iron, 'not badly fitted out, nothing to growl about really – a bit cramped for room – and sharing it with a lass I have not seen yet'.[2]

There was a mess room where the nurses drank their tea and coffee after meals, 'a fairly large room with the heater in the centre'. Then there was a dining room attached to that but there was no relaxation for the women who, following their long days of training, had to still sit up with 'cape and veil all complete'.[3]

One of the friends Viv met at Puckapunyal was Ballarat-born nurse Clarice Halligan,[4] who had enlisted the previous year, just short of her thirty-sixth birthday. She was from a big country family. Her father had worked at the Ballarat Brewery before moving to a lovely nineteenth-century home in Kew, Melbourne. Clarice told Viv about her days growing up in a happy home with a relatively carefree childhood, playing with her siblings beside the Yarra River and buying ice creams from a river punt, and holidaying at a sheep station in Deniliquin near the Murray River, where an older sister lived with her husband, a dashing young officer returned from World War I.[5]

Clarice had completed her nursing training at Melbourne Hospital in 1927 and was registered as an obstetric nurse in 1929.

She then completed the necessary training in Mothercraft and Infant Learning in order to take charge of a Baby Health Centre. She worked at Royal Melbourne for three years and earned a reputation for always giving back to others. In 1934 she heeded a call from the Anglican Mission and travelled to the wilds of New Guinea, treating villagers in remote locations.[6]

Back in Melbourne, Clarice had worked for the Grey Sisters, an order of Anglicans looking after the poor, and she was then appointed matron at a small hospital in Neerim South. There was talk of her marrying the doctor there, but her parents disapproved of him. Then Robert Menzies performed his melancholy duty and plans for Clarice to marry were put on hold. While she waited for her call to duty, she'd flitted about Melbourne in her smart Ford convertible motorcar.[7] She would leave it with her relatives when she was deployed overseas.

Also at Puckapunyal, Viv met Jim Austin,[8] a ruggedly handsome young army officer with the 2/15th Field Artillery. Jim was a strapping lad as tall as Viv's brother, John, with grey eyes and red hair.[9] Viv and Jim would regularly dine together, along with men from his battalion.

VIV'S FIRST MORNING in the wards at Puckapunyal was very different from what she had been used to recently, but it brought back memories of her training days at Broken Hill. At 11 a.m. there was an inspection, when the commanding medical officer, matron and a couple of sergeants did a round of the wards. The commanding medical officer appeared 'after much blowing of whistles' by the sergeants, and all the staff dropped whatever they were doing and stood firmly to attention. The patients were sitting up, not daring to move for at least fifteen minutes for fear of wrinkling their quilts. Viv told Eva in a letter:

> There are about twenty-five girls here and they all appear very nice and one of them I knew at Jessie Mac's ... It's so nice to be out in the wide-open spaces and to see a few green trees – it's so nice and fresh – will probably put on

weight and then my suit and uniforms won't fit which will be a pity because they look quite nice.[10]

She had no idea how long she would be there as 'mine [is] not to reason why'. John Bullwinkel, meanwhile, had received his airman pilot's commission after flight training on Gipsy Moth and Tiger Moth biplanes and Wirraways at Wagga Wagga in the Riverina in New South Wales. He was ready for overseas service.[11]

In August 1941 three of the staff nurses at Puckapunyal received their postings to the Middle East, but Viv was one of ten who were transferred to the Lady Dugan Red Cross Hostel and Convalescent Home for War Nurses in Domain Road, South Yarra.

The vast colonial mansion, built in 1865 and close to Melbourne's Royal Botanic Gardens, included a grand ballroom that had hosted the richest and most influential people in the country. It had been the family home of the wealthy Poolmans, but had been donated to the AANS by Jeannie Poolman[12] following the recent death of her husband, Ernest, one of Melbourne's most prominent businessmen and philanthropists.[13] The hostel was named for the Victorian Governor's wife. Sister Rosalind E. Ballard, who had served on hospital ships in World War I, was appointed the matron.[14] The property was to provide accommodation for army nurses assembled from Victoria, South Australia and Tasmania before they were shipped out on duty. Matron Ballard inspired the nurses staying there with her stories of saving lives in Victorian hospitals at Bairnsdale, Mildura and Wangaratta, and during the war, patching up the bullet wounds and shattered nerves of men at military hospitals in Bombay, Secunderabad and Bangalore, then on a hospital ship running between India and Egypt, and finally at military hospitals in England.[15]

With its rustic stone walls draped in ivy, rose-covered pergolas and manicured lawns, Viv's new home became something of a spiritual oasis for the women about to experience the horrors of war. Mrs Poolman had also donated a baby grand piano and left some of her expensive carpets and period furniture to make the nurses as comfortable as possible before they were given their new postings.

There were six large bedrooms, painted in soothing leaf-green, as well as two sleepouts. Some of the bedrooms had as many as six beds, and Viv never had any doubts that this was a hostel and not a hotel. There were staff nurses in the old mansion preparing to sail for a war zone, and she was one of them.

Viv was told she would be soon shipping out with the hastily formed 2/13th Australian General Hospital (2/13th AGH), which at the time included eight officers, forty-four staff nurses, twenty warrant officers and sergeants, 126 other ranks, three physiotherapists, then called masseuses, and a chaplain. Together they had the capacity to run a hospital with 600 beds. The 2/13th had been formed at Melbourne's Caulfield Racecourse on 11 August, its personnel and equipment brought together in the rush that war created.[16]

Viv passed her medical examination, was X-rayed, and inoculated against typhoid and smallpox. On 8 August 1941,[17] she swore that she would well and truly serve her Sovereign Lord, the King, in the Military Forces of the Commonwealth of Australia, signed her name on a pink attestation form and was issued with her uniform, pay book and identity disc, which was to be worn at all times. On the same day, the American and British governments warned Japan that they faced tough economic sanctions if they dared to extend their advance through South-East Asia into Thailand. The world watched on nervously.

While Viv stayed at the Lady Dugan after her stint at Puckapunyal, most of the 2/13th AGH awaited news of their new postings while camped on straw-filled mattresses amid the equine aromas of the horse stalls at Caulfield, 10 kilometres away. The hospital personnel at Caulfield only had two thin blankets and their greatcoats to repel the night chills.

The volunteers would soon be moving to more comfortable quarters, though, aboard a luxury ocean liner, the *Wanganella*, which had been completed in 1932 in Belfast by Harland & Wolff, the builders of the *Titanic*. For eight years the sleek vessel had cruised the Trans-Tasman route to New Zealand and then the Sydney to Fremantle run before being requisitioned by the Commonwealth for the war effort.

The *Wanganella* was completely refitted as a hospital ship and in that era of exaggeration and war propaganda, medical officers declared that working conditions on it were better than in a modern hospital on shore.[18]

The Minister for the Army, Percy Spender, told the press that he was grateful that almost the entire equipment for the ship's conversion had been made in Australia, from the fitments in the green-painted wards, which each had their own refrigerators, to the powerful X-ray plant and the apparatus in the air-conditioned, up-to-the-minute operating theatre, as well as the dental surgery and mechanics room. The ship was also carrying tonnes of Red Cross donations, ranging from portable gramophones to cigarettes, sweets and cakes. Recreational facilities on the ship included a deck cinema, a soda water machine, and electric lifts to service each deck.[19]

The *Wanganella* was berthed at Station Pier in Port Melbourne and, while a strike by dockworkers threatened the provisioning of the ship for its voyage,[20] Major Arthur Home, the new registrar of the 2/13th, sent a deputation of ten of his own men to load the ship with its equipment and supplies.

While the war raged overseas, Australia was consumed by political turmoil. Prime Minister Robert Menzies resigned and Country Party leader Arthur Fadden became prime minister, though the nation wondered how long that would last in such a time of unrest and uncertainty.

THE 2/13TH PERSONNEL BASED at Caulfield moved onto their gleaming white transport, now rechristened His Majesty's Hospital Ship *Wanganella*, awaiting its departure which was planned for 2 September 1941. On board the ship were permanent nursing staff assigned as the 2/2nd AGH to treat wounded combatants.

The ship had started its most recent journey in Brisbane a week earlier,[21] collecting six nurses before arriving in Sydney to collect another twenty-eight from New South Wales.

Among them was Ellie McGlade,[22] a deeply religious convent-educated 39-year-old originally from Armidale, New South Wales. Born to Catholic parents in Australia's New England region, her life had been difficult from the time her mother, Agnes, had died from consumption not long after Ellie's baptism at Armidale's Saints Mary and Joseph Church, where her parents were married. Ellie's father, Francis Aloysius McGlade, a well-liked solicitor, also died of consumption just two years later. The local Armidale newspaper painted a sad portrait of Ellie, their 'poor little child' who was 'being tenderly cared for by sympathising friends'.[23] From her kindergarten days, she would spend fifteen years as a boarder at St Ursula's convent in Armidale, winning awards for elocution and Christian doctrine.[24]

On leaving school Ellie had visited her grandfather, Colonel Archibald Hume, in Scotland, and then toured Ireland with a cousin to meet her late father's relations, some of whom were wealthy landowners.[25] As a young woman of independent means, she early on decided to devote her life to helping others and began training as a nurse at Sydney's Royal Prince Alfred Hospital in 1923. She graduated four years later before specialising as a mothercraft nurse in the Hunter Valley.[26]

Another of the Sydney nurses was Janet 'Jenny' Kerr,[27] a 31-year-old who had grown up in central New South Wales. Her divorced mother, Ida, was the matron of the small Woodstock Hospital outside Cowra, and Jenny had followed her example, graduating as a nurse from St George's Hospital at Kogarah in Sydney and working as a theatre nurse there for many years. She had enlisted only a few days before the *Wanganella* had left Sydney.

Jenny's colleague, 26-year-old Mona Tait,[28] who hailed from Booval, a suburb of Ipswich in Queensland, had for the last few months been based at Sydney's Victoria Barracks. The ever-smiling Mona had grown up in Newcastle and trained at the nearby Cessnock District Hospital. Prior to enlisting, she was the sister in charge of the X-ray department at Canberra Hospital for three years.

JUST AFTER DAWN ON 2 SEPTEMBER, Viv and the remaining staff nurses at the Lady Dugan rose and assembled in the grand ballroom. Their eager chat about what lay ahead was silenced when Matron Ballard entered the room. She told them to be ready to leave for the *Wanganella* at 09:00 hours. She did not reveal their final destination.

Among the nurses Viv travelled with were the livewire Mona Wilton[29] and the much more reserved Wilma Oram,[30] two nurses from country Victoria. Mona was born in the village of Willaura, near Ararat in western Victoria, a year after a great fire almost wiped out the few houses there. In 1933, when she was twenty, she joined her sister Amy as a nurse at Warrnambool Hospital, completing her training in general nursing and then midwifery. At Warrnambool, Mona met Wilma Oram, who was three years her junior and from Glenorchy in the Wimmera wheat country in central Victoria. The two became best friends and stayed in close contact, even though they were transferred to different hospitals over the next few years. Mona had worked with Viv at the Jessie McPherson, and in 1940 she had volunteered as an army nurse, persuading Wilma, who was working at Allansford, outside Warrnambool, to join too. Another of Mona's friends travelling on the *Wanganella* was 37-year-old Kit Kinsella,[31] who had trained with her at Melbourne's Alfred Hospital.

Viv and the other nurses loaded their heavy kitbags onto a bus and were driven the 6 kilometres to Station Pier. There, toting their gear over their shoulders, they walked the gangplank onto the *Wanganella* in single file.

On deck, Viv was met by a familiar face – Gavin Crabbe, now Captain Crabbe, one of the doctors she'd worked with in Broken Hill. Until a few days earlier, Dr Crabbe had been working at the Lachlan Park Hospital, a secure mental health facility in New Norfolk, Tasmania. That was until he enlisted. His colleagues had passed the hat around and farewelled him with gifts of a cigarette case and fountain pen, wishing him 'God speed and a safe return'.[32]

Dr Crabbe told Viv that her old boss at Broken Hill, Matron Irene Drummond, had enlisted in Adelaide almost a year earlier and was now matron of the 2/4th Casualty Clearing Station in Malaya.

Viv surveyed the brilliant-white hospital ship gleaming in the winter sunshine and listened to the nervous, excited chatter of the men and women on board. She was thrilled to be deployed in her country's service, but she also knew there could be many dark days ahead.

The nurses were given the ship's orders. While it sounded like a romantic thing to do, there were to be no messages in bottles thrown overboard into the sea, lest they fall into the hands of crew manning German submarines, better known as U-boats, and betray the *Wanganella*'s movements. To save fresh water, all ranks were permitted just one shower a day, but there was a hairdressing salon on board, open for business for two hours in the mornings and afternoons. It cost just nine pence for officers and nurses and was free for other ranks. There was also a library that was open for forty-five minutes every afternoon from which they could borrow books.

Some of the nurses thought they were about to sail for the Middle East to treat the wounded from the fighting against the Italians and Germans. But Viv had other ideas.

The Japanese onslaught in South-East Asia was continuing. They had taken Saigon (now known as Ho Chi Minh City) and were heading south and west towards Thailand and Malaya. In response, American President Franklin D. Roosevelt had ordered the seizure of all Japanese assets in the United States and, along with Britain and the Dutch government in exile, had placed an embargo on oil and gasoline supplies to Japan, which relied on America for 80 per cent of its petroleum products.[33]

That could only end badly, as there were oil fields aplenty in the Dutch East Indies (now known as Indonesia).

Viv suspected that she and her colleagues would be going to help the Australian forces in Malaya and Singapore.

Chapter 6

BASS STRAIT HAD A REPUTATION for wild weather but on their first day at sea, Viv and all on board relaxed as the *Wanganella* glided over glistening, calm blue waters. The ship was on course for Fremantle in Western Australia, almost a week away.

There were lectures in the men's mess and a bottle of beer for each recruit per day. Once the *Wanganella* was off the coast of South Australia, the skipper took the ship well south of the commercial shipping lanes to avoid any encounters with U-boats which were thought to be lying in wait. Now the ship was travelling at a latitude beyond 40 degrees south, deep in the Southern Ocean, amid howling winds and rolling seas. For hour after hour, great walls of water smashed over the ship's bow, and several lifeboats were damaged. Viv and most of the other passengers stayed below deck and out of harm's way until six days into the voyage, when the captain changed course to the north-west. As the ship approached the deep water sea channel called Gage Roads, in the outer harbour area of Fremantle, they again found themselves in more placid waters.

There the stunning white *Wanganella* stood in stark contrast to the grim grey of two giant passenger liners that had been repainted and converted into troop ships. The 80,000-ton *Queen Mary*, at 310 metres long, and the even bigger 83,000-ton *Queen Elizabeth*, at 314 metres, had become known as the 'Grey Ghosts', because of their camouflage paintwork and the speed they could travel to avoid enemy submarines.

Both ships were heading for Egypt via Ceylon (now Sri Lanka), with thousands of Australian troops on board.

While the *Wanganella* had been crossing the Southern Ocean, Nazi forces in Lithuania had started the mass murder of 100,000 Jews, Poles and Russian prisoners. At the same time, Japan was threatening war with the United States if President Roosevelt did not lift his embargo on oil.

But the mood off Fremantle was more euphoric than gloomy. The Australian troops on the Grey Ghosts whistled and called out 'Coo-ee!' to the nurses. 'Good luck, boys!' the nurses shouted in response. 'Give it to that mongrel, Hitler!'

As the two great liners steamed away towards the horizon, the nurses frantically waved goodbye, knowing that, like the men on the Grey Ghosts, they too faced an uncertain fate. As the *Wanganella* steamed into Fremantle's inner harbour, Viv heard more shouting. It was coming from the Australian warship HMAS *Canberra*, which had been operating around the southern coast of Western Australia and would soon be sailing back to Sydney for patrol work around New Guinea. At the sight of the *Wanganella*, and the nurses on deck resplendent in their starched and stylish uniforms, the 750 sailors on board were as enthusiastic in their cheering as the men on the Grey Ghosts.

Most of the crew and passengers on the *Wanganella* were granted shore leave, and many took the opportunity to travel into Perth to make expensive telephone calls back home to their families or to visit friends and relatives.

Viv got to see very little of Fremantle, though, the *Wanganella* only staying long enough for the Western Australian contingent to board.

Among those who joined the ship in Perth was the commanding major of the 2/13th, the remarkable Dr Bruce Hunt[1] who, not long after leaving Melbourne Grammar, had fought on the Western Front as a teenager before going on to study medicine. Dr Hunt, a tallish, studious-looking man of forty-two with greying hair, had set up the diabetes clinic at what would become Royal Perth Hospital.[2] He had served as a squadron leader in the medical branch of the RAAF from 1939, before being seconded to the medical staff of the AIF.[3]

The nurses who boarded the ship in Fremantle included fresh-faced 28-year-old Alma Beard[4] from the Western Australian wheat belt, and Perth's 33-year-old Minnie Hodgson,[5] and thirty-year-old Iole Harper.[6] From a prominent Perth family, Iole was a small woman just a tick over 5 feet tall (150 cm) but made of stern stuff. Two of her uncles had died in the attack on Gallipoli when she was four years old, while her father and two other uncles had become prominent Western Australian cricketers. Like Viv's brother, John, Iole's brother Bill[7] had joined the RAAF.

ON 9 SEPTEMBER 1941, the *Wanganella* sailed out into the Indian Ocean with its full complement of 216 personnel of the 2/13th. Major Home assembled his men and women and told them they were heading, not for the war zones of Northern Africa or the Middle East but for Singapore, as Viv had suspected. Many were disappointed, including Viv, who wondered why they were being shipped to a place so far from the war zones when she felt sure she'd be more useful in a hospital where there was actual fighting. But Major Home explained that many of the troops already based in Malaya and Singapore were suffering from malaria and other tropical illnesses.

For more than a decade, Australia had pinned its defensive strategy around a major naval base in Singapore and a British fleet that was expected to rule the waves in the southern hemisphere as it had for so long in the north. While most Australian soldiers had been deployed to save Britain and its shipping routes closer to England, the bulk of Australia's 8th Division, under the command of Major General Gordon Bennett,[8] had taken up positions in Malaya and Singapore, supported by four RAAF squadrons and eight warships.

The 2/10th AGH was already operating out of Malacca, and Major Home told Viv and the rest of the 2/13th that they would establish their medical headquarters in the three main brick buildings of the relatively new St Patrick's School for boys on the south-eastern side of Singapore island. The school had been constructed on six hectares on the East Coast Road, halfway between Singapore's central business district and the Changi Fortress, where a British coastal artillery battery had been established to guard the Straits of Johor, the narrow stretch of water between Singapore and the Malay Peninsula. The big British naval guns were designed to make Singapore the 'Gibraltar of the East'. The new commanding officer for the 2/13th was Melbourne doctor Colonel Douglas Pigdon,[9] who had served as a medical officer with the Australian Army Medical Corps in Palestine in World War I and had been in Singapore since May awaiting the rest of his team.[10]

As the *Wanganella* sailed north along the Western Australian coast, Viv attended lectures on tropical medicines and taught first-aid and other medical practices to the orderlies and stretcher bearers in their unit.

The sea was endlessly fascinating, with flying fish darting about the ship like arrows. A few days into the voyage there was the stunning sight of smoke and ash rising from the volcanic archipelago of Krakatoa in the Sunda Strait between Sumatra and Java. At night, the lava created an astonishing orange light that caused the ship's white hull to glow. The phenomenon was mesmerising and terrifying at the same time.

The next day, the nurses of the 2/2nd permanently assigned to the *Wanganella* plunged the new chums – including Viv – into the time-honoured humiliations that had been part of crossing the line – the Equator – for centuries of sea travel. The veteran nurses who had crossed the Equator before used mosquito netting, lobster shells and cotton wool to transform themselves into mermaids of the deep who, at Neptune's behest, rubbed their victims with a hideous concoction and dunked them into the ship's swimming pool.

It was all good, dirty fun and, after cleaning up, Viv and some of her pals enjoyed a sherry in the cabin of nurse Edna Mounsey before they all moved on to the wardroom to celebrate their imminent arrival in Singapore.

THE *WANGANELLA* REACHED Singapore's Keppel Harbour on the morning of 15 September 1941. The great expanse of water and boats was unlike anything Viv had ever seen. The entrance to the inner harbour was crowded with small, lush, green islands and everywhere she looked were sampans and junks, boats common to the area, their crews flitting about dressed in blue cotton trousers and shirts and almost hidden under their wide-brimmed Chinese hats.

The sun was scorching and the humid air hot and sticky with the aroma of spices and sandalwood. There were warnings from the officers about the myriad of fatal tropical diseases here, as well as admonitions to not drink the local water or eat fruit with broken skin. They were told that venereal disease was rampant in Singapore and Malaya. One of the chaplains on board warned the nurses that Singapore was the 'sin city' of the Orient and that wickedness waited at every corner. A second chaplain told his audience that they were all adults and to go out and enjoy themselves.

From the deck, Viv could see the great port and the city beside it, full of grand colonial buildings. She knew the streets were full of markets and adventure and that there would be a warm welcome for all the Australians in the restaurants and nightspots. The gorgeous white bungalows of Singapore looked stunning against the deep green foliage all around. Viv thought she'd be very happy amid the bustle and excitement of this new world, especially under the protection of the fighting men of the British Empire.

VIV AND THE OTHER NURSES had no idea of the cracks in the British defences around Singapore. The island was guarded by a military force of about 60,000 British and Commonwealth troops, including Australian, Indian and Malay soldiers under the command of Lieutenant General Arthur Percival,[11] who for years had been protesting about the lack of investment in Singapore's defences.[12] Though touted as one of the ramparts on which the British Empire stood, Singapore was no fortress.

Britain had built a large naval dockyard on the island's north coast in the 1930s and planned to dominate the Asia-Pacific region with warships. But under this ill-conceived 'Singapore Strategy' British naval vessels would not be based at the island but rather, in times of crisis, rushed there at full speed from Europe. There was a dearth of modern aircraft and the airfields in the jungle were remote and hard to defend. Few of the soldiers posted to Singapore had experience with jungle warfare and tanks were so scarce as to be almost non-existent. The Governor of the Straits Settlements, Sir Shenton Thomas, refused to allow the building of air-raid shelters lest it send his population into panic and damage business. Digging slit trenches, he said, would be a waste of time, because they would only become filled with water when it rained and cause mosquito plagues.[13] There were heavy guns facing the water in Singapore and even more confronting was the thick wall of Malayan jungle to the north. How could the Japanese, portrayed by the British military as physically and intellectually inferior to Europeans and sometimes disparagingly depicted as dimwits with glasses and buckteeth, possibly find a way through all that?

Viv noted in her diary:

Monday, 15th September 1941. Arrived Singapore 11 a.m. glorious view. Harbour & shipping very pretty with lots of canoes, sampans & barges. Very warm. Drew up to the wharf. Coolies [labourers] running tow rope around pole. Three Aussies welcomed us with much horn blowing.[14]

Viv and the other passengers were ferried to the docks along with their luggage and equipment. Singapore revealed itself to be a great mass of humanity, Sikh soldiers in turbans, British officers in crisp white uniforms, Australian fighting men in khaki and local workers all rushing around with an urgency borne from being part of one of the most important trading centres in the world. Everywhere cars and rickshaws fought for space on the streets.

Colonel Bill Kent-Hughes, World War I hero, Olympic hurdler and prominent Melbourne politician before this war and now the Deputy Quartermaster General for the Australian forces,[15] welcomed Viv and the other Australians to the city. He told them he had organised buses to take the 2/13th to their new home at the St Patrick's School.

Viv would have to wait, though, to experience the excitement of Singapore. Major Home announced that, while the other nurses were headed to their lodgings at St Patrick's, Viv and nine other nurses from the 2/13th had been seconded to the 2/10th at Malacca and would board their transport for the 250-kilometre journey that night. Among the nurses to accompany Viv were Mona Tait, Jenny Kerr, a tiny Tasmanian named Maisie Rayner,[16] and Nancy Harris,[17] twenty-eight, who had been born to a prominent doctor in Guyra, New South Wales, but who had grown up on McLaren Street, North Sydney. Nancy had attended Pymble Ladies College in the 1920s and, in between holidays at the remote coastal spot Byron Bay, had graduated in nursing from Sydney's Royal North Shore Hospital. She was a slim young woman with wavy brown hair and hazel eyes, a beautiful smile and calm demeanour.

As most of the nurses rode off in trucks and ambulances to the St Patrick's School, Viv and the other nine nurses felt forlorn as they waited on the dock with their bags. Young doctor Clem Manson[18] strolled over with some words of comfort. Clem had come from Gippsland to Melbourne's Scotch College as a student before graduating in medicine at Melbourne University in 1933. He had been a resident medical officer at the Alfred Hospital for two years, and then opened his own practice in Hawthorn before he enlisted.

Clem was only thirty-one but he gave the young nurses some fatherly advice, telling Viv and the others not to behave like silly girls but to remember they were representing their country as army nurses in a great fight. He knew they felt abandoned but said they'd all be laughing about the separation in a few days.

Later that night Viv was with a party of nurses that left the dock by ambulance for the railway transport office at Singapore's main station. It was only a short journey but an air-raid drill caused all the lights of the city to be extinguished so it took much longer than it should have. When Viv and her companions arrived at the train station they realised that two of the Tasmanian nurses, Mollie Gunton[19] and Harley Brewer,[20] were missing. The lights were still out in Singapore and there were fears for the safety of the two young women. As the 'All Clear' was given and the power came back on, military policemen and several assistants took off to retrace the path of the nurses. But nurses Gunton and Brewer were hale and hearty. Confused over their orders, they were still on the *Wanganella* singing up a storm at a party.

Reunited, Viv and the other nine nurses were finally underway, chugging on a steam locomotive across the kilometre of causeway to the bustling city of Johor Bahru and then on into the Malayan jungle, bound for Malacca.

They reached the halfway point of the journey at 4 a.m. on 16 September when a detachment of the 2/15th Field Regiment escorted the tired but excited women to a group of trucks parked near the railway platform. An hour earlier, one of the captains had asked for volunteers to accompany him to the railway siding to pick up a group of Australians arriving from Singapore. There were no volunteers, not one, but when he said it was a party of Australian nurses, a forest of hands reached for the sky. The soldiers commandeered the most comfortable chairs they could find from the officers' mess. Viv was both startled and amused by the sight of the small utility vehicles, each with cane chairs on the tray to make the journey by road as pleasant as it could be for the passengers.

Once settled in their cane chairs, the nurses were driven to the commanding officers' quarters for a welcome breakfast of bacon and eggs washed down with hot tea.

While the nurses were breakfasting, the Australian soldiers set up umbrellas over the cane chairs to protect the women from the fierce equatorial sun on the second leg of their journey. On they drove for hours through the Malaysian jungle. Now and then they would pass a small village with waving children and every

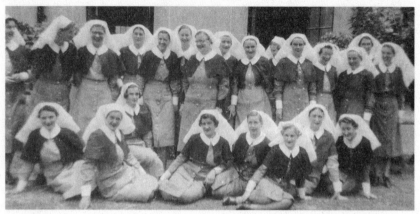

Viv, centre, back row, and some of the nursing staff from the 2/13th Australian General Hospital in Singapore. Standing from left: Gladys Hughes, Merle Trenerry, Lorna Fairweather, Jean Ashton, Bessie Ellen Muldoon, Viv, Irene Drummond, Maude Spehr, Bessie Taylor, Marie Hurley, Ellie McGlade, Flo Casson, Veronica Clancy, Harley Brewer. Front row: Maisie Rayner, Ada Bridge, Minnie Hodgson, Nellie Bentley, Betty Garood, Loris Seebohm, Jenny Kerr, Elvin Minna Wittwer.
Australian War Memorial P01344.001

so often a vast rubber tree plantation. In the heat and humidity, surrounded by the calming green of the jungle all around, many of the nurses took the opportunity for some shut-eye.

They didn't know that this would be a time of calm before the biggest storm to ever hit the region.

MATRON OLIVE PASCHKE, who had been in Malacca for seven months, had a warm greeting for her ten new nurses, especially Viv, who she remembered from the Jessie McPherson Hospital. Viv also met Olive's second-in-command, the tiny but dynamic Nesta James,[21] who at just 4 feet, 11 inches (150 cm) made up for her lack of height with a giant spirit and huge smile. Nesta was Welsh-born and had recently been nursing at the Shepparton Base Hospital in northern Victoria.

Viv and the others turned in early after their long journey, but the next day took a tour of their new temporary home. The main section of the hospital at Malacca was a five-storey building just north of the city on a hill overlooking the Malacca Straits, where cargo ships plied the busy waterway between Singapore and the Andaman Sea and beyond it to the Bay of Bengal and the Indian ports of Madras and Calcutta. The hospital's top balcony afforded Viv spectacular views to the east coast of Sumatra in what was then still the Dutch East Indies.

The hospital had 1200 beds and a number of specialty departments.[22] The Australian medical team was primarily involved in fighting malaria, treating skin diseases and repairing injuries sustained by the Australian infantry battalions stationed nearby. Viv was wearied by the stifling humidity of Malacca and one of the 2/10th nurses, Betty Jeffrey,[23] told her it was one of the hottest places in the world. Born in Hobart but raised in Melbourne, Betty – often called 'Jeff' by her friends – had worked as a secretary and schoolteacher before taking up nursing at age twenty-nine. She graduated, specialising in midwifery, in 1940 when she was thirty-two. She was sent to Malaya with the 2/10th, arriving in Singapore on the *Zealandia* only three months before she met Viv at Malacca.[24] She and Viv became firm friends, sharing a zest for life.

Later in the day, Viv took a tour of the wards and attended a welcome address from Lieutenant Colonel Glyn White,[25] a young Melbourne doctor. Small and wiry, with seemingly boundless energy, he was known as 'Splinter' White[26] and was the Deputy Assistant Director of Medical Services for the 8th Australian Division under Colonel Alfred Derham,[27] a World War I veteran who had been wounded on Gallipoli.

INITIALLY, VIV WAS ASSIGNED to Ward C-11, where her colleagues included her old friend from Puckapunyal, Clarice Halligan. Before long, though, she was working in the hospital's blood bank led by Melbourne doctor Charles Osborn,[28] who had worked at the Orthopaedic Hospital in seaside Frankston before the war. Osborn told Viv that he was setting up a blood bank for the 2/13th in Singapore and needed her to learn everything she could about blood transfusions as quickly as possible because she was going back there with him. Viv relied heavily on two colleagues for instructions in using blood: Flo Trotter,[29] a devout Christian who had worked at the Brisbane General Hospital, and

Jenny Greer,[30] a Sydney nurse known for her sense of humour. Jenny was always whistling and singing, perhaps because she'd met a dashing Scotsman in Sydney named Duncan Pemberton. He was on holiday from his oil job in Singapore at the time and Jenny had no idea then that she'd be in Singapore, too, before long.

It took Viv only a couple of weeks to learn all she needed to know about blood banks and on 5 October 1941, she and the other nine nurses from the 2/13th set out on motor transports to meet the train to Singapore. Before Viv left, Olive Paschke told her that she hoped they would meet again soon.

After a delay over some misplaced luggage, Viv and the other nurses finally arrived back at the St Patrick's School in Singapore the following night. Matron Irene Drummond was waiting for them, her kindly eyes shining behind her glasses.

The next day, with the support of two independent parliamentarians who had previously backed Australia's Coalition government, Labor's John Curtin,[31] the member for Fremantle in Western Australia, became the fourteenth Prime Minister of Australia.

Ill winds were blowing a gale and Curtin and the rest of Australia were about to face a harrowing time.

Chapter 7

THE WORK WAS TOUGHER in Singapore than it had been in Malacca and constant air-raid drills shattered the nerves, disrupted the daily routine, and required the constant shifting of patients.

Still, St Pat's was in a stunning location and it smelt divine, a mix of hibiscus, frangipanni and bouvardia. The nurses' quarters were in the south wing of one of the main buildings and although there were sublime views of swaying coconut palms and the blue sea and islands beyond, landmines dotted the foreshore and beach across the road. The military had made that area out of bounds and erected barbed-wire fences and signposts that warned 'DANGER KEEP AWAY'. Almost as dangerous were the monsoon drains more than a metre deep that ran throughout St Pat's and which were potentially lethal during air raids and blackouts. Many of the nurses such as Brisbane's Phyllis Pugh[1] were nauseated by the smell of the canals along Singapore's streets. Phyllis was well used to scorching Queensland heat, but Singapore's cloying humidity was at first unbearable and 'any worthwhile sleep was impossible'.[2]

For extra training, the nurses visited nearby Alexandra Hospital, which had been renamed the British Military Hospital, the Tan Tock Seng Hospital and Singapore General Hospital to attend lectures on the treatment of malaria, beri-beri, typhoid fever and other tropical diseases.

It wasn't all work though. The nursing staff was supplied with Chinese servants – amahs – for domestic chores. Viv and her colleagues were given every second night off, with free time starting at 2 p.m. and concluding at midnight. Phyllis Pugh reckoned that for breakfast the army served the women 'goldfish – herrings in tomato sauce – morning after morning' but Viv and her friends were often invited to dine on more satisfying fare at functions held by the officers of the various Australian units.

All Australian officers including Lieutenant Vivian Bullwinkel were made honorary members of the elegant Singapore Swimming Club, where there was not only a spectacular pool surrounded by beach umbrellas, but a live orchestra, fine dining with immaculately dressed waiters, darts, billiards and card games. There were popular nightspots, too – the Adelphi and Airport hotels and the lavish Raffles, which hosted regimental dinners where officers in smart uniforms with chests covered in medals would dance cheek to cheek with nurses in beautiful evening gowns and exotic perfumes to the strains of the band of the Argyll and Sutherland Highlanders.

There were coffee shops and cinemas and invitations to relax at private homes, including those of the wealthy Dodd and Hanson families. The Dodds had magnificent gardens where the nurses could play tennis or swim and then drink cocktails served by waiters in smart white jackets. On one night, soon after Viv's arrival back in Singapore, Richard and Peg Hanson took her and Nancy Harris out for a formal dinner on one of the ships berthed in Keppel Harbour. The group had been invited by the ship's engineer Jimmy Miller,[3] a charming young Kiwi-born officer keen to meet two bright and attractive Australian nurses.

The visitors boarded a sampan for the short trip across the water to their evening's entertainment, Richard Hanson dressed in a dinner suit and Peg Hanson, Viv and Nancy resplendent in evening dresses. They arrived at their destination, a 77-metre-long white steamship that was used both as a cargo vessel and as the royal yacht of Sarawak, on the north-west of Borneo island.

It was called the *Vyner Brooke*. When it had been launched in Scotland in 1927, the ship's upper deck cabin could accommodate forty-four first-class passengers and featured a large, ornately furnished dining saloon with mahogany wood panelling on the walls and exquisite leather chairs.[4] The ship's main deck had accommodation for crew as well as a refrigerated storeroom for its work as an island trader sailing between Singapore and Sarawak's capital Kuching.

Once on board, Richard Hanson introduced Viv and her companions to Jimmy Miller and the ship's second officer John Thomas. The ship's captain and first officer were ashore on business and Jimmy explained that the ship was the first word in luxury. It now generally carried only twelve passengers in its exquisite suites, in addition to its crew of forty-seven. The ship was owned by the 'White Rajah', Charles Vyner Brooke,[5] a London-born Cambridge graduate whose family had ruled Sarawak for a hundred years as a reward for helping the Sultan of Brunei fight pirates and civil unrest. The family had become fabulously wealthy through developing the rubber and oil industries.

Viv could hardly believe the opulence, but she found Singapore frustrating. She felt she was wasting her time there and could have been used to much better effect in a war zone. The distractions of the city's night life were little compensation.

In her diary on Saturday, 18 October, Viv wrote about going on a double date with Nancy Harris and two soldiers.

Went around to Amber Road for drinks and then to Raffles for dinner. Rather disappointed in Raffles but still had a very nice dinner out in the courtyard. Frank is an amusing young English lad, and we danced at Raffles for a time. Then we went onto Coconut Grove for more dancing and back to Amber Road for a night cap.[6]

Viv's friends Mona Wilton and Wilma Oram attended a lavish ball at the Johor Bahru palace of the ardent Anglophile Sir Ibrahim,[7] the Sultan of Johor. They had met His Royal Highness by chance while waiting for a taxi at a club between Singapore and Johor Bahru. The Sultan was sixty-eight but he had an eye for attractive women and it was a magical evening for Viv's friends, who were taken to the palace in one of the royal limousines. They danced with charming army officers until 3 a.m. The Sultan's sixth wife, Marcella Mendl, a Romanian model forty-two years his junior, had everyone at the ball talking.

But the good times would soon end. On 20 October, with the Japanese advance through South-East Asia continuing, the British Defence Committee agreed to send the new battleship *Prince of Wales* and the ageing battle cruiser *Repulse* to Singapore. The aircraft carrier *Indomitable* was to have accompanied the ships but it ran aground on a sandbar near Jamaica, meaning the two warships had little fighter-plane protection.

VIV'S BROTHER, JOHN, now twenty-one, had been on the move ever since his first flight lessons in Wagga. In October 1941 the young pilot was in Canada continuing his flight training. He bought his sister a Christmas present he thought would amuse and delight her – a pair of silk pyjamas. In those more reserved and modest times John had the poor shop assistant blushing over the purchase of such a delicate item.

John moved on to England, preparing to battle the Nazis in aerial combat, but he was relieved that the voyage across the Atlantic was uneventful and they didn't see a hostile craft the whole time. After a few weeks in England, he'd added 3 kilograms to his spare frame and as soon as he was granted six days' leave he went to visit his father's people in London, including his 'Old Gran' Eliza Bullwinkel,[8] George's mother, and his uncle Dudley,[9] George's younger brother, who had served as a captain with the Royal Field Artillery on the Western Front in World War I.

John wrote a letter to Viv. Unsure of where she was in the world at war, he addressed it to her unit, hoping it would find her alive and happy. 'Old Gran', was a dear, he told his sister. Eliza was nearly ninety and crippled by rheumatism, but her brain was still nimble and she point-blank refused to budge from her house during the blitz by German bombers.

Dudley was a livewire chap 'and broadminded', John said. Dudley, who was in his late fifties, said John and his mate Tom Worley were welcome to stay at his house in Ilford but that being a young, single man he might prefer the bright lights of the big city because he was sure to have a good time in London. John and his mate heeded the advice. They met a couple of nurses. 'We took them everywhere we could find,' John wrote, 'of course [we] spent some cash but we certainly enjoyed spending it.'[10]

'By gosh' the nurses they met were 'jolly nice girls', he said, just like the nurses at Broken Hill when Viv was there. 'They are so easy to get on with and speak to. They made our London stay quite enjoyable, with dances and dinners and luncheons.' John told Viv that together with the nurses he had visited a few of the historical sites he'd read so much about and was leaving the others for another time. He saw the 'Changing of the Guard at the Palace but without all the colour it was nothing to speak about'. He'd had a quick look through Westminster Abbey, visiting the tombs of some of the great figures of British history. He saw the Tower of London but was mortified by the brutality that went on there. How could people be so cruel? They spent an hour or so at Madame Tussaud's waxworks, and while some of the figures were 'exceptionally well done' others, particularly that of Robert Menzies, were 'very poor'. Together they saw a couple of stage shows including the *Black Vanities*, starring the popular radio comedy duo Flanagan and Allen.[11] It reminded John of comedy shows he'd seen at the Sydney Tivoli. They also saw 'a real good play' called *No Time for Comedy*, starring Rex Harrison and Diana Wynyard. John had seen the Hollywood version starring Jimmy Stewart and Rosalind Russell but thought the stage performance to be much better.[12]

There was a war to be won, though, and John and Tom were sent to different postings. John had been sent to Wales to train on the single-seat Supermarine Spitfire fighter planes, which, together with the Hawker Hurricane, had helped turn back the German attacks during the Battle of Britain in 1940.

John was in awe of the Spitfire, which was so much more advanced than anything he had flown before. The magnificent throbbing Rolls-Royce Merlin V-12 engine produced almost 1500 horsepower and a top speed of more than 360 miles (580 km) per hour. Not only was it one of the fastest fighter aircraft of its time but the design of its wing allowed it to turn with all the control of a sports car. 'Believe you me,' John wrote, 'they're the goods.'

John told Viv that he much preferred the English countryside to the cities.

> The country we passed through certainly came up to my
> expectations. The lovely green fields, gentle undulating
> hills and little streams lined with trees, with little hamlets
> tucked away in the hills, is truly gorgeous. I suppose you
> are in the middle of sand desert, or else in the middle of
> the jungle with all its accompanying discomfort. Cheer up
> kiddo … We are at present stationed miles from anywhere
> and in the middle of mud. Still our quarters are quite nice
> … Plenty of food and beer so really when we get settled
> down properly we should be fairly comfortable …
>
> Well old dear afraid I'll have to leave off. Drop me a line
> at the address on this letter and it will be forwarded on to
> me sometime.
> All the very best.
> Love John[13]

At the same time as John was coming to grips with the speed and power of the mighty Spitfire in November 1941, Japan's new Prime Minister General Hideki Tojo[14] appointed Lieutenant General Tomoyuki Yamashita[15] to command Japan's 25th Army, stationed on Hainan Island, the largest and most populous island of China.

At fifty-six, Yamashita, a burly, round-faced doctor's son with close cropped hair, had commanded the Kwantung Army in China. In 1940, with Japan continuing to seize territory, he led a military mission to Germany to study the Nazi war machine in detail and, after meeting Hitler and Mussolini, had watched Spitfires dogfighting with German Messerschmitts over the English Channel off Calais.

ON 7 NOVEMBER 1941, Viv and Maisie Rayner, along with four doctors, were transferred to Tampoi, a suburb of Johor Bahru. The 2/4th Australian Casualty Clearing Station was converting an asylum into a casualty hospital for Viv's unit before heading further north into Malaya, where most of the Australian troops were stationed. A few weeks earlier, Kit Kinsella, who had taken over running the unit from Irene Drummond, had led a team of nurses there that included Bessie Wilmott,[16] Peggy Farmaner,[17] Millie Dorsch[18] and Mina 'Ray' Raymont.[19] Bessie and Peggy were friends from Perth Hospital. Bessie was not only a strong swimmer but a keen theatre goer and devoted parishioner at her local Church of England.[20] Mina and Millie were from Adelaide. Millie was the granddaughter of a Lutheran pastor who had trained at a bible college in America. Mina's father had died not long after being invalided out of the army, a physical and emotional wreck, suffering from what was termed 'Delusional Insanity' caused by 'active military service'[21] in Egypt and on Gallipoli during World War I.

Kit's team told Viv and those coming after her that they would be kept busy. In the few days after Kit's nurses arrived there, 257 soldiers were admitted, most of them suffering from malaria.

The Tampoi asylum was surrounded by thick jungle, and presented an ideal layout for a military hospital, its many wooden buildings distributed over extensive grounds making it a difficult target for aircraft. More than 700 tonnes of equipment had to be carted in to make the hospital ready for casualties and surgery.

The windows in all the buildings were barred, and Viv and her colleagues borrowed sledgehammers to smash them out.[22] The nurses' tents were almost 2 kilometres from the wards, which were open and airy with thatched roofs. Within those wards there were more than 10 kilometres of corridors, and Viv and the rest of the staff were given bicycles.

Viv was appointed the Sister in Charge of Ward C-1, where those suffering with malaria were housed. The ward had no sinks, running water or electricity, and driving rain flattened Viv's tent. Still, she and the others pressed on, doing their best in the conditions.

On 17 November, while the nurses were busy caring for the sick at Tampoi, the Australian battle cruiser HMAS *Sydney* and its 645 men, having escorted the *Zealandia* into the Sunda Strait off Java on its way to Singapore, turned back for Australia. The *Sydney* was a mighty warship, 171 metres long with twelve heavy guns, twenty-one machine guns and eight torpedo tubes.

Two days later the *Sydney* was off Carnarvon and heading south towards Fremantle, 800 kilometres away. Just before 4 p.m. the ship's crew spotted through the haze a suspicious-looking vessel about 30 kilometres away, heading north.

The *Sydney*'s signalmen immediately began sending messages by flashing lights and, when they were closer, also by signal flag, demanding the mystery ship identify itself. The ship signalled back that it was the Dutch merchant ship *Straat Malakka* and hoisted a Dutch flag.

It was in fact a German raider called the *Kormoran*, a freighter that had been requisitioned by Hitler's navy and had undergone the installation of concealed weapons. It carried 399 men and would masquerade as a cargo ship to blow unwary Allied vessels out of the water.

By April 1941, the *Kormoran* had sunk seven ships in the Atlantic and was on its way to wreak havoc in the Indian Ocean. In the Bay of Bengal, between India and Burma, it destroyed the Australian freighter *Mareeba* and a Yugoslavian cargo ship. Then it sank a Greek freighter in the Indian Ocean, before setting off to mine shipping lanes off the Western Australian coast.

Now the *Kormoran* opened fire on the *Sydney*. Within five minutes the Australian battle cruiser had been hit by at least eighty-seven shells and hundreds of explosive bullets, the barrage killing or disabling about 70 per cent of the ship's crew, including most of the officers.

A return salvo hit the *Kormoran* in the funnel, engine room and electrical installations, starting uncontrollable fires. The *Kormoran*'s crew abandoned ship. Over the next few days, 318 of the German crew were rescued by a troopship, a British tanker and an air and sea search.

All 645 men on the *Sydney* perished.

VIV WELCOMED THE REST OF THE 2/13th nurses and staff to Tampoi on 23 November because more hands were needed to bring the hospital up to an acceptable standard, especially if the Japanese caused trouble in the area, which was looking more and more likely.

Wards and operating theatres were equipped and work began to install taps, telephones and electricity. The old Sultan, Sir Ibrahim, donated vital medical equipment including a portable X-ray machine.

On 25 November, Viv was granted leave and headed back to Singapore. She found the St Patrick's School almost deserted. But as she was walking down the long ground-floor corridor, a young Australian army lieutenant approached. He looked familiar and he gave Viv an admiring glance. It was Jim Austin, the young officer she knew from Puckapunyal. Jim still cut a fine figure, though he was pale and perspiring. He had been suffering from what he called a 'tropical bug' and was visiting the hospital as an outpatient.[23]

Jim might have been in a weakened state but he still had the gumption to ask Viv on a date. So that night in Singapore's Anzac Club, the pair enjoyed a round of drinks before moving on to the Adelphi Hotel, where they caught up with another of Viv's friends, Beryl Woodbridge,[24] a Melbourne nurse with the 2/10th.

Viv and Jim moved on to dinner at Singapore's Airport Hotel and then took a taxi to Raffles. On this night, the hotel's ballroom was decorated in stunning style. The floor had been inlaid with glass squares that reflected dazzling colours projected by floodlights above. Viv and Jim waltzed on the dance floor, as musician Dan Hopkins and six other members of his band in dinner suits created the music of love.

Viv wrote in her diary later that she had the time of her life, and that when Jim dropped her off at St Patrick's just before midnight he promised to visit her at the new hospital across the causeway as soon as he could get leave. As she made her way back to her comrades at Tampoi, a Japanese fleet of thirty-three warships and auxiliary vessels, including six aircraft carriers and more than 350 aircraft, was getting ready to sail for the Hawaiian Islands.

AT TAMPOI, VIV HAD TO LOOK after two wards at night, C-1 and C-2, with the help of orderlies Ernie Ward and Jim Carmody.[25] One night early in December, with her patients sleeping soundly, Viv kicked off her shoes and put her feet up for a well-earned break. Just across the Johor Strait the lights of Singapore blinked as a shining beacon to the power and wealth of British colonialism. Although everyone at the hospital suspected the Japanese might eventually cause a few problems, British Prime Minister Winston Churchill had given his assurances to both Australia and New Zealand that defending Singapore would

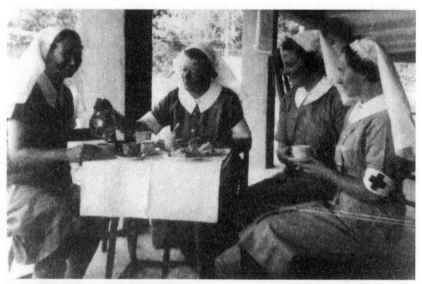

Viv (left) enjoys a cup of tea with Irene Drummond, Margaret Anderson and Margaret Selwood at the Tampoi hospital outside Johor Bahru. *Australian War Memorial P01 344.008*

take precedence over the British defence of the Mediterranean. Even though Britain was facing fierce opposition from both Germany and Italy, there seemed no way that Churchill would let Singapore and Malaya fall into Japanese hands. The great warships *Repulse* and *Prince of Wales* were on their way, too.

Viv couldn't wait for two days off to visit the restaurants and clubs of Singapore with Jim Austin again. Then, out of the corner of her eye, she saw something that made her heart jump. It was like a long, polished piece of opal from the Australian Outback, its brilliant colours glistening in the moonlight. Viv had never seen a snake quite so exquisite. For a moment, she wondered if she was imagining it. The serpent's thin metre-long body was a shimmering royal blue and its tail and head a vivid orange, the colour of the finest citrus grown in Australian orchards.

Viv was transfixed by the creature's hypnotic beauty. She had seen plenty of snakes growing up in Broken Hill and was not afraid, but she knew it would be better for everyone at the hospital if the snake was back in the jungle and not under the feet of her patients. She grabbed a broom, planning to hurl the snake into the trees, when suddenly one of the local Malay domestic servants – an amah – appeared and cracked the snake across the back with a thick stick. As the snake writhed in fierce contortions the amah cracked it again before lifting the wriggling, dying mass of scales and coils with the end of her stick and tossing it back into the darkness.

Viv protested that such a fascinating creature had to die so brutally, but the amah told her that the blue Malayan coral snake was the deadliest of all the snakes in the jungle.

Suddenly Viv did not feel so safe anymore. The amah brought her a pot of tea to calm her nerves, and Viv's hand shook as she poured herself a cup.

It had been a close call. But an even more ominous threat was on the horizon.

On Hainan Island, General Yamashita was learning everything he could about the Malay Peninsula and the British positions. Yamashita came to believe that the best way to overcome the

British strongholds would be invading the Malay Peninsula from the north, charging south down the main highway along the peninsula's west coast, and taking the fortress of Singapore from the rear.[26]

Offered five divisions for his attack, Yamashita said he would need only three. A lean force, he said, would accomplish more than a heavy one. His men planned to confiscate thousands of bicycles, which would let them move swiftly and silently along jungle pathways.

Yamashita also had an ample supply of warships to escort his transport convoys south and there would be 564 aircraft flying in support – fighters, bombers and reconnaissance planes that were far superior to the British machines in the area.

Senior officers drilled into their men again and again the religious mantra that they were fighting for the freedom of Asia against the western devils, and that, if needed, they would sacrifice their lives in honour of Emperor Hirohito, a descendant of the Gods.

Yamashita had more than 60,000 ruthless, merciless, well-trained, brainwashed men ready to kill anything or anyone that stood in the way of the ravenous Japanese war machine.

Chapter 8

HEART POUNDING AND IN A HOT SWEAT, Viv leapt out of bed to the sounds of shouting and the rattle of metal helmets. Air-raid sirens screamed eerily through the warm night air. She heard boots pounding. As she tried to wipe the sleep from her eyes, the ground shook. BOOM, BOOM, BOOM.

Viv and the other nurses bolted from their tents to the hospital's open grounds facing the Johor Strait and Singapore beyond, as men rushed about, arming themselves with their .303 rifles. Viv found two Queensland comrades leaning on a railing. Blanche Hempsted[1] from Brisbane and Val Smith[2] from the Atherton Tablelands were gazing out over the water and up at the sky, transfixed by what they were seeing.

Blanche had a big heart and a foul mouth. She 'could drink and swear with the best of the cattle drivers'.[3] 'They're bombing bloody Singapore,' she said dryly.

Val pointed to the night sky, where the silver beams of searchlights pierced the blackness as aircraft sped about like moths. 'I think it's the Japs!' she exclaimed. 'See the red dots on the planes?'[4]

If it hadn't been such a menacing spectacle it might have been a marvellous light show. The ghostly machines burst in and out of the lights as tracer bullets danced around them like fireworks to the constant 'ack-ack' of anti-aircraft cannon fire.[5]

Flames began to erupt in the darkness over Singapore. Viv and the other nurses all looked at each other despondently. 'War,' they uttered almost in unison.[6] They all knew that now they would be thrown into trauma nursing. And the casualties would be high.

It was 8 December 1941. Japan had just unleashed what would be the deadliest storm ever to hit the Asia-Pacific region. Coordinated bombing missions involving attacks in the air, on the sea and on land had been launched within hours over an area covering thousands of kilometres from Singapore to Hawaii. The air strike on Singapore was made by Japanese bombers that had flown more than 1000 kilometres from their base at Thu Dau Mot in what is now Vietnam. General Arthur Percival, the English military commander of the region, was stunned that Japan's military aircraft could fly so far.

Despite air-raid sirens sounding the alarm at 4 a.m., Singapore's streets had remained brightly lit and the Japanese navigators found their targets easily. A formation of nine bombers flew over the city at 3600 metres to draw the searchlights and anti-aircraft fire away from the other eight machines, which flew at just 1200 metres and released their deadly cargo with devastating effect on Singapore's RAF (Royal Air Force) bases at Tengah and Seletar, the Sembawang Naval Base and Keppel Harbour.

When the bombs began landing, the Allied anti-aircraft guns immediately opened fire, assisted by the gun teams on the warships *Prince of Wales* and *Repulse*. But the Japanese caused mayhem at the airfields.

The area around Raffles Hotel took an even heavier bombardment. World War I hero Hudson Fysh, in Singapore to expand the business of his growing airline Qantas, had checked into the hotel the night before. At a quarter past four the following morning, Fysh was shocked from his slumber by the unmistakable bark of anti-aircraft guns and the roar and shudder of bombs falling nearby. He managed to escape Singapore quickly.

After an hour's onslaught, and despite concerted ground fire from the two British ships, the Japanese aircraft headed back to their base at Thu Dau Mot undamaged. They had left sixty-one people dead and more than 700 injured. But it could have been much worse. The attack was originally assigned to sixty-five bombers, which had taken off late on the night of 7 December. However, thick clouds and high winds over the South China Sea caused the six squadrons to become separated, and most of the aircraft were forced to turn back. In the end, only seventeen of the Mitsubishi G3M bombers known as 'Nells' continued on to Singapore.

They left behind heartbreaking scenes of rubble and ruin. Clouds of smoke filled the sky as women wept over dead children. The attacks had only just begun.

THE NEXT DAY, VIV and the other nurses learned the full extent of the Japanese offensive. The series of coordinated attacks started at Kota Bharu on the north-eastern coast of Malaya. Kota Bharu, 730 kilometres north of Singapore, was the base of operations in Northern Malaya for British and Australian airmen, and its beaches were guarded by artillery and criss-crossed with barbed wire and pillboxes. Just after midnight on 8 December, Indian soldiers patrolling the local beaches noticed three huge shadows about 3 kilometres out to sea. They were Japanese transport vessels[7] dropping anchor to disembark 5200 troops, most of whom had been blooded in the brutal Chinese campaigns.

As the landings began, they were supported by covering fire from Japanese warships but III Corps of the Indian Army and several British Army battalions offered grim resistance. There were fierce gun battles on the shore, particularly around the Kota Bharu aerodrome, and then a twin-engine Lockheed Hudson from No. 1 Squadron RAAF became the first Allied aircraft to make an attack in the Pacific War. Brisbane pilot Oscar Diamond,[8] whose name sounded like a call-sign, dropped a pair of 250-pound bombs on the Japanese transport *Awazisan Maru*, and on his second run dropped two more bombs. He strafed the ship with machine-gun fire and left it burning.[9] Gunfire from one of the other Japanese ships blew out one of Diamond's engines but he made it back to Kota Bharu with one remaining propeller.[10]

Artillery fire from Japanese ships shot down two other Hudsons and badly damaged three others. One crippled aircraft crashed into a fully laden landing craft.

The Japanese suffered about 300 deaths among 800 casualties in the early assault but the British and Indian forces were poorly equipped and despite their postings, largely untrained in jungle combat. The Japanese quickly surrounded the defenders and forced their capitulation.[11]

The landings in Malaya preceded a furious drive down the eastern side of the Malay peninsula towards Singapore, while the troops who had landed in Thailand advanced down the western side. The speed and the savagery of the Japanese troops in this 'Bicycle Blitzkrieg'[12] quickly earned General Yamashita the nickname the 'Tiger of Malaya'.

The Japanese also landed at Pattani and Singora on the south-eastern coast of Thailand and had launched simultaneous attacks on Hong Kong, the Philippines, Shanghai, Guam and Wake Island.

Meanwhile, just forty minutes after the landing at Kota Bharu and while it was still 7 December on the other side of the International Date Line, 353 Japanese aircraft rained fire on Pearl Harbor in Hawaii, killing 2400 people and destroying much of America's Pacific fleet. The Japanese hoped they had rendered the United States impotent as a fighting force.

The headquarters of the British Far East Command issued a communique to military personnel that played down the danger the Japanese posed:

> ... a formation of Japanese aircraft attacked targets in the Singapore area, but no damage was done to military installations. Some damage to property and casualties are reported from bombs which were dropped on Singapore Town. Daylight attacks were made against aerodromes in northern Malaya but reports so far indicate that little damage was done.[13]

Viv and the other nurses all knew that the damage in Singapore and the loss of life had been colossal. A few hours after the raid, the two great ships *Prince of Wales* and *Repulse* had left Singapore to attack the Japanese forces in northern Malaya. Two days later,

Japanese bombers swooped on the ships in the South China Sea, destroying both vessels with the loss of 840 lives.

At Tampoi, Matron Irene Drummond told her staff that Australia was now at war with Japan and it was battle stations for everyone. Nurses were instructed that there were to be minimal lights at night-time, that slit trenches would be dug outside each ward in readiness for more air raids and that the nurses were to wear their metal helmets at all times and carry gas masks and emergency kits. They were also to always wear Red Cross armbands, though Colonel Pigdon warned them that they might not be much protection since 'the enemy we are fighting does not play cricket'.[14]

There would be 166 patients from Tampoi evacuated to other hospitals. Bed capacity was dramatically increased from 359 to 1183, mirroring the size of the hospital at Malacca, as the Australian troops would soon be moving north to tackle the hordes of Japanese who were in trucks and on bikes heading south, killing anyone who stood in their way.

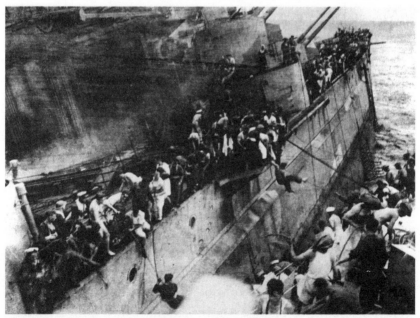

The sinking of HMS *Prince of Wales* by Japanese aircraft off Malaya in December 1941 was a devasting blow for the defence of Singapore. *Imperial War Museums HU2675*

Viv and the rest of the 2/13th worked around the clock to make the hospital ready, fitting out operating theatres, intensive care and surgical wards; hauling tonnes of equipment; erecting mosquito netting over beds; sorting out thousands of medical instruments; cataloguing boxes upon boxes of drugs and medicines; and stocking every ward with hundreds of plates, cups and sets of cutlery. Their work was often interrupted by the scream of the air-raid sirens as Japanese reconnaissance aircraft made it through the ring of defence to scout out more targets over Singapore. The nurses would have to hurriedly collect the sick and injured and carry them into the slit trenches in case the reconnaissance planes were leading squadrons of bombers. Those patients too sick to be moved were fitted with helmets and placed under the beds as some sort of protection against the fire raining from on high.

The Japanese had more than 600 aircraft at their disposal, including the state-of-the-art Zero Fighters and Betty and Nell bombers. The British had just 158 aircraft, including relics such as the Vickers Vildebeest biplane and the Brewster Buffalo.[15]

Viv and the others kept abreast of the Japanese advance through daily wireless briefings from Far East Command, while newspapers at home in Australia outlined the grim toll that the Japanese were taking.

On 11 December, Viv's mother, Eva, was met with news that the two British ships had been sunk and that Malaya was in flames.

In Northern Malaya the Japanese forces continue heavy attacks ... British troops and the R.A.F. are attacking another Japanese force trying to land at Kuantan. Reports filtering through to Singapore to-day from stations up-country, however, indicate that the position of the defending forces leaves no ground for complacency. The Japanese are demonstrating a faculty for imitation, which proves that they have well learnt the German blitz methods. Northern

Malayan aerodromes are being constantly attacked by large forces of enemy planes, which are dive-bombing recklessly.[16]

That night, in an attempt to put her mother's mind at ease, Viv wrote home to the anxious widow whose only two children were now thousands of miles from home and facing deadly risks every day. She told Eva not to worry. The curfews meant she was in bed by 9.30 every night and she had her tin hat and respirator with her as 'constant companions'.

I don't think any of us will ever forget the last air raid, we were all woken by the anti-aircraft guns and so congregated outside making up our minds whether it was the real thing or just the practice. Then we saw the planes approaching and they flew over us in the searchlights and all remarked what a pretty sight it was. Nothing else to see so all retired once again and some 20 minutes later heard the 'all clear' signal and it wasn't till 10 a.m. next morning when we were about to have another air raid that we realised we were at war. So all that day we played at air raids which really was a jolly nuisance as we had to drag our veranda patients inside and put tin hats on our sick boys who muttered 'a fellow would be ill when the fun starts'.

I don't suppose it's much use telling you not to worry but really we are quite safe and all as happy as sandbugs. We are opening up new wards in anticipation and in our off-time duty we have all been madly working in an effort to equip a mobile theatre as soon as possible.

The quarters are just a hive of industry. This morning we had a spot of bad luck – the autoclave in the theatre blew up sending it right through the roof, scattering bricks everywhere and flames flying. I think everyone thought the Japs had arrived. Unfortunately one of our boys was badly burnt about the face and arms.

When you send the next parcel would you include that floral linen frock of mine – that is if it's not in use –

the pink and blue flowers in rows – if I remember rightly – we are allowed to wear them about the quarters and as we are in a brown-out we don't have to dress for dinner, so if you wouldn't mind?

Jim Austin is much better and I was seeing quite a bit of him before all the leave was stopped and as his camp is only a couple of miles away notes arrive periodically per ambulance driver. He expects to join one of the artillery units at a moment's notice.

Well I must away and do a spot of sewing. Matron Drummond wishes to be remembered to you.

Lots of love.

Viv.

P.S. The boy that was burnt yesterday died this morning and the entire unit is very upset.[17]

Viv tried to remain optimistic but two days after she had written to her mother, the Japanese swamped the 11th Indian Division at Jitra, which the British had established as a defensive bastion. Japanese aircraft killed more than 2000 civilians in bombing raids on Penang and destroyed most of the Allied aircraft at Alor Setar.

On the night of 16 December two Japanese heavy bombers attacked RAF Tengah again. Everyone knew there would be more coming. Viv was reassigned to a ward that was run by Dr Bruce Hunt, a ward that was mostly focused on treating malaria cases.

Matron Drummond insisted every one of her girls put on a brave face for the sake of the patients and for each other, and that despite the threat of air-raid sirens drowning out the carols, Christmas dinner would go ahead at the hospital with all the trimmings and with a guest list that included Major General Bennett and Lieutenant Colonel Glyn White.

The wards were decorated and the Red Cross and Salvation Army provided additional food for both staff and patients, who dined on succulent chicken and ham. The Sultan of Johor arrived too and invited Irene Drummond, Colonel Pigdon and as many of the staff who could be spared to a formal dinner at the palace, where the guests dined off golden plates using golden cutlery.

Mona Wilton, who had been having a wonderful time double dating with Wilma Oram and different army officers, both British and Australian, wrote home that a lovely tea plantation owner she'd met would likely come back to Victoria with her when hostilities had ceased.[18]

The Japanese continued their charge south, though, capturing Ipoh, 560 kilometres north-east of Singapore, on the day after Christmas, following more than a week of relentless bombardment and the strafing of its streets by fighter aircraft. Jim Austin arrived in Tampoi to see Viv just before New Year's Day. His health had improved dramatically and he told her that recently he'd been serving as an AIF liaison officer with the air force.[19] Grimly he told Viv that their reunion was to be short-lived as he would soon be back with the 2/15th Field Regiment, and he was certain that they would be racing north to meet the Japanese onslaught.

He was not sure when he might see her again. In war you were always saying goodbye, never knowing if you would ever again see the people you cared about.

Ever since the Japanese had first landed in Malaya, Yamashita's men, better equipped, better trained and more merciless than the defenders, had constantly outmanoeuvred the British and Indian forces, surrounding whole units and killing thousands of men. Rumours abounded that the Japanese did not take prisoners, but only left bodies in their wake.

There was an uneasy silence between Viv and Jim[20] until Viv asked if they could exchange letters. Jim said that would be a great idea but he didn't know if Viv's would reach him in the jungle, wherever he might land. So they returned to the officers' mess for a farewell drink and then it was time to say goodbye. Jim walked down the path from the hospital and disappeared into the night.

THE ALLIED COMMAND WAS staggered by the level of fanaticism among the Japanese forces, which led to rape, torture and mass murder, according to eyewitnesses. The Japanese invaders were part of a system in which every day the necessity for absolute obedience was drilled into the fighting men. The soldiers were often beaten by their superiors, who in turn lived in fear of the officers above them. It created a culture of shameless cruelty.[21]

The Japanese government had signed the 1929 Third Geneva Convention, which guaranteed prisoners of war minimum rights and humane treatment. However, they refused to observe its requirements.[22] Under the Japanese Combatants' Code a soldier was expected to fight to the death, 'not to survive to suffer the dishonour of capture'.[23] The opportunity to die for the emperor was considered an honour. Prisoners of the Japanese would be treated with the utmost contempt.

Reports were emerging that several hours before the British surrendered at Hong Kong on Christmas Day, Japanese soldiers entered St Stephen's College, a private school that was now being used as a military hospital. Two doctors from the Royal Army Medical Corps protested and were marched away, killed and mutilated. Japanese soldiers burst into the wards and used bayonets to kill all the British, Canadian and Indian troops who were too sick or injured to hide. Some of the nurses were dragged away and gang raped.

More than 100 people were killed.[24] The day after the atrocities, while searching the hospital grounds, Sergeant Major Stewart Begg found among the mutilated corpses the naked bodies of his wife, Eileen, and two of her friends.[25]

It would later emerge that the soldiers from the 1st Battalion, 229th Regiment of the 38th Division of the Japanese Army, had been involved in the rapes and murders. They were under the command of a small and heartless young officer from Kagoshima, a seaside city on Japan's Kyushu Island, in the shadow of the active volcano Sakurajima.[26]

His name was Captain Orita Masaru.

Chapter 9

LIKE ANGELS OF DEATH, twin-engine Japanese bombers attacked Singapore again on the night of 29 December 1941. At the same time, the advance of the Japanese Army through Malaya was proceeding with few checks from outgunned defenders.

In order to free up more hospital beds in Singapore, the first evacuations of convalescent patients – mainly those with tropical diseases – started on New Year's Eve, when 114 Australian patients sailed for home via Batavia (now Jakarta, Indonesia) accompanied by several AANS nurses. Their escape vessel was a flat-bottomed Yangtze River boat that had been hastily converted into a makeshift hospital ship and painted white with red crosses on its sides. It was the *Wah Sui*.

Plans were also made for other, more seriously injured Australians to be relocated to the 2/12th AGH, based at Colombo in Ceylon (Sri Lanka).

By New Year's Day, the Japanese were near the town of Slim River about 100 kilometres north of Kuala Lumpur. They killed thousands of Indian soldiers guarding the area. The Japanese were now broadcasting warning messages to the Allied forces, using female announcers who spoke English to tell the nurses at Malacca to get out of their hospital because it would soon be bombed.[1] The female broadcasters were eventually given the generic nickname of Tokyo Rose for their barbed messages. That day, a truck loaded with twenty of Olive Paschke's nurses from Malacca arrived at Tampoi, telling Viv and the others that more nurses were following behind as the 2/10th had been ordered to evacuate.

They were to set up a new hospital at a former Methodist boys school inside Oldham Hall on the main road north out of Singapore leading to the causeway. Olive Paschke sent seventy-six patients and more than 700 tonnes of equipment 200 kilometres south in a huge convoy to Tampoi before starting work on Oldham Hall, which had been deserted and ransacked by looters. Olive and her nurses worked tirelessly to turn the dump into a 200-bed hospital, boiling surgical instruments in billies on portable spirit stoves in readiness for a high number of casualties. Viv's 2/13th AGH was now the only Australian hospital in Malaya and the front-line facility to treat the wounded when the AIF went to battle.

On 11 January 1942, the Japanese entered Kuala Lumpur with only minor skirmishing, the British troops having already retreated. The invaders continued rolling down the highway now known as Malaysia's Federal Route 1. The Japanese transferred their aerial operations to southern Malaya and the following day launched their first daylight raid on Singapore.

On 14 January, Yamashita's army finally faced General Bennett's Australian 8th Division, and found stubborn resistance from the Australian fighting men. Yamashita experienced the first major setback in his campaign with savage fighting around Gemas, the railway junction between the Malaysian west- and east-coast rail lines.

B Company of Australia's 2/30th Battalion launched an ambush against the advancing Japanese as they raced south on their bicycles. The Australians blew up the Gemencheh Bridge and opened fire with machine guns, rifles and grenades.

The Japanese suffered more than 1000 casualties in the battle,[2] which eventually lasted for thirty-six hours. The Australians suffered eight deaths and eighty wounded, but the numbers would mushroom over subsequent days. The Japanese repaired the bridge and forced the Australians to retreat.

At Tampoi, Viv listened stony faced as Matron Drummond told the nurses to be prepared for an influx of wounded patients who would first be treated by the Field Ambulance Unit before they would be moved on to the Casualty Clearing Station, where they'd be stabilised for the 200-kilometre journey south to Tampoi.

Irene tried to keep the spirits of her girls buoyant, visiting her nurses every day, either in the wards or in their rooms, sharing cups of tea or gossip or amusing stories that made her kindly eyes shine.

Writing to her sister at the time, she quipped: 'I heard a good story the other day. Have you heard it? What did the brassiere say to the top hat? You go on a head, and I'll give the other two suckers a lift.'[3]

At the same time, all the nurses congratulated Olive Paschke, who received the second-highest award for service in nursing, the Royal Red Cross, First Class.[4] While there were celebrations for her honour, they were muted.

DOCTOR BRUCE HUNT TOLD Viv and the others not to worry about normal, detailed procedure but to simply record the name and number of each wounded soldier so that he could get to them more quickly. It was vital, Hunt said, for the nursing staff to get them in, cleaned up, fed and bedded down for the night because the men were most likely traumatised and wouldn't have slept for days. In the early afternoon of 14 January ambulances caked in mud and misery began arriving at Tampoi with their bloodied and battered cargo. Orderlies carefully stretchered the wounded men into the admission building before racing out to bring in more. Ambulances continued to arrive, some ferrying emergency cases. Viv had seen terrible injuries in mining accidents at Broken Hill, but she had never seen anything like this. She was moved by the sight of men with bullet and shrapnel wounds lying quietly as they waited for their turn to be assessed, neither crying out in pain nor complaining about delays.[5]

The nurses raced about tenderly, carefully removing mud- and blood-soaked bandages from the soldiers. Dr Hunt moved between the wounded, assessing the injuries of each man before giving instructions to his staff.

Matron Drummond, who the nurses looked upon as an unflappable and inspirational leader, gave advice and comfort to both nurses and soldiers as wet and bloody uniforms were swiftly but gently cut from broken, bleeding bodies. The nurses sponged them down and dressed them in clean pyjamas, then helped lift them into beds with crisp white sheets. Those who needed it were spoon fed before lights out and the comfort of sleep, if it came.

The procession of casualties continued through the night and by next morning Dr Hunt and the nurses were exhausted after the busiest, bloodiest twelve hours of their lives. Dr Hunt told the nurses that they had produced 'a magnificent effort that had saved the lives of many fellow Australians. But get some sleep for the happenings of this day could well be frequently repeated in the days to come.'[6]

In fact, it would get much worse.

On the next night, 15 January, the Australian artillery briefly turned back a Japanese attempt to land and seize the harbour at Muar on the west coast of Malaya, about 160 kilometres north of Tampoi, but the Japanese eventually moved in and continued their charge south. Over the next week the Australians were engaged in some of the most savage jungle fighting of the war.

Australia's South African–born Lieutenant Colonel Charles Anderson,[7] a grazier from Young, New South Wales, led his men on repeated bayonet charges against enemy positions. Anderson was awarded a Victoria Cross for his heroics, but the Battle of Muar cost the allies an estimated 3000 casualties

While Anderson and his men fought desperately for survival, Japanese Field Marshal Hisaichi Terauchi[8] sent orders to the 38th Division, which was still in Hong Kong after their murderous spree at St Stephen's College. They were to invade and capture the city of Palembang on Sumatra and the adjacent Bangka Island. A plan of operations was prepared involving eight transport ships.

The commander of the Muntok landing unit – the 1st Battalion of the 229th Infantry Regiment – would be the merciless Captain Orita Masaru.[9] He was to lead a surprise landing on the shore south of the Muntok airfield around 3 a.m. on 16 February. After seizing the airfield, he was to then secure strategic points on Bangka Island.[10]

VIV AND THE OTHER NURSES were run off their feet at Tampoi as more and more wounded men arrived every hour from battlefields now just to the north. Not only were they carrying war wounds but increasing numbers were presenting with symptoms of typhus, a disease spread by bacteria in fleas and lice. Many of the soldiers had high fevers, headaches, chills, muscle aches and exhaustion. And they were the lucky ones who hadn't been shot or bombed. Some of the typhus patients experienced hallucinations; others fell in and out of comas.

Under the bright lights, the operating theatre became like a furnace, doctors and nurses dripping in sweat over their blood-soaked patients. At night some of the wounded men would scream in shock and terror. South Australian nurse Lainie Balfour-Ogilvy[11] would often sing them to sleep with her beautiful, lilting voice.

On 20 January, with the Japanese artillery raining bombs all day on Singapore, sometimes from more than eighty aircraft at a time, and with reports of rapes and murders in Hong Kong fresh in his mind, Alfred Derham, the 8th Division's chief of medical services, called for an immediate evacuation of the 130 Australian nurses. However, the Division's commander, Major General Bennett refused, saying it would damage the morale of the soldiers preparing for the Japanese invasion.

As the Australian forces retreated towards Tampoi, Nancy Harris, the nurse from Guyra, told Viv that she'd heard Tokyo Rose spruiking on the wireless again, telling the 2/13th Australian General Hospital to get out of Tampoi while they could because the Imperial Japanese Army would be taking over all the buildings on 26 January 1942.

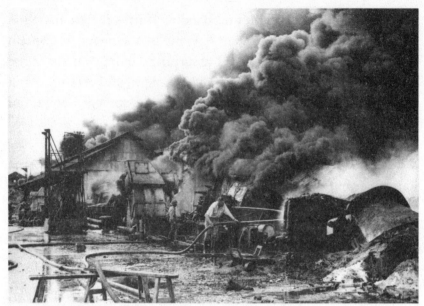

Firefighters battle blazes at naval yards in Singapore after a Japanese bombing raid.
Australian War Memorial P01182.010

Because the hospital was already over-crowded with the sick and wounded, Lieutenant Colonel Pigdon, Viv's commanding officer, decided to send 200 patients to Olive Paschke and the 2/10th now at Singapore's Oldham Hall. After meeting with his senior officers, he then decided to move the 2/13th back across the causeway, as Singapore seemed to offer more defences. The horror stories coming out of the battlefields north of Tampoi were chilling even for some of the grizzled war veterans among the Australian leaders.

It was decided that Viv and the other nurses, together with their patients would begin evacuating to Singapore on 23 January.

Three days earlier Lieutenant Colonel Anderson and about 200 men of the 2/29th Australian battalion, in addition to two Indian detachments, had begun a fighting retreat from the town of Bakri, which the Japanese had surrounded. Anderson knew that the only way any of his men could escape with their lives was to fight their way out. They left the area in fifty trucks and ambulances heading south carrying their wounded men towards Viv and the nurses at Tampoi.

At the first roadblock, Anderson personally put two machine-gun posts out of action with grenades. At the second roadblock, the Australians routed two companies of enemy troops. On the Muar Road, Japanese soldiers with six heavy machine guns had pinned down 'C' Company of the 2/19th. With a platoon from the 2/29th, Lieutenant William Picken Carr led a forward attack through a swamp. In an attempt to divert gunfire from their comrades, who were being massacred, Carr's platoon charged. It was an impossible task, but Carr and his men rose as one and rushed at the enemy, 'bayonets fixed, guns blazing' while singing 'Waltzing Matilda' at the top of their voices.[12]

On the following morning, 21 January, Anderson's men reached the outskirts of the village of Parit Sulong. It had been an English stronghold, but to the horror of the retreating men it was now held by the Japanese Imperial Guards and the only way across the river was blocked by their troops.

Under a flag of truce, Anderson asked the Japanese if two ambulances with dying men could be allowed to pass but the request was refused and the Japanese again opened fire. Anderson told his men that those who could run should head south through the jungle as quickly as they could.

He had no choice but to leave Captain Rewi Snelling with more than 150 Australian and Indian soldiers who were too badly injured to move. Anderson hoped the prisoners would be treated as humanely as the British treated those Japanese who were captured. Instead, the Japanese began killing all the wounded. Those who could stand upright were clubbed to the ground with rifle butts and kicked senseless. Indian soldiers were beheaded or shot.

Viv would later hear that some of the Australians were tethered together with wire and machine-gunned in the street. The Japanese poured petrol over the bodies and set them alight. Some of the shot men were still alive when the petrol caught fire.[13]

ON 23 JANUARY, JAPAN ATTACKED Australian territory for the first time, with a bombing raid on New Britain, an island off the west coast of what is now Papua New Guinea. On the same day, the move from Tampoi to Singapore began, with thirty-one operating-room staff and forty patients going to Oldham Hall.

Two days later, Viv crossed the causeway for St Patrick's in an ambulance and was directed to a stately house just down from the hospital that a wealthy Englishman had donated to the Allies as staff accommodation. Soon another 198 patients and 108 staff left Tampoi, and a fleet of thirty or so trucks with local Malay drivers were brought together to carry 1100 hospital beds and hundreds of tonnes of equipment.

Singapore was drowning in fear and the military hospitals were overwhelmed with casualties. Many of the roads had disappeared in bombing raids and some of the drivers, fearing the Japanese advance, had discarded their uniforms and trucks and returned to their families.

'Place in a terrible mess,' Viv scrawled into her diary. 'All patients were evacuated by 3 a.m. Terrible job sorting out and looking for patients and charts. Beds and boxes all together. Meals very scratchy.'[14]

St Pat's was reconfigured to house 700 beds, including 100 in the school's concert hall, and provisions were made inside the school's chapel and nearby buildings for more wounded, who would undoubtedly soon arrive. The operating theatre was set up in a large room in the basement that had previously served as an officers' mess.

The new theatre was in use twenty-four hours a day, with surgical teams working in shifts, trying to stay focused on their life-saving work as the city shuddered from what now seemed like a ceaseless barrage of bombs. Major Hunt insisted that every possible receptacle – baths and buckets, spare pots and pans – be filled with water, as he suspected the Japanese would cut the supply to the island at their first opportunity. The nurses also began cleaning up the abandoned homes around the school for use as accommodation for the medical staff because they figured all the room at the school – and then some – would soon be needed for the wounded.

Viv was given the role of assistant to 36-year-old South Australian–born sister Jean Ashton[15] in caring for the patients in the chapel, which had filled with wounded in just one morning. One of the young men was barely alive, having sustained a series of bullet holes to his chest from a Japanese machine gun. Orderlies lifted him onto an operating table as he asked the surgeon if he could have a last cigarette. There was little chance of him surviving so his wish was granted. After the young man inhaled deeply on his durry, Viv and the others in the operating theatre were staggered to see wisps of smoke spiralling towards the ceiling from the bullet holes in his chest.[16]

Every night, screaming air-raid sirens were followed by bombs. Sleep was fractured and nerves were frayed. Everyone was exhausted and anxious. Not long after she had assumed duties in the chapel, Viv was once more jolted awake by nearby explosions and screams coming from St Pat's. She raced from her quarters to the school grounds to find some of the nurses comforting soldiers who had been admitted earlier with war wounds. A Japanese aircraft had dropped a bomb near the officers' mess next to the school before scoring a direct hit with another bomb that crashed through the roof of one of the wards. The explosion had destroyed an outer wall and much of the roof. Water gushed over beds and furniture from a shattered pipe. Fortunately, the ward was unoccupied but the catastrophe it created only added to the shock and pain of the badly wounded patients.

On 30 January, a Japanese shell destroyed the kitchen at the Oldham Hall hospital, despite it displaying a large red cross. In just fifty-five days the outnumbered Japanese had advanced more than 700 kilometres through Malaya, losing only 4500 men compared with 25,000 British and Commonwealth casualties.[17]

Chapter 10

THE ALLIES HAD BEEN fighting on the retreat for more than six weeks when General Percival made the inevitable decision that Malaya was lost. He ordered all troops in Malaya to cross the causeway and begin a fight to the death to save the 'Lion City'.

The thousands of troops that crossed the Johor Strait ready for a final confrontation were sad, weary and forlorn men who had spent a month and a half fighting losing battles against better-equipped, better-trained and better-prepared soldiers.

The final detachment of Allied troops, the Argyll and Sutherland Highlanders, crossed over to Singapore on 31 January 1942. The sound of a lone piper was soon drowned out by the explosions, as engineering teams blew up a 60-metre section of the causeway in the hope of slowing the Japanese advance.

One of the Australian soldiers to return to Singapore was Jim Austin, who came to see Viv at St Pat's. She was tending to a wounded patient when Jean Ashton told her that there was a young officer waiting to see her.

Exhausted, unshaven and wearing a battered, mud-splattered helmet, Jim told Viv that he'd been posted to the General Base Depot, as the allies prepared to defend the island[1] against the Japanese invasion that was expected within days. 'God bless,' he said to Viv before hurrying off to prepare for an enemy that fought to a different set of rules.

Before long there were a million people trapped on the island in a city being blown apart. Many of the shops boarded up their windows and stacked sandbags against their walls. The Japanese began firing anti-personnel bombs called 'grass-cutters' that, on explosion, would propel hundreds of pieces of white-hot shrapnel at body height to shred human beings. Large concrete pipes became temporary bomb shelters, though many civilians preferred to shield themselves in monsoon drains, which at that time of year harboured a multitude of deadly water snakes.

Irene Drummond told her sister in Adelaide: 'There is nothing to write about as usual, except bombs and more bombs ... A good many of the officers I knew at Port Dickson [on Malaysia's west coast, south of Kuala Lumpur] have been killed or are wounded. The two Scotchmen who taught us to do the eightsome [sic] reel on the *Queen Mary* have both been killed.'[2]

The arrival of Britain's 18th Division from England bolstered Percival's fighting strength to more than 70,000 men in comparison to just 35,000 Japanese troops, but the Japanese turned off Singapore's water supply from the reservoirs across the strait. It would only be a matter of time before they raised the Rising Sun battle flag across the Johor Strait.

As the Japanese established artillery batteries at Johor Bahru, the bombing of Singapore intensified. Soon the city was enveloped by plumes of thick, acrid black smoke from the burning oil supplies beside the docks that were targets for the Japanese big guns. Citizens and the military who weren't blown apart choked together from the thick pollution, and when it rained, buildings were covered with a thin black film.[3]

Kath Neuss,[4] of the 2/10th, 'a tall, fun loving and gregarious woman with brown eyes, dark hair, and a wicked sense of humour',[5] wrote home on 6 February to quip, 'Guess you will be thinking I've gone up in smoke. There is plenty of it about.'[6]

At a meeting of the leading military officers in Singapore on 8 February, a British nitwit even volunteered the suggestion that the Australian nurses should stay and that if, God forbid, the Japanese forced a surrender and all looked lost, Allied soldiers could shoot the nurses to stop them falling into enemy hands.

Alfred Derham was appalled and kept pressing Bennett to let the nurses go, arguing so forcefully that Bennett made an order, instead, that they definitely stay.

Wilma Oram heard all the reports and later recalled in an interview: 'We were conscious of the danger we were in. We knew. Some of our officers said they'd never let us fall into the hands of the Japanese; they'd shoot us first. I thought, *Hang on, I'm twenty-five years old. I'll take my chances, please.*'[7] A friendly pharmacist offered Pat Gunther[8] a phial of morphia 'just in case' she decided to choose a painless death rather than fall into Japanese hands. Pat was a tough and resourceful young woman, a descendant of the convict turned entrepreneur Mary Reibey, and she had left school at twelve because she was needed on the family farm. She declined the morphia.

Derham wasn't finished though. He decided that he would get around Bennett's directive by telling his deputy, Glyn White, to evacuate as many of the wounded men as possible. They would need nurses to travel with them. Lots of nurses.

THAT NIGHT, 8 FEBRUARY, after fifteen hours of sustained fire from Yamashita's heavy guns, when 88,000 shells hit Singapore and its trapped hostages, the first Japanese troops set out across the Johor Strait in barges and collapsible boats. As the 22nd Australian Brigade, now just 3000 men after having been devastated by casualties in Malaya, waited nervously in their positions along the north-western coast of the island, the first wave of 13,000 Japanese troops from Japan's 5th and 18th Divisions approached in the darkness. Another 10,000 were ready to follow them at first light.

Spotlights had been set up on the beaches to illuminate invaders but many had been damaged by artillery fire. As the landing craft came close to the Australian positions in a mangrove swamp, the soft splash of paddles in the dark water was a sinister prelude to the roaring storm about to begin. From their fox holes, the Australians took aim at the shadowy figures through the mist and mosquito swarms, working the bolts and bullets into the barrels of their .303 rifles, their fingers rested in readiness on the triggers.

Before they could fire, though, teams from Australia's 2/4th Machine Gun Battalion, interspersed among the riflemen's fox holes, opened fire. Rubber dinghies were shredded and bullet-riddled Japanese infantrymen splashed dead into the water. More boats came to replace them. The machine-gun fire continued along with rifle fire.

Australian grenades exploded among the Japanese, too, and there were cries of anguish. But still the Japanese kept coming. There were sixteen Japanese battalions in the attack and just two Australian battalions to repel them. Much of the first wave of the Japanese was cut down and the second was decimated, but another wave began landing around the mouth of the Murai River. They were met with bayonets. An hour's battle of intense hand-to-hand combat followed, and Jim Austin's 2/15th Field Regiment fired almost 5000 rounds from their rifles. But the Japanese had landed in numbers.

The procession of Australian wounded and dying accelerated. All the pews were removed from St Andrew's Cathedral, near Raffles, as the 2/9th and 2/10th Field Ambulances converted the cathedral into a hospital for troops and civilians.

Across the road in a park near the sea, a battery of Australian guns blazed away on the Japanese positions in what would prove to be a last desperate fight. Inside the cathedral, hundreds of sick and wounded men and women were lying in every available space. One onlooker remarked that 'in a small vestry-like room, improvised as an operating theatre, doctors were performing remarkable feats of medical skill; civilians here and there were administering to the wounded soldiers and civilians'.[9]

'Monday 9th February,' Viv wrote in her diary, 'Shelling and raids, busy as hell. Operating theatre going day and night ... the boys are marvellous.'[10]

Palls of black smoke continued to billow from burning warehouses full of rubber, blazing offshore oil depots and the abandoned naval base. Air-raid sirens wailed as Japanese planes circled high above. Cars packed with evacuees and luggage crawled towards the waterfront, past rubble and burnt-out vehicles, fallen telegraph poles and tangled power lines.[11]

That day, the Japanese captured four men from Australia's 2/9th Field Ambulance at Sarimbun Beach on Singapore's north-western coast near the aerodrome at Tengah. The Australian ambulancemen were William Lewis, Alf Woodman, Harold Ball, a 21-year-old who had played for Melbourne in the 1940 Australian rules grand final, and their medical officer, Captain John Park, who had won a silver medal as a hurdler at the recent Empire Games at the Sydney Cricket Ground. The Japanese soldiers tied their captives' hands behind their backs and then cut their heads off.

The following day, Japanese soldiers marched twenty Australian soldiers into the jungle at nearby Kranji and ran them through with bayonets and swords.

MAJOR GLYN WHITE SAW a glimmer of hope for his nurses and some of the wounded men. Just as the British had done in evacuating their troops from Dunkirk in France in 1940 as the Nazis closed in, White wanted to use any vessel he could to help women, children and wounded soldiers escape to what was still seen as the relative safety of the Dutch East Indies.

On 10 February, Winston Churchill sent a telegram to General Percival's boss General Archibald Wavell, commander of American-British-Dutch-Australian Command saying:

> There must at this stage be no thought of saving the troops or sparing the population. The battle must be fought to the bitter end at all costs ... Commanders and senior officers should die with their troops. The honour of the British Empire and of the British Army is at stake.[12]

But there was no way the Allied forces could hold off the Japanese. Glyn White knew the situation was hopeless and wanted the women away from Singapore as soon as possible. Bennett and

Percival finally ordered the evacuation of all Australian nurses.[13] White chose eighty patients to be among the first evacuees, and Olive Paschke chose six nurses to travel with them on the *Wah Sui*. Given just an hour to collect their things, the six nurses begged to stay to help with the casualties but Olive told them orders were orders and it was out of her hands. Many tears were shed as they said their goodbyes.

Bundaberg nurse Pearl 'Mitz' Mittelheuser[14] from the 2/10th was determined to stay with her friends and the wounded. Fellow nurse, Sister Molly Campbell, was assigned to leave on the *Wah Sui* but was upset that her close friend, Sister Thelma McEachern, had not been given a berth as well. Mitz offered to gamble her place on the *Wah Sui* with Thelma, with a coin toss to decide their fate. Pearl tossed the coin and without revealing the result, told Thelma she had won, and that she could travel with Molly on the *Wah Sui* while Pearl stayed behind. It proved a bad toss to lose.

Mona Wilton scribbled a note to one of the wounded men to deliver to her parents. It read: 'In a terrific hurry to get the boys on a ship – to home & safety. Goodness knows when we will follow. Don't worry – will you? We can dodge bombs with the best of them.'[15] It was the last word her parents ever received from her.

The wounded and the six nurses were driven from Oldham Hall by a fleet of ambulances to the docks on Keppel Harbour. From there they were ferried by launches out to where the *Wah Sui* was anchored, well away from the other ships in the harbour. Despite its dilapidated condition, and despite their reputation for savagery, the Japanese recognised the little rust bucket as a hospital ship. They had even asked for it to be moved away from legitimate shipping targets that they were bombing.

The little converted riverboat left Singapore with 300 passengers, mostly Australian and British wounded. It was bound for Batavia, three days away. To the horror of all on board, the *Wah Sui* was buzzed by Japanese aircraft but, perhaps because of the red cross painted on its side, it was not fired upon.

Not all the Japanese were heartless. It seemed a simple matter of luck in these times as to whether you encountered men or monsters. Later, the little vessel was challenged and stopped by a Japanese cruiser. A boarding party came on board to examine the passengers and cargo but, remarkably, they let the ship go. The *Wah Sui* safely reached Batavia, where the passengers were disembarked and hospitalised. The six Australian nurses were transferred to the troopship *Orcades*, and they reached Adelaide a few weeks later.

THE AUSTRALIAN NURSES still in Singapore were told that half of the 130-strong Australian staff would leave immediately. However, when Irene Drummond assembled Viv and all the other sisters of the 2/13th and called for volunteers for evacuation, no one stepped forward. There were more than a thousand casualties in the hospitals, and every nurse wanted to stay to help the wounded. Irene had just learned that one of her friends, a young soldier, had shot himself. Badly wounded, he did not want to be a burden.[16]

At St Pat's, the wards were overflowing so, as the Japanese kept up a constant barrage with artillery and mortar shells, some of the casualties were placed on stretchers in rows on the lawn.

The city had crumpled into chaos. People were running, screaming, pushing their way over the dead and dying, begging for salvation to a soundtrack of explosions and machine gun fire. But even with the Japanese now within 5 kilometres of St Pat's, the women who had devoted their lives to caring for the sick and injured did not want to leave their patients. Viv's colleague in the 2/13th Jessie Simons,[17] a tall bespectacled kindly woman from Launceston, noted that 'there was a good deal of sulphurous protest against the distasteful order to evacuate'.[18]

Olive Paschke had the same response when she asked nurses of the 2/10th, as did Kit Kinsella with the 2/4th Casualty Clearing Station.

Colonel Derham warned that any nurses who refused to be evacuated would be court-martialled, and so, on the following morning of 11 February, the matrons chose half of the sisters to leave immediately by boat. Betty Jeffrey, who desperately wanted to stay with the sick and wounded, kept out of sight, remaining in one of the wards to change a poultice on one of her patients.

The nurses chosen were to sail on the *Empire Star*, a refrigerated cargo ship that, in its seven years on the ocean, had been used mostly to transport frozen meat from Australia and New Zealand to England. It had arrived in Singapore on 29 January as part of a convoy bringing 17,000 reinforcements from Britain's 18th Division. The ship's skipper, Selwyn Capon,[19] of the Royal Navy Reserves, had received an OBE for his service in World War I and knew Singapore well, but he had never seen it like this. The exotic city of spices and languid, lazy humidity that he regarded as a second home now appeared like a nightmare vision of hell. From the bridge of his ship, he watched soldiers rolling abandoned cars and trucks to the edge of the pier and pushing them into the sea to ensure the Japanese didn't get their hands on them.

Captain Capon was well used to escape missions, as he had helped British sailors get away in the great evacuation of Dunkirk two years earlier. The *Empire Star* generally carried only twenty-four passengers but on 11 February it was overflowing with more than 2000 evacuees. Capon was only awaiting the arrival of fifty-two Australian nurses and seven masseuses.

Viv was among those nurses chosen to stay in Singapore until the last moment. With tears, kisses and hugs, she and the remaining sisters gave an emotional farewell to their colleagues, who were ordered to leave with whatever they could carry in a small haversack and a tiny kitbag.

Matron Drummond hugged each of the women of the 2/13th. 'Good luck, kids!' she said as she waved them off.[20]

The departing nurses took off as fast as they could in ambulances, disappearing into the night to St Andrew's Cathedral to collect the women from the 2/10th, who would be sailing with them on the *Empire Star*. Along the way, another air raid forced the women to seek shelter in the cellar of the Adelphi Hotel, but they managed to collect their colleagues and make their way to the dock, where the great refrigerated cargo ship was anchored.

With bombs exploding all around, the nurses and wounded diggers joined the heaving mass of terrified evacuees. The dock was littered with abandoned cars and slippery with oil. A large Chinese junk was burning, from which people, also on fire, were jumping into the sea. Military police pointed guns at anyone trying to get on the ship without authorisation, but one group of Australians – army deserters dressed as civilians – pushed desperate women and children aside to climb on board.

Here and there lay the detritus of shattered lives. Someone had dropped their life story in photographs like a discarded hand of cards. Others had dropped personal belongings, cherished right up to the water's edge only to be cast off as too much to carry with so many lives on the line.

As Sister Kathleen McMillan of the 2/10th boarded the ship she picked up an abandoned toy rabbit with a bow tie. It was eyeless and nameless, a symbol of the chaotic, shambolic evacuation.[21]

Among his passengers, Captain Capon counted 1573 RAF, British Army and Royal Navy personnel, many of whom would continue the fight against the Japanese from Java. There were 139 Australian soldiers, mostly wounded, and 133 army nurses and signalling personnel. Altogether there were 160 women on board and thirty-five children.[22]

The nurses were given a tin of bully beef or baked beans and biscuits and allotted an area in the hold. They settled in as best they could for what they suspected could be a voyage they might not complete. The Japanese had announced by radio from Tokyo that the British were not going to be allowed to escape Singapore in the way they had fled Dunkirk. All ships attempting to leave would be attacked.

There were few comforts on the *Empire Star* and the vessel smelt of old, stale meat and blood, but the nurses could open their hold to the night sky. When the Japanese aircraft weren't flying over, the stars glittered with the promise of freedom. The gentle throb of the ship's two diesel engines was somehow reassuring. Some of the army boys threw cartons of cigarettes and abandoned toys to the nurses in the hold. Maude Spehr of the 2/13th caught a teddy bear and called it 'Blitzer'.[23] All around them storage tanks were going up in flames.

By 6 p.m. it was dark but the harbour was bathed in the eerie glow of the burning fuel dumps. The night buoys that marked the sea minefields around Singapore had been destroyed,[24] so the captain moved his ship out into the harbour and waited until he could see a safe passage by the first rays of dawn on 12 February. He finally set off with the cargo ship *Gorgon*, escorted by the cruiser HMS *Durban* and anti-submarine vessel *Kedah*, a converted Singapore–Penang ferry. The nurses came upstairs and crowded together on what little deck space there was, and watched as Singapore, blazing with fires and rocked by explosions, disappeared into the distance.

It was a hot and humid morning, and about to get hotter. Captain Capon threaded his ship through the myriad islands south of Singapore in an effort to avoid detection by Japanese aircraft, but about four hours into the journey, at 9.10 a.m., the convoy was just south of Batam Island when a lookout spotted six Japanese dive-bombers in the distance. Capon gave the order to man the machine guns and anti-aircraft cannons.

Physiotherapist Bonnie Howgate later recalled that she and some of the other nurses had just eaten a breakfast of biscuits and cheese when they heard the machine-gun fire getting closer 'with their "rat-tat" and our bodies went flatter than ever'. She heard orders being bellowed to 'Take cover! Get right inside and keep away from doorways! Keep down!'[25]

Men lined the railings, blasting away with their .303 rifles at the low-flying aircraft, which returned fire with machine guns and bombs. The *Durban* was firing at the aircraft too, but they kept coming in swarms. One plane was hit as it came in low. It spiralled into the sea, trailing black smoke and flame.

Children screamed as terrified mothers tried to comfort them. A few people passed out, either from the broiling heat or abject fear.

A second plane was hit and broke off over the horizon, pouring smoke.

All around the *Empire Star* huge spurts of water rose heavenward as bombs hit the surface. Capon tried as best he could to steer the ship out of the way of direct hits. Then a bomb struck the starboard side, opening a jagged hole, and in a flash of brilliant light and a great rushing force of energy, people were smashed against the ship's metal walls, their ears almost bursting from the noise of the blast.

As Japanese Betty Bombers came in again and again, the exploding bombs caused cascades of water to rain over the ship. Two of Viv's friends from the 2/13th, Margaret Anderson[26] and Vee Torney,[27] saw that some of the evacuated patients were being smothered by smoke and fumes. Thinking the raid had passed, they helped drag the men to the deck. But the bombers returned and machine-gunned the decks.[28]

More bombs exploded around the ship as men rushed about with hoses, trying to douse the flames. There were two more hits on the *Empire Star* and Margaret and Vee were hurled about alongside the soldiers. Blood made the floors slippery.

Capon's every move could save or kill the more than 2000 souls under his care. There were three fires raging but as the men rushed to put them out, below deck some of the nurses started a singalong – stirring tunes such as *There'll Always Be an England* – to calm the petrified children.

On the main deck, Margaret and Vee worked on as many wounded men as they could, though some, the ones missing limbs or with other deep wounds, were beyond help.

Someone screamed 'Look out' as a Japanese bomber hurtled towards them again, machine guns blazing. Without a moment's concern, Margaret and Vee threw themselves across the bodies of the wounded men they were ministering to. Bullets slammed into the deck, ricocheting in all directions as the bomber passed so close the crew could almost touch it. But then, all their ammunition spent, the Japanese aircraft flew away.

They returned at 1.10 p.m., having reloaded and refuelled. But the covering fire of the *Durban* and Capon's brilliant manoeuvring of the *Empire Star* – zigzagging and often throwing the engines

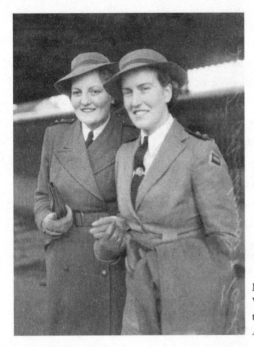

Margaret Anderson (left) and
Veronica Torney were lauded for
their astonishing courage under fire.
Australian War Memorial 136836

into full reverse to dodge the attacks – meant that only one more
bomb landed on the ship. It hit a cabin next to an engine room
and did little damage.

The Japanese dropped two 1000-pound (450 kg) bombs, one
on each side of the vessel, and the *Empire Star* was literally lifted
out of the water. When it righted itself, the nurses heard only one
of the two engines working. One of the lifeboats had also been
destroyed.

In total, the Japanese had sent more than fifty twin-engine
bombers in four separate attacks over four hours, but the *Empire
Star* was still afloat and the passengers were cheering their escape,
tears of joy running down their faces.

Fourteen people had been killed in the raid and seventeen
wounded, but Selwyn Capon reckoned he had never seen bravery
like Margaret and Vee showed that day. He rewarded the bravery
of the Australian nurses by granting them the use of his bathroom,
where some of them washed their delicates. Phyllis Pugh later
wrote that the *Empire Star* 'became the only ship in the British
Navy with smalls waving gaily from the bridge'.

The next day, the fourteen dead were buried at sea, their bodies slipping into the brine to the hymn 'Abide with Me'. Then, after another forty hours at sea, the ship and its precious human cargo arrived at Tanjung Priok, the port of Batavia.

The Australian deserters on the *Empire Star* were placed under guard. Though there were calls for them to be executed, they were allowed to rejoin the Australian forces in Java.[29]

Repairs were made to the ship and the Australian nurses eventually reached Fremantle a week later on 23 February, where the local Red Cross met them with fresh clothes and hearty meals. Margaret Anderson was presented with the George Medal for bravery, and Vee Torney was made a Member of the Order of the British Empire (Military MBE).

Selwyn Capon, a crusty old salt and now veteran of two world wars, wept as he asked all the nurses to do two things every day of their lives: to thank God they were alive and to never forget the Merchant Navy.[30] Captain Capon was awarded the CBE to go with his OBE from the Great War, but eight months later, sailing the *Empire Star* from Liverpool, England, towards Cape Town, his ship was attacked by a U-boat in the North Atlantic. Most of the crew and passengers climbed into three lifeboats that drifted for two days in heavy rolling seas. Two boats were rescued by the Royal Navy, but the third – carrying Capon, and thirty-seven others – was never seen again.

THE NURSES ON THE *Empire Star* wondered every day what had happened to the friends in Singapore they'd farewelled – Vivian Bullwinkel, Irene Drummond, Olive Paschke and all the other nurses. Even though they had been reluctant to leave, from the safety of Australia they knew they had been fortunate to have escaped the bloodbath in Singapore. They prayed for those brave and beautiful souls left behind.

Chapter 11

IT WAS THE MORNING OF 12 FEBRUARY, just hours
after the *Empire Star*'s departure. Exhausted and almost in a
daze, Viv was doing her rounds when Major Bruce Hunt grabbed
her by the arm and told her to quickly collect her things. She and
the rest of the Australian nurses were to be evacuated immediately,
no arguments. Viv found her boss, Jean Ashton, preparing a young
soldier's leg for amputation,[1] and in a whisper lest she alarm the
wounded men Viv uttered the words that they were being forced
to go.

Overcome with feelings of guilt and shame, Viv hid her face
in case of tears. It tore her up to leave the soldiers, whom Betty
Jeffrey called 'those superb fellows',[2] to the mercy of the Japanese.
'We felt we were letting them down badly and couldn't even look
them in the eye,' Viv recalled later.[3]

All of the patients needed attention, but none of them, nor
the doctors who desperately needed help with the wounded, ever
complained.

An hour after the order to leave was given, the nurses were all
smartly dressed in their grey uniforms, though some were sobbing
uncontrollably. To console them, some of the soldiers, barely able
to move in their sickbeds, told them they were glad the nurses
were going because it was a relief to know that they would be safe.
The soldiers smiled but Viv knew they were 'sad at heart'.[4]

Then to cries of 'Good luck' and 'Godspeed', Viv and the other
nurses climbed into a fleet of waiting ambulances to negotiate the

nine hazardous kilometres of ruined roads and crushed rubble of what had, until recently, been a jewel in the British Empire. As the nurses left St Pat's the orderlies and officers formed a guard of honour and saluted. Viv and the other nurses returned their salutes by waving their white handkerchiefs out the windows.

The ambulances arrived at the makeshift hospital that was St Andrew's Cathedral to see an anti-aircraft gun inside the church grounds blasting away at a Japanese bomber above. Wounded soldiers lay in stretchers all about the lawn. Viv could hardly believe that this area, where she had once strolled with her girlfriends and male companions towards the nearby elegance of Raffles, was now a war zone. Inside the cathedral, the nurses of the 2/13th gathered around the altar with their colleagues from the 2/10th and 2/4th to begin the convoy home. There were sixty-five of them and Glyn White and Olive Paschke ticked their names off from White's list. Olive then gave all the nurses a Red Cross armband, hoping it might be some protection if they fell into Japanese hands. They carried all their possessions in small kitbags. Some of the Australian soldiers preparing for one last rear-guard action against the Japanese made their way to the cathedral to farewell the nurses and wish them a safe passage home.

Then the final contingent of the Australian sisters to leave Singapore headed for the docks. They were only a couple of kilometres away, but the route was so crowded with panic-stricken citizens, abandoned vehicles, burning debris and rubble, that the ambulances had to stop and let the women make the rest of the journey on foot.

The smell of death and decay in the streets was nauseating. Smouldering, dismembered and decomposing bodies were strewn everywhere among the sad remnants of scattered, burst-open suitcases. The Japanese had cut Singapore's water supply and the sewerage system had been destroyed in the bombing. Raw sewage oozed into the streets and gutters.

AT HER NEAT LITTLE home in peaceful, suburban Adelaide, a long way from the fighting, Viv's mother had just posted a short letter to her in a sky-blue airmail envelope complete with a nine-penny stamp. It was addressed to the 2/13th AGH in Singapore.

Eva Bullwinkel was replying to a letter Viv had sent on 5 February and a cable the next day in which she reassured her mother that everything was fine in her neck of the woods. Eva was worried, nonetheless.

My dear Vivian,

… I listen to the wireless for every bit of news about Singapore. In this morning's paper it says the Japs have secured a foothold … I am worried. However, when I receive your letters things always seem a little brighter, when your letters do not come my hopes go down to zero again.

Adelaide is all blacked out at night now so I do not go out after dark.

I received a cable from John a few days ago with birthday greetings and saying he is well. He sent the cable from some place called Woking. Thanks awfully darlingist [sic] for your kind wishes for my birthday, fancy you thinking of it when you must be frightfully busy and so much for you to think about.

How is your pal Jim Austin, I do hope he is well and quite himself again. I am looking forward to your letters – if you have time to write letters there should be quite a lot to write about.

Well darling I must stop now. Sincerely hoping that Singapore will be able to hold out until reinforcements arrive, which I hope will be very soon.

Hoping and praying you will come through safely.
With fondest love to your dear self from
Mum

THE HEAT FROM THE OIL FIRES all around Singapore was so intense that Viv and the others had to shield their faces with their bags. The naval base at Seletar had been set alight when it was abandoned. Black rain from the oil and showers of sparks covered Viv's clothes.

Thousands of distressed parents carrying small children swarmed at the gates to the docks waving documents and passports in the faces of the military guards, begging for a berth on the ships. The guards ushered the nurses through but thousands of others began to realise there was no escape from the Japanese, who were snapping at their heels. One group of terrified men began rushing through the crowd, knocking everything in their path out of their way in a mad, desperate scramble to board a ferry bound for the ships in the harbour, but the military police drew their revolvers and opened fire. Viv could hardly comprehend the carnage as some of the men were shot dead and the others with them, perhaps brothers, stood stunned and mortified.

Others in a panic stepped over the bodies and started waving their passports again.

Then a Japanese aircraft came hurtling across the sky just above the huge crowd and dropped bombs into their midst, tearing bodies apart and ripping away large pieces of timber and concrete from the wharf.

Viv saw frantic mothers holding pieces of what had been their precious babies, and small children wandering around as though in a trance calling for mothers and fathers who had likely been killed. As if under remote control, Viv and the other nurses rushed into the sea of bleeding humanity to do what they could, ripping apart clothes from abandoned suitcases to use as bandages and tourniquets to treat severed limbs and shattered bones. All the time they knew that with the Japanese so close and the hospitals already overflowing, most of these wounded people would die.

Viv was ministering to a young woman who had been wounded in the air attack when she saw a well-dressed young man only a few metres from her sitting forlornly beside the body of a dead woman. Gently he rolled the body over and from underneath it picked up a baby the mother had been shielding from the Japanese blasts. With tears rolling down his face he cradled the baby to his chest and, without a backwards glance, left the dead woman where she lay and joined the queue hoping to find a place on one of the boats.[5]

Over the next two days, forty-four ships fled Singapore with evacuees on board. After dodging the mines around the island city, the ships would try to hide by day in the shallow bays of the jungle-covered islets along the labyrinth-like route to Batavia and then sail by night, all the while trying to avoid Japanese aircraft.

But a large Japanese naval force was anchored at the head of the Bangka Strait directly in front of the ships carrying evacuees. Despite the best efforts of the skippers leaving Singapore, all but four of the ships would be bombed and sunk. There were not only ships fleeing Singapore but every type of craft that floated – two-man canoes, 12-foot skiffs from the Singapore Yacht Club, sampans, open cargo boats called tongkangs that were powered by oars, sails and punt poles, private launches, junks, pleasure yachts, tugboats of every description, and small coastal vessels.

Most of them never made it to safety either. Thousands of men, women and children would die before any could reach land.[6]

AT THE DOCK, OLIVE PASCHKE pleaded with some of the medical unit's top brass, Colonel Derham and Glyn White, that the situation on the water was too dangerous for her girls and, that, in any case, they all wanted to stay with the wounded troops in Singapore and take their chances with the Japanese. But the officers told her that General Gordon Bennett, the commander of the 8th Division, remained resolute in wanting the nurses evacuated.

And so, in the late afternoon of 12 February 1942, accompanied by jeers and catcalls from civilians still crammed into the long queues, Viv and the others marched towards a waiting tugboat.

All around Viv her colleagues were crying. Turning back for one last look at a city in flames, Viv thought of the men at St Pat's trapped in the old school wings and out on the lawns as the invading army drew ever closer. Who would tend to them now?

Overhead, the Japanese aircraft still circled menacingly and in the water all around the tugboat were the burning shells of bombed craft. In the half-light in the distance, illuminated by the fires on Singapore, Viv could see a small coastal steamer, now painted battleship grey, that she had known in happier times.

It was the royal yacht of Sarawak, the *Vyner Brooke*. Four months earlier, Viv and Nancy Harris had dined on the ship in the lap of luxury with the yacht's engineer Jimmy Miller and some friends.

Now the little ship had been requisitioned by the Royal Navy. As the nurses entered the ship through a steel door in its side at 5 p.m., Jimmy Miller was there to greet them once more. This time, however, his mood was grim and resolute, given the clear and present danger. So different from when they first met.

Jimmy took Viv and Nancy below deck and told them they could use his cabin while he was on duty and they should help themselves to his stash of cigarettes and whiskey.[7]

Lieutenant Arthur Mann, who was in charge of the ship's radio, offered the use of his cabin to Adelaide nurse Mavis Hannah,[8] but she declined under orders from Matron Paschke, and instead the room was used by an elderly couple among the evacuees.

The other nurses had made their home forward of the upper deck, and Jimmy then led Viv and Nancy upstairs to join them.

Although the *Vyner Brooke* normally only carried twelve passengers it now had more than 200 people on board. There were seven officers and forty-five crew,[9] mostly Malays who were members of the Straits Settlements Volunteer Naval Reserve. The sixty-five Australian nurses brought the number of passengers up to 181, most of them women and children. They included Olga Neubronner, an English-born nursing sister who was seven months pregnant. She was the wife of a Malayan rubber plantation owner and had been fleeing south from the Japanese for weeks.

Stephen and Cevia Warman were Polish Jews who, having fled the Holocaust in their homeland, had travelled through the Ural mountains in Russia, on to Siberia, across to war-ravaged Shanghai and then on to Singapore, where they thought they might be safe with their little hairdressing business.[10] They had their three-year-old son, Isidore, with them, who the Australian nurses called 'Mischa'.[11] Another passenger was Canadian-born

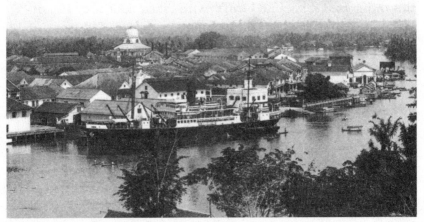

The *Vyner Brooke* was the Royal Yacht of Sarawak.

master brewer Eric Germann,[12] who was in Singapore working for Malayan Breweries, a Heineken subsidiary, as the company had increased beer production for all the thirsty Allied troops, without foreseeing the rapid fall in demand. Germann climbed on board the ship wearing high leather boots and a fireman's helmet after having just come from a day fighting the blazes caused by the Japanese bombers.[13]

Nurse Jessie Simons was angry and frustrated at the number of children on board. She felt so sorry they were in such danger but could only be 'coldly angry' with their parents, who for many weeks had known of the approaching peril and time and time again had put 'off the day of reckoning until now when it might be too late'.[14]

The *Vyner Brooke* also carried military personnel – code breakers, intelligence officers and radar experts, including Major Bill Tebbutt,[15] a World War I veteran who had landed on Gallipoli on the first day of the attack[16] and had been a Sydney solicitor before this conflict. All were deemed too important to risk capture by the Japanese.

The crew handed out life jackets to the nurses, and Olive Paschke and Irene Drummond told their girls they were to put them on immediately and keep them on.

Viv wrestled her life jacket over her broad shoulders. 'I hope this thing works, because I can't swim,' she told Nancy Harris.

'Don't worry about it, Bully. I'll look after you,' Nancy replied.

Up on the bridge deck, Jenny Greer, the Sydney nurse known for her perpetual sense of good cheer, began singing 'Wish Me Luck as You Wave Me Goodbye'.[17]

Viv and Nancy turned to look back at the city they were leaving.

Viv later took a pencil and into a small diary with a mock snakeskin cover she scratched out her thoughts about the carnage all around her.

Feb 12th Thurs ... looking back at Singapore the place just a mass of flames along the waterfront and the island burning on the other side ... terrible sight.[18]

THE *VYNER BROOKE* FLEW the white ensign of Britain and now had a four-inch cannon mounted on her bow, two old Lewis machine guns either side of the bridge and racks of depth charges. The cannon and machine guns were relics from the last world war, and everyone knew they would be little protection against the Japanese bombers or naval patrol boats.

The ship's skipper, Richard 'Tubby' Borton,[19] was a 54-year-old Yorkshireman who was employed by the Sarawak Steamship Company and had been given the temporary rank of lieutenant in the Royal Naval Reserve. Borton was at home in the Far East, having married in 1927 the daughter of a British doctor at Sarawak, with whom he'd had four children. His family had already been evacuated to India on the first leg of their journey home to Leeds, leaving their smart cottage on Singapore's Orchard Road behind.

Borton had spent years threading the *Vyner Brooke* and other vessels through the maze of islands around Singapore, Malaya, the Netherlands East Indies and the Philippines. Young Jimmy Miller was his engineer, and his first officer was thirty-year-old Welshman Bill 'Ginger' Sedgeman,[20] who had survived the sinking of the *Prince of Wales*. Borton and his crew had been attacked several times by Japanese aircraft as the *Vyner Brooke* travelled on Royal Navy duties, and the skipper was experienced in zigzagging his vessel to avoid their bombs.

Food was short on the ship, and while the nurses had meagre rations, it was an abundance compared to most of the passengers and crew, many of whom had fled to the docks with just the clothes on their backs.

Betty Jeffrey and some of the other nurses went up to the galley and prepared a stew of bully beef and tinned vegetables that all on the ship could share. There were army biscuits and cheese as a second course. Matrons Paschke and Drummond had decided that the nurses would share all their food and that for the voyage to Batavia they would ration their provisions and prepare two meals a day for everyone on board.

About an hour after sunset, sometime around 8 p.m., when the bombing had subsided for a while, Borton began moving the *Vyner Brooke* slowly across Keppel Harbour towards the Java Sea.

Viv retired early to an awful, fretful night of disturbed sleep. There was much shouting on board and ringing of bells as Borton cautiously steered his way through the mines adrift in the water, but in the darkness it was hard to find his way, and for a time the *Vyner Brooke* was lost among the deadly hazards.[21] While the fires of Singapore had illuminated the water for a time, drifting clouds of smoke obscured many of the buoys that marked safe passage. In a few hours it would be Friday the 13th, and who knew what that might bring?

The next morning, Viv woke agitated and alarmed. Only Bill Sedgeman's 'good navigating' had got them through the mines, she was told.

The food situation had become even more grim as someone had looted army rations during the night.[22] But as the rays of a fiery orange sun broke over the blue sea that morning, Viv couldn't help but gasp at the beauty of the tropical islands around her. Borton brought the *Vyner Brooke* into what he thought was a good hiding place in the lee of one of the Lingga Islands, an islet covered with thick jungle and with a hill that he believed would conceal the ship from Japanese patrols. Many of the passengers lazed about on the deck, trying as best they could to shield themselves from the blazing sun until nightfall when Borton planned to continue sailing towards the Javanese coast and Batavia.

Jessie Simons recalled:

> Some of us dozed, drugged by the sun; a few admired the feathery beauty of palm-crowned islets, or idly watched the effortless sweep of snowy gulls; the gloomy and the anxious scanned the sky for planes, periodically stirring their neighbours to emphatic protests with false alarms; and the phlegmatic settled down to books which they had the foresight to stuff into bulging luggage.[23]

For Viv and the other nurses there wasn't a lot of downtime. They had the communal cooking with their biscuits and bully beef, and there were lifeboat drills. Olive and Irene told Viv and the other nurses that in the event of an attack by the Japanese 'if necessary all civilians to boats first whilst girls to go overboard and swim … fingers being kept [crossed]'.[24] There were six lifeboats, enough to carry 180 people at most, and nowhere near enough for everyone on board.

Olive told the nurses: 'Remember, remove your shoes, hold your life jackets down firmly and jump into the water feet first. If you don't hold your jacket down it can come up and hit you under the chin with the possibility of breaking your neck.'[25]

Matron Drummond reminded her girls that organisation and discipline were the keys to them all overcoming what might be a trying time.

For the remaining hours of daylight, the *Vyner Brooke* remained in the lee of the island, while Viv and the other nurses secreted supplies of morphine-filled syringes inside the pockets of their uniforms and prepared field dressings, hoping against hope that the Japanese did not spot their little ship in its hiding place.

Borton still had a long way to go before reaching the safety of

Batavia. So, at 8 p.m. on 13 February, he raised anchor and set a course south-west for the coast of Sumatra and the Bangka Strait, a stretch of water that had become known as 'Bomb Alley'.

It was dark when the *Vyner Brooke* was hit by a dazzling shaft of bright light. Then other beams of light criss-crossed around it.

Borton ordered complete silence and cut the ship's three-cylinder, twin-screw engine. There was a cacophony of distant explosions and the unmistakable roar of heavy naval guns. Borton steered for the safe cover of another island in the Tudjuh Archipelago.

No one dared make a sound. Viv would later write: 'Almost ran into a naval battle. Much searchlights just reaching over in the shelter behind our island.'[26] The Japanese had been attacking another ship in the darkness, and Borton, more than half a day behind schedule, decided to make a run for it.

VIV COULDN'T SLEEP after the close call with the Japanese, but the dawn of 14 February revealed what she called a 'beautiful sunny morning' and 'calm sea'. However, this peacefulness would soon be 'disturbed'.[27] Borton anchored in the lee of what Viv called 'a very pretty island', where on that hot, still day they again waited for the cover of darkness. Viv stood on the bow of the ship as Jimmy Miller pointed into the distance towards Sumatra and told her the Bangka Strait was the gateway to freedom.

A little further south was Batavia's port, which had not yet fallen to the Japanese but was surrounded by their ships and aircraft.

Later, below deck, the nurses organised a small birthday party to lighten the mood, using whatever meagre rations could be scrounged, for Vi McElnea,[28] one of many McElneas from a pioneering family in Ingham, North Queensland, who had enlisted for this war.[29] No one was much in the mood for a party, though.

Olive levelled with the nurses and told them that Borton believed it was inevitable they would be spotted by Japanese aircraft and that they would be bombed. She went through the procedures for when the command came to abandon ship, as it would almost certainly be happening soon. Two of the lifeboats had been allocated to mothers with children and passengers who couldn't swim. All the nurses who could swim were told to give up their seats on lifeboats for non-swimmers and rely on their life jackets in the water.

At 11 a.m., Viv heard a distant engine on the darkening horizon, and the lookout on the bridge pointed to black specks approaching low across the sea. Some of the machines flew over the ship but as all on board watched in horror, a single-engine fighter dropped almost to sea level and flew in a direct line towards the *Vyner Brooke*.

There was no time for anyone to man the cannon or machine guns, and Viv watched, stunned, as flashes of gunfire from the aircraft's wings caused jets of water to rise from the sea. Soon the bullets were ricocheting off metal into the soft wood of the lifeboats and spraying the ship's bridge.

With a deafening roar the Japanese plane hurtled just over the heads of those on deck before returning for another burst of machine-gun fire. Everyone, Viv recalled, took to the lower decks and manned their battle stations as pre-arranged, but the raid was soon over.

Somehow all those on the ship had escaped serious injury but some had suffered cuts caused by flying wood splinters. Some of the lifeboats on the starboard side had been badly damaged.

Captain Borton said that schools of sharks were everywhere in these waters. And it would not be long before the ravenous sharks of the air returned in a feeding frenzy.

Jessie Simons seemed stoic. She and Viv had shared one of the pre-arranged battle stations below deck with Lorna Fairweather,[30] a bespectacled Adelaide nurse who specialised in paediatrics. Jessie had staggered Viv and Lorna with her courage under fire. She'd appeared unconcerned by the Japanese machine-gun bullets and far more interested in reading her book,[31] the Ethel Mannin anti-war novel *Cactus*,[32] about the futility of countries fighting and the sacrifice of all those poor souls caught in the middle.

'Peacefulness disturbed as planes flew over and machine-gunned boat,' Viv wrote in her diary. 'All took to lower deck as pre-arranged, but raid all over and much discussion on planes sinking us and enemy aircraft'.[33]

That discussion, between Borton, his officers and Major Tebbutt, the senior military officer on board, resulted in Borton deciding that the *Vyner Brooke* and its precious cargo were sitting ducks if they stayed where they were. Viv scratched in her diary that Borton 'took up anchor and steamed along'.[34]

Tebbutt later wrote: 'The captain stated to me that he considered it suicidal to remain anchored close to land, that the ship could easily be picked up from the air and would provide a sitting shot for bombers. From his experience he believed that he might be able to avoid bombs in the open fairway. Accordingly, he did not obey his orders to anchor in the daytime.'[35]

BACK IN SINGAPORE, the Japanese had been shelling the British Military Hospital (now known as Alexandra Hospital) all day. By 1 p.m., Japanese soldiers had surrounded the hospital and over the course of about an hour three large groups of them went from room to room shooting and bayonetting doctors, orderlies and patients. They even killed an anaesthetised patient who was still lying on the operating table. Large groups of prisoners were locked in tiny rooms overnight with no air or water. Some perished. The next day those who had survived the ordeal were murdered with bayonets. At the end of the slaughter as many as 200 patients and staff had been butchered.

Meanwhile, Tubby Borton pushed the *Vyner Brooke* as hard as it could go – 25 kilometres per hour – towards the entrance of the Bangka Strait between Bangka Island and Sumatra.

A deathly quiet again descended over the ship and some of the nurses, such as Betty Jeffrey and Pat Blake[36] fell asleep through sheer exhaustion.

Then just before 2 p.m., Viv heard a noise that made her tremble.

Chapter 12

THE DISTANT SOUND of another Japanese aircraft approaching caused Betty Jeffrey and Pat Blake to wake from their slumber in shock. Everyone leapt to their feet. As the aircraft approached, they knew the Japanese pilot had seen the ship and recorded its position. The plane flew off without firing a shot, but Tubby Borton said it was only a matter of time before the big guns, and many of them, arrived.

Borton decided to run for Bangka Island about 20 kilometres away, which afforded more chance of hiding. Some of the Royal Naval Reservists on board manned the cannon and the old Lewis machine guns, hoping they might somehow land a blow on the speeding Japanese dive-bombers. Viv and the nurses donned their helmets and life jackets and made sure the other evacuees were prepared to abandon ship.

Soon the ship's lookout spotted six dots in the distance flying towards them in two V-formations.[1]

'2 p.m. air raid siren,' Viv scrawled into her diary. 'All down to lower deck and flatten down.'[2]

Brisbane nurse Flo Trotter[3] swallowed hard. She could see the red dots of the Rising Sun symbol on the bombers and knew what they were in for.[4] She thought momentarily that, if worst came to worst, she could inject herself with one of the morphine syringes in her pocket.[5]

The approaching aircraft were twin-engine Nell bombers. From a height of a few hundred metres, they dropped three bombs at the little ship, but Borton managed to dodge them and they exploded in the water. Below deck, Viv and the other nurses were lying flat, at the ready to help evacuate the mothers and children, many of whom took cover under beds and mattresses.

Two more aircraft dropped bombs, but again, steering this way and that, Borton avoided them, though his passengers were tossed about and became increasingly traumatised by the nearby explosions. Then dive-bombers strafed the sides of the ship with machine-gun fire. More aircraft dropped bombs.

'Six planes attacking once more,' Viv wrote. Again the Japanese fired machine-gun salvos into the hull and bridge. Betty Jeffrey lay flat with the foot of a little girl under her. The child's mother had four little ones on board and the mother prayed aloud for all of them.

Our Father, who art in heaven
Hallowed be thy name
Thy Kingdom come ...[6]

For five minutes, the bombers dropped bomb after bomb, but Borton managed to dodge them all. Then, deciding to hunt in a pack, the Japanese pilots formed a line so that if Borton changed course suddenly he would still steer straight into the path of an explosion.

'Bombs hit', Viv scrawled, 'second, third time, third bomb below the water line. Whistle for all on deck to take to lifeboats.'[7]

One of the first bombs to find its mark – possibly the first – plunged straight down the ship's funnel and exploded in the engine room at 2.10 p.m., killing or badly injuring all the crew there. Viv watched gobsmacked as Wilma Oram, who had been lying next to her on the floor, was lifted into the air before coming down with a sickening thud. The blast had torn away a large section of bulkhead and Viv could see the ocean through the gaping hole.

A second bomb destroyed many of the state rooms, killing most of the elderly passengers there and blowing apart many of the life rafts, poorly built craft about a metre and a half square made of wooden pallets and canvas. A third bomb landed on the forward deck, destroying the cannon and its crew and killing an elderly couple who were sheltering in the radio operator's cabin. There was smoke everywhere and the smell of terror. Even experienced nurses such as Viv, well used to combat wounds, were sickened by the unfolding horror. Passengers, many of them babies and small children, suffered cuts and burns so bad that some of the nurses gagged.

During the next few frantic minutes, a period that seemed to Viv like a hellish eternity, many of the civilians collapsed into a blind panic, pushing each other out of the way in a scramble for the stairs. Little Mischa Warman's father, Stephen, who had apparently endured months of torment and terror, suddenly left his wife and son behind, ran out onto the deck and jumped into the water. He disappeared below the waves and was never seen again. His wife, Cevia, collapsed in shock.

Five minutes after the first explosion, three more Japanese bombers attacked again, and even though their bombs missed, machine guns sprayed the port side of the ship, damaging more of the lifeboats.

Borton gave the command to abandon ship, and the nurses followed the procedure that had been drilled into them: women civilians and their children first. Viv, Jessie, Iole Harper and a gregarious Western Australian nurse Vima Bates,[8] who had flaming red hair, groped their way along the unlit passages, looking for anyone who was trapped, opening cabin doors and calling out to survivors. All the while, they could feel the ship breaking apart beneath them.

Viv and the other nurses began administering to the wounded. Viv saw Wilma and Queensland nurse Sylvia Muir[9] giving comfort to an old man with a gaping, bloody stomach wound. They knew he had no chance and so did he. As Sylvia patted his hand he looked with dimming grey eyes directly into hers and began to sing 'Rule Britannia'. Sylvia had suffered shrapnel wounds to her arm, and she ripped up her petticoat to bandage them.

Jessie Simons, always cool in a crisis, had a shrapnel wound to the arm but didn't notice it until one fearful passenger grabbed it tightly, asking for help. Viv noted that her friend, the Ballarat nurse Beth Cuthbertson,[10] had also been badly injured.

Betty Jeffrey and Caroline Ennis,[11] a nurse from Swan Hill, Victoria, emerged on deck, each carrying a small child before going back to help more of the wounded. More Japanese bombs exploded off the ship's port side as those on deck sheltered from yet another spray of machine-gun bullets.

Viv saw that two of her friends were covered in blood from the waist down. Rosetta Wight,[12] a cheeky farmer's daughter with a mischievous smile from Fish Creek, Gippsland, and Clarice Halligan, the Ballarat girl Viv had met at Puckapunyal, had both suffered deep cuts to their thighs. Rosetta's wound was down to the bone. Flo Casson,[13] the former matron of a hospital on the South Australia–Victoria border,[14] was cut on both her legs and reckoned one of them was fractured.

Viv and the others stopped the bleeding and half-carried their injured colleagues and some of the civilians – mostly the frail elderly and mothers with children – onto the deck to await the lifeboats.

Kath Neuss had been hit in the hip by shrapnel and had to be helped to the lifeboat by Wilma Oram and Mona Wilton, who had both suffered deep gashes to their legs from flying glass. Pat Gunther gave Kath her tin hat in case she needed to bail water from the lifeboat. 'We'll see you on shore,' she said.[15]

Many of the passengers were already dead. Veronica Clancy,[16] a tall, strapping, assertive South Australian–born nurse, realised that many of the wounded would soon die in agony or drown from their horrendous wounds. She gave them extra injections of morphia to ease their suffering.

The lifeboats on the port side had been rendered useless by the Japanese machine guns but while the three on the starboard side had also been blasted by bullets and shrapnel, they still looked likely to float.

Irene Drummond and Olive Paschke oversaw the loading of about twenty of the wounded civilians into a first lifeboat that

Bill Sedgeman would command. Irene climbed in to lead the way and look after the wounded.

As Jimmy Miller directed operations from the deck, the boat was lowered safely into the water and sailors threw down blankets and greatcoats to cover those who had been badly injured. But the lifeboat was immediately caught by a strong current and began drifting away from what was left of the ship. It was full of bullet holes and Viv watched it floundering about, Irene Drummond facing forward at the front, Bill Sedgeman in the rear facing the ship, and in the middle two sailors using their helmets to bale water out of the flimsy vessel for all they were worth.

Eric Germann, who had been a lifeguard in New York, had also helped to lower the first lifeboat before jumping into the water to assist some of the women struggling to reach it and the life rafts. Wanting to help some more of the terrified women descend from the ship, he shucked off his boots and life jacket and climbed back on deck using the ship's ladder. On his way up he met some of the civilian passengers coming down in high heels. Some used his head as a stepping stone to the sea, while others accused him of only creeping up the ladder so he could look up their dresses.[17]

A Japanese aircraft made another strafing attack on the ship but a second lifeboat was soon filled with about thirty of the badly wounded,[18] including Rosetta Wight, Kath Neuss and Flo Salmon,[19] a young sister from Punchbowl in Sydney. But as the lifeboat was being lowered to the sea it overturned. The nurses, their gouged flesh giving them horrendous pain in the salt water, would have to cling to its side for the next eight hours.

Eric Germann was back on deck. A soldier helped the now widowed Cevia Warman over the ship's railing and into the water, while a passenger thrust three-year-old Mischa into Germann's arms and asked him to save the child.

'Don't be afraid,' Germann told the little boy. 'We're just going to jump into the water for a nice, cool swim'. Germann held his hands over Mischa's mouth and nose and jumped. They hit the water together and both laughed as they bobbed to the surface. Germann placed the boy in the third lifeboat and, after helping others into it, climbed in himself. Crowded and ringed with people grasping the looped handlines on the sides, the boat was barely afloat. Three empty life rafts floated into sight. Men swam after them and attached them to the boat with a long line. Everyone except rowers were then transferred to the rafts, and the long pull began to Bangka Island, just visible in the distance.[20]

The *Vyner Brooke* was now tilting so badly that some of the sailors feared it would keel over onto the third lifeboat. Oil from the sinking vessel floated around it for about 200 metres, coating both the living and the dead. Debris cascaded down from the tilting deck, while sailors tossed objects out into the sea that they thought might help survivors remain afloat.

Jean Ashton, Wilma Oram and Mona Wilton had been helping passengers into the third lifeboat when Olive Paschke told them: 'It's time to go, girls. We have treated all the wounded we can. Now please take off your shoes and jump in the water.'[21] The nurses dived, jumped or fell into the sea. Betty Jeffrey was scared of heights and lowered herself down on a rope, shredding the skin on her hands so badly that she had to let go while still a few feet above the waves. When she hit the water, she screamed in agony from the cuts.

Having treated so many wounded on board, Viv and a small group of other nurses were among the last to leave the ship. Viv took off her shoes and again was faced with the sad fact that she couldn't swim. She knew her survival in the shark-infested waters would come down to luck and the life jacket. The ship had rolled so much that it was now only a short drop from the ship's railing to the water. Viv climbed onto the railing and, remembering Olive's advice to hold the life jacket firmly down, leapt into the blue-green water and down into the enveloping darkness. It was quiet down there and no one could hear her scream.

For a brief moment, she felt a calming coolness. The day had started out as a beautiful morning and now, just fifteen minutes after the bombs had hit the ship, Viv wondered if this would be the last moment of happiness in her life.

She had seen so much death that day she momentarily doubted that it was worth fighting the overwhelming odds stacked against her. Perhaps she should surrender to the cool, calm quiet blackness. But the thought was fleeting, and she pushed herself hard to the surface of the water.

Viv was so close to the *Vyner Brooke*'s hull that she could almost touch it. The ship seemed immense. She could hear a voice crying out, telling her to save herself and get away before the ship toppled over. Even though Viv had never learned to swim, with the life jacket keeping her afloat she dog-paddled as best she could away from the immediate danger.

Pat Gunther and Win Davis,[22] a young Sydney nurse who had grown up on the Clarence River near Grafton, had seen where Viv and some of the others had exited the *Vyner Brooke*, and they entered the water from the same place only a few seconds later. Now the ship was so low in the water they simply stepped silently into the sea.

Olive Paschke had seen most of her nurses leave the ship when she finally took off her shoes, climbed onto the railing and called out boldly, 'Here I come, girls! Look out for me. Remember, I can't swim.'[23] She held the collar of her life jacket down as she had instructed the nurses, then jumped. She sank deep into the water.

Jean Ashton, Wilma Oram and Mona Wilton were also in the water. Jean swam away strongly from the sinking ship but Mona and Wilma, the best of friends for years, were propelled deep underwater. 'Mona couldn't swim at all,' Wilma related later, 'and I couldn't swim much …'

We jumped out to try and get away from the ship but the ship tipped over on top of us. I said to Mona, 'Aw, we're sunk this time.' I came up through the [ship's] rails, put my hands up above my head and caught the rails and came up through them, but when I came to the surface Mona was nowhere about and that was it. I never saw her again. I can only think that the ship dragged her down.[24]

Mona's life, and their years of friendship, were gone in an instant.

As Wilma looked this way and that, desperate for any sign of her friend, she heard a shout from above. Looking up she saw a life raft hurtling down towards her, but it was too late to avoid it. The heavy raft struck her a glancing blow, knocking the senses from her and forcing her back under the water. When the buoyancy of Wilma's life jacket lifted her out of the water again, she was badly dazed and bleeding from a deep head wound. She barely had time to take another gulp of air before a second raft, flying like a lethal projectile, crashed onto her. More life rafts and debris rained down from the ship, and Wilma was hit four more times in rapid succession. Barely conscious, she came up out of the water again and managed to clamber onto one of the rafts. She pushed the raft away to give herself distance to avoid more catastrophe as the *Vyner Brooke* slowly 'tipped up on its end' and went under the waves.[25]

Wilma figured she'd need twenty stitches to seal the hole in her head, and in the fog of her jumbled mind she thought she'd had a conversation with Kit Kinsella as she drifted past. Perhaps she imagined it because no one else saw Kit after the *Vyner Brooke* went down. Wilma recalled there was a woman on another raft, Mrs Dot Gibson:

> She called out, 'Do you mind if I get on your raft with you?' So we got on the raft together and that was at 2.15 in the afternoon. We spent all that night until 6 o'clock the next morning in the Bangka Strait trying our very best to get to the shore.[26]

All the time Wilma had her eye on the other survivors clinging to rafts and lifeboats and debris. She continued to call out frantically for her friend Mona, but no one had seen a trace of her.

Flo Trotter recalled that the nurses had to jump from the ship and swim away as hard as possible to avoid being sucked under as the *Vyner Brooke* rolled in its death throes. 'I remember jumping in,' she recalled, 'and thinking how funny it was I still had my tin hat on.[27] Our tin hats came in handy! The Japanese came back and machine-gunned us in the water.'[28]

Some of the Japanese aircraft that had destroyed the *Vyner Brooke* and killed many of its passengers came back yet again to finish off the survivors. Hurtling along at what seemed just metres above the waves, the dive-bombers had their machine guns blazing, as bullets rained down on all those trying to stay afloat amid the carnage. To avoid being shot, many tried to sink below the surface, but the buoyancy of the life jackets kept bringing them up and into the line of fire.

For many of those sheltering in lifeboats or clinging to life rafts and debris, there was no escape. Having thought that they had escaped a sinking ship, many were now blown apart by the Japanese guns, and blood mixed with oil among the devastation. Satisfied that they'd killed everyone they could, the Japanese finally flew away.

Flo Trotter and four other nurses – Jenny Greer, Brisbane's Joyce Tweddell,[29] Beryl Woodbridge and Jessie Blanch[30] from northern New South Wales – were all hanging onto a plank that had been part of the ship's railing while they tried not to vomit, having swallowed so much oil. They were literally hanging on for dear life. 'One of the girls was quite a wag,' Flo recalled. '[She] started singing "We're off to see the wizard".'[31] That was Jenny Greer, trying everything she could to keep everyone's spirits afloat when so many souls had gone down during a day of savagery unlike anything any of them had ever experienced.

VIV DOG-PADDLED HER WAY across to the upturned lifeboat and grabbed onto the rope that ran around the boat's gunwales. Also hanging on were Rosetta Wight, Flo Salmon and Kath Neuss, along with eight other nurses.[32] There was also Louise Beeston, a 34-year-old Englishwoman who had been teaching at the St Andrew's School in Singapore, and an elderly couple who were desperately clinging to each other.

Jimmy Miller was also there, exhausted and covered with so much oil he looked like a fur seal. So much had happened since

Viv and Jimmy had dined together in evening wear on the *Vyner Brooke* just a few months earlier.

'Viv!' Jimmy exclaimed with all the energy his battered body could muster. 'Thank God you're safe!'[33]

DEAD BABIES AND THEIR mothers floated beside dead fish, oil drums, and the contents of suitcases that had been burst open by the explosions. About fifty people had died in the attack, though no one would ever be really sure, because the ship had fled Singapore crowded with desperate people and there was no time to keep an accurate record of the passengers' names.

While the Japanese bombing raids had ceased, there was the ever-present threat of attack from below. Sharks, including aggressive bull sharks and huge tiger sharks, hunted the seas around Sumatra. Blood in the water and the constant movement of the shipwreck survivors' legs could only mean trouble. Jimmy Miller tried to put everyone's mind at ease by saying there wouldn't be a shark within 20 miles of the area, given the number of bombs the Japanese had dropped. Still, everyone was sure they'd be much safer on Bangka Island if only they could get there.

Vima Bates, the vibrant redhead, who had helped Viv look for wounded passengers only an hour or two earlier, was floating alone on a life raft, but in the powerful currents that seemed to change direction rapidly, she drifted away from the main groups of survivors and was never seen again.

Betty Jeffrey swam past Win Davis and Pat Gunther, who were clinging onto a canvas stretcher. She saw that a number of life rafts had been lashed together, and Olive Paschke was among a group of oil-soaked nurses on them. Olive told Betty that she was delighted that despite being a non-swimmer she had managed to stay afloat, bobbing about in the oil for an hour until several of the other nurses had grabbed her and dragged her onto their life raft so she could sit beside them. Olive was sitting next to Iole Harper and Millie Dorsch. Another on the combined rafts was Merle Trenerry,[34] who was from a pioneering Cornish tin-mining family and had spent much of her career in South Australian bush hospitals. There was also Gladys McDonald,[35] from Brisbane, and Mary Clarke[36] from Rylstone, on the western side of the Blue Mountains in New South Wales. Caroline Ennis was sitting on the rafts too, looking after a small, distressed English girl who she guessed was about three years old. The little girl had already started to call her 'Aunty Caroline'. Betty grabbed a Chinese boy of about four years as he floated by and passed him up into Caroline's arms. There were also two Malay sailors on the combined rafts, one of them badly burned, and Olive organised for some of the nurses to relieve them of their paddling duties, which they were trying to do with the slats from a smashed packing case. Olive showed the nurses the best way to kick their feet to help push the makeshift craft towards Bangka Island.

Win Davis and Pat Gunther abandoned their stretcher and grabbed onto a raft with Jessie Simons that contained three injured crew members from the *Vyner Brooke*. One of the British sailors told them that it was the fourth time he'd been on a sinking ship during this war – twice in European waters and just two months earlier on the *Prince of Wales*.

ABOUT NINETY MINUTES after the destruction of the *Vyner Brooke* and so many lives, a Japanese spotter aircraft flew over the scene yet again. The view below, 20 kilometres north of Bangka Island, would have been one of utter devastation. About a hundred survivors were scattered across a square kilometre. There was a wide, thick oil slick on the surface of the water, with dead bodies and detritus all mixed up in the muck. Here and there black heads bobbed about, and groups of bedraggled, barely alive humans huddled together around life rafts or lifeboats, which looked like they might sink at any time.

Down in the water, an elderly couple were floating together, holding hands. The wounded were in excruciating pain due to the effect of the oil and salt water on their injuries. Even the few who had escaped the carnage physically intact, such as Viv, were in great difficulty. The cumbersome life jackets slowed their progress as they could only swim breaststroke. The canvas rubbed the skin under their chins and around their armpits almost raw,[37] while the water just added salt to the wounds. Viv's legs felt like jelly from kicking to stay afloat. As the sun sank on a rotten day, some of the exhausted survivors fell asleep, drifted away from the others and drowned.

Mavis Hannah could hear her friend Lainie Balfour-Ogilvy calling out to her to join her group on Irene Drummond's lifeboat but chose not to risk swimming the distance towards her friend. She would later reflect on the fact that 'fate plays many strange tricks in life'. The decision not to swim to Lainie saved Mavis's life.[38]

Viv, Jimmy Miller and the others clinging to their upturned lifeboat had been dragged by the current towards land all afternoon. Now, in the darkness, they could see the glow of a bonfire, and Viv guessed that it had been lit by people on Bangka Island as a beacon for survivors of sinking ships in the area. Viv and Jimmy couldn't control their wrecked craft, but they held on as the current carried them closer to land. At about 10.30 p.m. on 14 February,[39] after having been in the water for almost eight hours, Viv felt something reassuring under her feet. Sand.

The survivors who could still walk let go of the boat and stumbled onto a beach, where their rubbery legs collapsed beneath them. Those with enough strength helped carry the three with the worst injuries – Rosetta Wight, Kath Neuss and Flo Salmon – onto the shore.

For a long time they all lay together and the only sounds were their gasps of relief that the ordeal in the water was over. Lying on her back, Viv looked up at the starry heavens above. What had become of the rest of her friends, she wondered.

STRONG OCEAN CURRENTS were pushing the other survivors, boats and life rafts in all directions. Some of those in the water had seen the bonfire in the distance and had done their utmost to steer towards it with varying degrees of success. Other survivors thought they could hear distant cries and shouts coming from land. No one could be certain if they were real or imaginary.

Sylvia Muir was clinging to a life raft with fellow nurses Mitz Mittelheuser, Jean Ashton, Mina Raymont, Veronica Clancy, New Zealand–born Gladys Hughes[40] and Tasmanian Shirley Gardam.[41] Also hanging on was Mrs Anna Bull and her three-year-old daughter, Hazel. Mrs Bull was the forty-year-old wife of an English police magistrate in Singapore. She was in great distress because her two other children, eight-year-old daughter, Molly, and seven-year-old son, Robin, had drifted away from her. The nurses told Mrs Bull not to fret because, if the kids were wearing life jackets, they would no doubt be rescued by the strong swimmers among the nurses. Little Hazel was in tears. Not only had she seen horrors no human, let alone a small child, should ever see, but while holding onto a rope in the water she had let go of her teddy bear, which had drifted away. Jean Ashton swam after it and brought it back to the delighted little girl.[42]

Before long the life raft started sinking and the nurses moved to another collection of rafts tied together. There were now twenty-three people huddled on the makeshift craft, and to ease overcrowding, it was decided that everyone would take turns on the rafts and in the water. The only ones who could permanently stay on the craft were Olga Neubronner, the British nurse who was seven months pregnant, and 58-year-old Mrs Evelyne Madden,[43] whose husband of thirty years, Lewis, had died in her arms after several hours in the water. Mrs Madden's hands had been ripped raw as she slid down the rope from the *Vyner Brooke,* and she was in great physical and emotional turmoil.

The only person on the raft who refused to have a turn in the water was imperious German Annamaria Eleanor Goldberg who, despite being a medical doctor, seemed to have little sympathy for the sick and injured. She and her husband had been interned as enemy aliens in Singapore and accused of spreading anti-British propaganda.[44] With a heavy German accent, Dr Goldberg told the others on the raft that she would not budge. 'I am more important than any of you,' she said. Veronica Clancy lifted herself out of the water and half onto the raft and punched Dr Goldberg as hard as she could in the middle of her back. Goldberg screamed defiance but still refused to move. Blanche Hempsted decided to go tag-team with Veronica and grabbed Dr Goldberg in a headlock, dragging her backwards into the water, and telling her to kick with her feet like everyone else.[45]

ON ONE OF THE RAFTS, Pat Gunther applied lipstick as a salve to the rope burns on Jessie Simon's hands and was delighted that it gave some relief. She could do nothing for a badly burned British sailor, though, who sometime after sunset died and disappeared from the raft without a sound.

Just before dawn on 15 February, Jessie's raft was surrounded by a flotilla of Japanese landing craft that were carrying troops and equipment from a large transport ship as part of the invasion of Sumatra. Jessie had removed her uniform during the night to use it as bandages and to plug holes in the raft so she was now dressed only in her petticoat and underwear. Her heart almost stopped and everyone else on the raft held their breath as some of the craft peeled off and wheeled around. One came alongside, and a Japanese soldier told the nurses they had to climb onto his vessel. Having heard all the horror stories about the Japanese soldiers, Jessie and the others thought the end was nigh, but they did as they were told. A rope was secured to the raft and it was towed to shore. The Japanese kept the women on the beach under guard.

But while so many of the Japanese troops had proved to be monsters, these were not only human beings but sympathetic ones. They gave the nurses water and cigarettes. Jessie was a tall, lanky woman, with short hair that was now plastered against her head by a combination of oil and salt water. One of the Japanese soldiers grabbed Jessie, pulled at the front of her petticoat, and peered down at her breasts. Given the atrocities the nurses had heard about, Jessie was petrified, but it seemed he was only checking to make sure she wasn't a male soldier in disguise. As the soldier walked away, a radio operator gave Jessie his shirt to wear.[46]

Around mid-morning, the Japanese marched this group of survivors that also included Win Davis and Pat Gunther down to the water's edge and into the port town of Muntok, which had a population of about 10,000 and a huge tin smelter worked by teams of Chinese labourers. The nurses were taken to an old cinema on the main street. Inside the cinema were about 200 captives – mostly European – who all looked as shattered as Jessie and her band of survivors.

OLIVE PASCHKE'S RAFT, with its passengers hanging on the side, made it to within 100 metres of Bangka Island but the fast-flowing, ever-changing current carried it away. Before dawn on 15 February, Olive's raft also drifted through a convoy of small Japanese transport vessels carrying soldiers and equipment. The raft bumped into some of the vessels, but there was no response. When dawn finally broke, Olive and the rest of her nurses could see that they had drifted many kilometres offshore. In the distance they could see a Japanese warship lobbing shells onto a small coastal town.

Betty Jeffrey and Iole Harper volunteered to lighten the raft and joined two Malay sailors swimming beside it. But then the raft was caught in a powerful cross-current and was quickly swept away from them. 'Jeff' and Iole cried out to their friends to turn the raft around but there was nothing anyone could do. 'Jeff' and Iole would eventually be washed up into a mangrove swamp, but for now they watched forlornly as Olive's raft was pushed further and further away. The dejected figures of Mary Clarke and Gladys McDonald were sitting either side of Olive, with Millie Dorsch and Merle Trenerry in the water alongside, hanging onto the raft's trailing ropes. Sitting back to back with her matron was Caroline Ennis cradling two small children.

Viv would never see those dear people again.

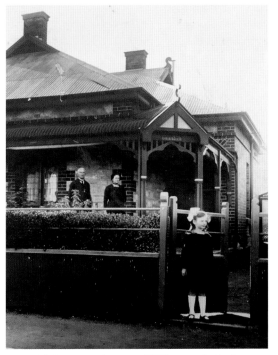

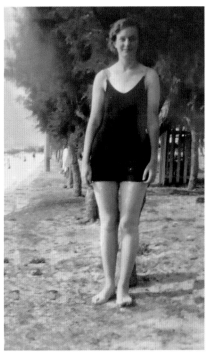

Viv with her grandparents William and Emily Shegog in Adelaide in 1922. *Vivian Bullwinkel collection*

The beach was Viv's favourite holiday destination as a teenager.
Vivian Bullwinkel collection

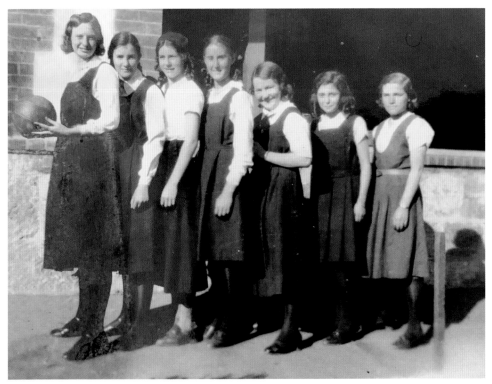

Viv (left) towered over the sporting landscape at Broken Hill High. Here she is with the tunnel ball team that included her great pal Zelda Treloar (third from right). *Vivian Bullwinkel collection*

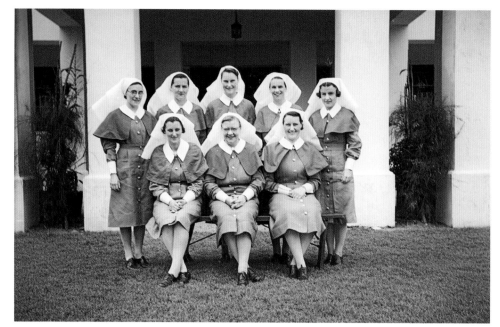

Sisters of the 2/4th Australian Casualty Clearing Station. Left to right, back row: Millie Dorsch, died off Sumatra; Bessie Wilmott, murdered Radji Beach; Mina Raymont, died as a POW; Lainie Balfour-Ogilvy, murdered Radji Beach; Peggy Farmaner, murdered Radji Beach; Front row: Shirley Gardam, died as a POW; Irene Drummond, murdered Radji Beach; Mavis Hannah, the only survivor from the group. *Australian War Memorial 120518*

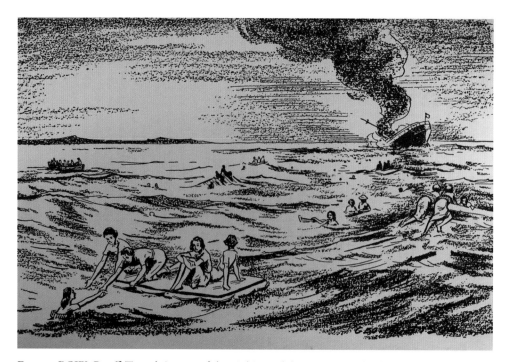

Former POW Geoff Tyson's image of the sinking of the *Vyner Brooke*, from the book *While History Passed* by Jessie Elizabeth Simons.

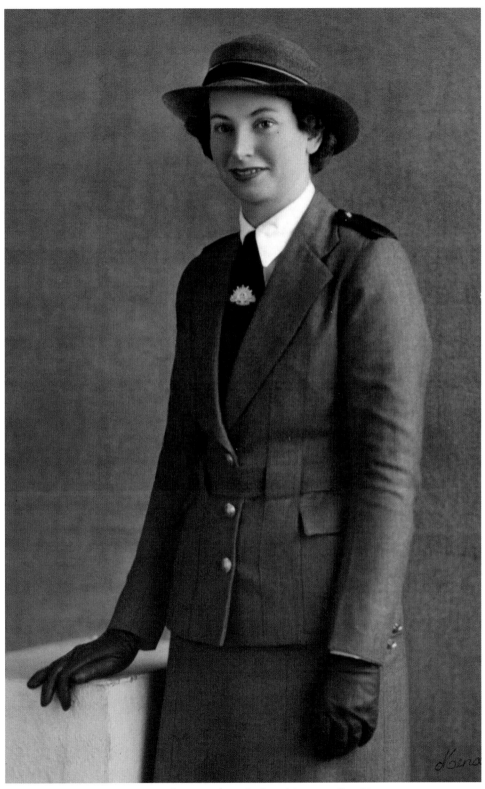

Viv in her new army nurse's uniform not long before shipping off to Singapore.
Australian War Memorial P03960.001

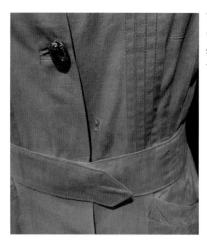

Vivian Bullwinkel's uniform on display at the Australian War Memorial in Canberra, showing the bullet wound just above the waistband. *Grantlee Kieza*

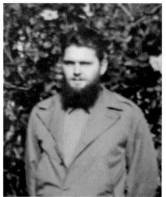
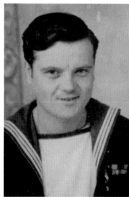
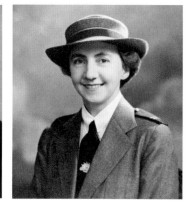

The two other survivors from the massacre on Radji Beach. Eric Germann (with beard) and Stoker Ernest Lloyd.

Matron Olive Paschke was loved and respected for her courage and kindness. *Australian War Memorial P02426.001*

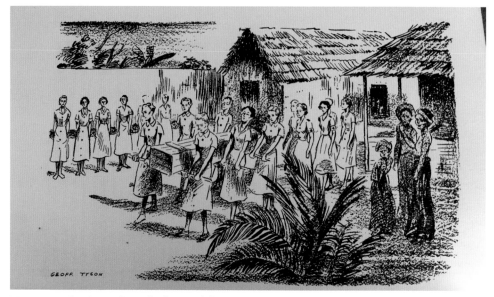

Nurses conducting a funeral of one of their own as depicted by former POW Geoff Tyson.

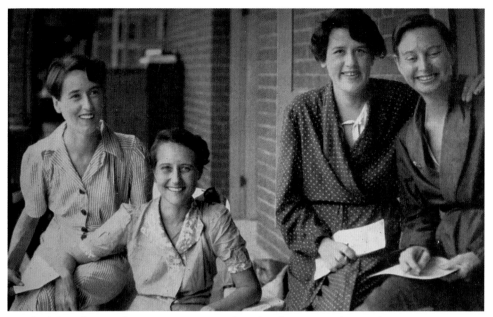

Viv (right) with Jessie Simons, Mavis Hannah and Wilma Oram during their recovery in Singapore.

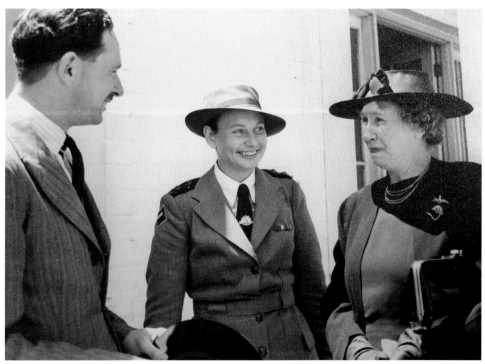

Viv's brother, John, and mother, Eva, celebrate her survival in Melbourne two days after the hospital ship *Manunda* docked there.

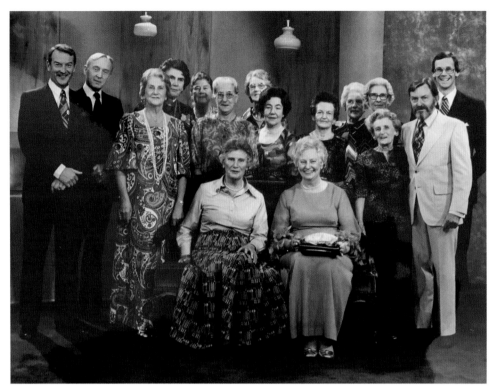

Viv and some of the participants in her *This is Your Life* episode, 1977. Left to right: Roger Climpson, host; Dr Harry Windsor, who flew on the Dakota to collect the dying nurses on Sumatra; Betty Jeffrey; Veronica Turner (Clancy); Jean Ashton; Sylvia McGregor (Muir); Jessie Hookway (Simons); Zelda West (Treloar); Mickey Syer; Wilma Young (Oram); Jess McAuley (Doyle); Nesta Hoy (James); Ken Brown, the pilot who flew to Sumatra; and Viv's nephew John Bullwinkel. Seated next to Viv is Dame Margot Turner, a celebrated British POW.

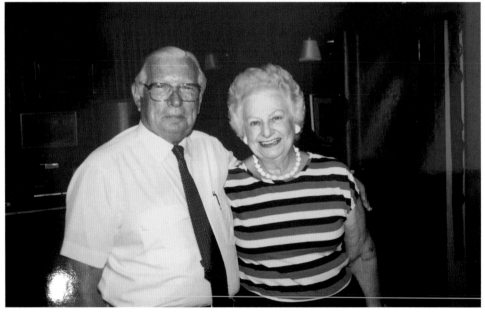

Frank and Viv had more than 20 years of happy marriage.

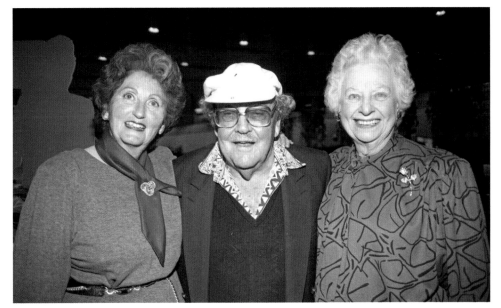

Viv and Edie 'Little Bet' Leembruggen (Kenneison), welcome former Royal Marine Gideon 'Jake' Jacobs to Perth in 1992. He was the man who led the mission to find the lost nurses in the Sumatra jungle. *Joe Wheeler/Westpix*

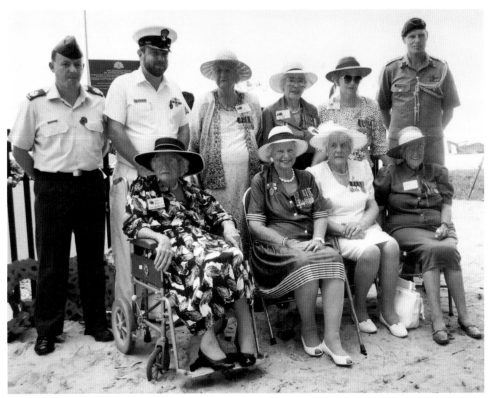

Some of the nurses at the unveiling of the memorial at Muntok in 1993. Seated front row: Mavis Allgrove (Hannah), Vivian Statham (Bullwinkel), Wilma Young (Oram), Joyce Tweddell. Standing: Jean Ashton, Flo Syer (Trotter), Pat Darling (Gunther). Colonel (later General) Jim Molan is on the far right.

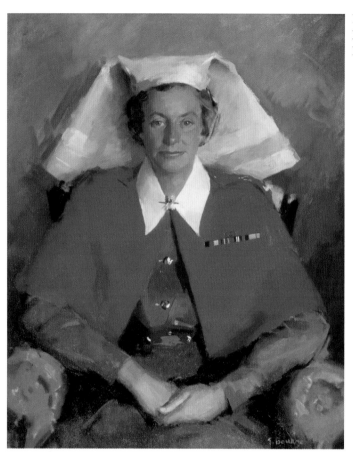

Portrait of Matron Vivian Bullwinkel by Shirley Bourne, 1965. *Australian War Memorial ART28389*

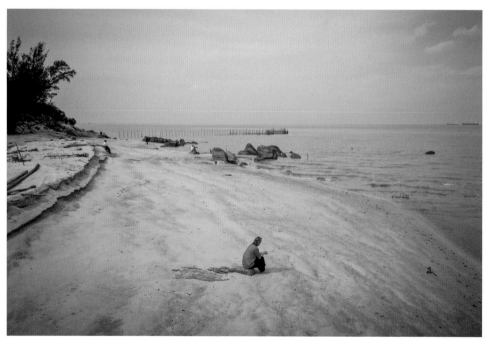

Wing Commander (Ret'd) Sharon Bown takes a quiet moment on Radji Beach during a commemoration ceremony there in 2023. *Justin McManus/Fairfax*

Chapter 13

EVEN WITH THE THREAT of Japanese everywhere, Viv felt far safer on the sand of Bangka Island than she had in the South China Sea. She guessed that the large bonfire they had all seen from the lifeboat was about 3 kilometres from where they had washed ashore.[1]

The shrapnel injuries to Flo Casson, Kath Neuss and Rosetta Wight were severe, worsened by eight hours of a life-and-death struggle in the sea, and they would require hospital treatment or, at the very least, pain relief, antiseptics, sterile bandages and stitches. The elderly civilians were in a state of shock.

When Viv and Jimmy Miller finally caught their breath and their legs were back in order, they decided to investigate whether there were other survivors on the island. Two other nurses agreed to go with them, and the four set off down along the dark beach towards the orange fire in the distance.

It was about 10.30 p.m. on 14 February[2] when Viv and the three others reached the blaze. They were all elated to find it had been lit as a beacon by Irene Drummond and the nineteen others who had made it to shore in the first lifeboat launched from the *Vyner Brooke.*

Matron Drummond and her group had spent a little more than three hours in the water, next to no time compared to the others. The sun was just starting to sink below the horizon when their lifeboat washed up on a long and narrow crescent-shaped stretch of sand that they would later learn was Radji Beach, a few kilometres north-west of Muntok. Over the next few hours more survivors had found their way out of the sea and beside the fire, so that by the time Viv and her party arrived, there were also about forty British servicemen there as well as civilian men, women and children. Another group of survivors arrived[3] in a holey lifeboat that had been lashed together with some rafts. It was the boat containing Eric Germann and little Mischa Warman, along with the nurses Peggy Farmaner, Lorna Fairweather, Brisbane-born Esther 'Jean' Stewart[4] and South Australian Nell Keats.[5] Jean Stewart was the daughter of a Coolangatta widow and had started nursing at Toowoomba, and subsequently trained at the Diamantina Hospital in Brisbane and the Royal Prince Alfred and Crown Street Women's Hospitals in Sydney.[6] Nell Keats had finished her training at Adelaide Hospital.

Sadly, not all on the boat had lived through the ordeal. A Malay sailor who had been burned by a bomb-flash on the *Vyner Brooke* was brought ashore but died shortly afterwards. He was buried in the sand, after what Germann called 'much tugging and pushing', because rigor mortis had stiffened his outflung arms and legs and he wouldn't fit into the narrow trench scooped out for him.[7]

Viv told Matron Drummond all about their time in the water and the need to get treatment for the most pressing cases, who Viv and Jimmy Miller had left behind on the other beach.

More and more survivors washed up at different points on Bangka Island, and Mischa Warman was eventually reunited with his mother.[8] Viv would later learn that twelve nurses, people who had become like family to her, had died in the water.

They were:

Olive Paschke, 36
Vima Bates, 31
Ellenor Calnan, 29[9]
Mary Clarke, 30
Millie Dorsch, 29
Caroline Ennis, 28
Kit Kinsella, 37

Gladys McDonald, 32
Lavinia Russell, 32[10]
Marjorie Schuman, 31[11]
Merle Trenerry, 32
Mona Wilton, 28

Fifty-three of the Australian nurses made it to Bangka Island, however, in a variety of ways. The raft containing Veronica Clancy, Blanche Hempsted, Gladys Hughes, Sylvia Muir, Jean Ashton and the heavily pregnant Olga Neubronner was a couple of kilometres off the island on the morning of 15 February. After bringing Dr Goldberg into line, Jean had been pushing and pulling the raft all night. She could see a fire on shore near a lighthouse. Jean and two of the others began swimming towards the shore to summon help for their drifting craft. A motor launch raced across the waves to meet them. To their astonishment, it was piloted by two RAAF airmen who hauled the swimmers and the women on the raft aboard. The airmen were shocked to discover that most of the nurses were almost naked, their uniforms having been torn up for use as sails, and their bra straps broken from having been struggling in the water for hours. The airmen warned them all to keep as quiet as possible since there were Japanese soldiers everywhere.

The launch arrived at a long jetty and the RAAF men lifted the women onto it, where, screaming in agony, Mrs Neubronner delivered a stillborn child. One of the airmen went off to look for help but in almost no time came sprinting back. His eyes were as wide as dinner plates and he leapt onto the launch with his comrade and roared away. A group of Japanese soldiers came racing down the jetty after them, firing shots at the fleeing vessel but apparently to no effect. Nearby was the body of a Chinese man recently beheaded. The women feared the worst, but with two nurses helping to carry Mrs Neubronner, the group found themselves with some of the other nurses under guard at the Muntok cinema, a building that was soon crowded with more than a thousand prisoners, many of them survivors from other ships the Japanese had just sunk.

The group of nurses who had been listening to Jenny Greer's hit songs from *The Wizard of Oz* spent all night hanging onto their narrow plank at the mercy of the unpredictable currents. They supported each other with renditions of popular tunes of the time and stories of their lives. During the night and into the next morning they bobbed about, watching both a lighthouse and a bonfire on Bangka Island, though the currents would not let them get close for hours. Finally, after eighteen hours in the water, they washed up in a sandy cove. It was wonderful for the women to feel the sand beneath their feet.[12] After flopping onto the beach in exhaustion, they removed their life jackets and waited to make their next move.

A local climbed up a coconut palm and gave the nurses milk to drink but they had swallowed so much oil during the night that they were all violently ill. Flo Trotter told the local man that they wanted to get to the other girls but it was impossible to travel through the dense tropical growth. He suggested that they go in the other direction to Muntok.

The nurses set off, and were walking through a small stream when Japanese soldiers came marching towards them. The nurses froze in fear. The soldiers ordered Flo and the other four nurses, Jenny Greer, Joyce Tweddell, Beryl Woodbridge and Jessie Blanch, out into a clearing. 'Obviously they intended to shoot us.' Flo recalled.

> They lined us up, our backs turned. Suddenly they changed their minds, walked us into Muntok, herded us into the Customs House and took us prisoners. Some girls were already there as well as civilians and naval men. Apparently, many ships had been sunk in the Bangka Strait on the same day as the *Vyner Brooke*. Many more people were brought later and soon overcrowding forced them to move us. As we went out the gates they gave us a little cold rice in the palm of our hand and enough meat to fit on a sixpence. There was still nothing to drink and we were all feeling dehydrated.[13]

On the same day, 15 February, Wilma Oram and Dot Gibson also drifted into the middle of a flotilla of Japanese landing craft – 'great big black boats'[14] – and they also became prisoners of the Japanese. On another beach nearby, Cecilia Delforce,[15] a nurse from Stanthorpe in Queensland via the outback town of Augathella, was also washed ashore. Walking along a jungle track she heard a rifle blast and to her horror saw that a Japanese soldier had just shot a prisoner and that there were several other local men with their hands tied behind their backs. The soldier was as shocked to see Cecilia as she was to see him, but rather than turn his rifle her way, he pointed to a small hut nearby and motioned for her to enter it. Inside, Cecilia saw there were several other women, including some nurses wearing uniforms she didn't recognise. Cecilia did not hear any more gunshots and did not know the fate of the other prisoners. She and the other women were eventually marched off into Muntok.

VIV TOLD MATRON DRUMMOND that her immediate priority was to get medical help for her group of survivors at a beach 3 kilometres away. Taking Viv with her, Matron Drummond went in search of a Chinese medical man, Dr Tay Soon Woon, who had travelled with her on the lifeboat.

The women found the doctor and asked him to accompany them to the other camp to treat the injured nurses. They were astounded when he refused, saying he was needed on the beach. If the Australians wanted help they would have to come to him, he said. Viv explained to the doctor that they were in great difficulties and needed treatment as soon as possible.

But still the doctor refused.

After the day she'd just had, Matron Drummond was especially furious. She turned on her heel and strode off down the beach in the direction of Viv's group, moving so fast for a small round woman that Viv had to run to catch her.

'Calls himself a doctor,' Matron Drummond snapped. And then for emphasis added: 'Indeed!'[16]

The two women asked some of the other survivors beside the bonfire for assistance, and Eric Germann and an English teenager fashioned a stretcher together out of two oars and two shirts. They followed Viv, Miller and Bill Sedgeman back to the other beach where the wounded women, including one of the nurses whose left breast had nearly been torn off by shrapnel, were resting.[17] They were distressed and the 3-kilometre journey to the main group beside the bonfire added to their pain, as they were half carried and half dragged. By the time they had finished transporting the wounded, Eric Germann was so weary he felt like vomiting.

By midnight all of those from Viv's boat were having their wounds treated beside the fire on Radji Beach.[18] As many of the survivors stared into the flames after the worst twelve hours of their lives and contemplated what fate had next in store for them, the sky over the sea constantly lit up as though consumed by an electrical storm. It was in fact Japanese guns causing more mayhem on the water.

Just before dawn, another lifeboat landed on the beach, after the Japanese had sunk yet another evacuation vessel from Singapore off Bangka Island. Among the men, women and children on board were several wounded servicemen and a Royal Navy officer, Lieutenant Commander James White, who had been picked up as he drifted on a life raft after the sinking of the *Vyner Brooke*. Viv, Matron Drummond and the nurses who could still walk helped make all the survivors as comfortable as possible and settled down to catch some sleep in the dark minutes that remained.

VIV WOKE ON THE MORNING of Sunday, 15 February, and listened as Bill Sedgeman, Jimmy Miller and Irene Drummond made plans for a coordinated search for food and assistance from local villagers. There were now more than seventy survivors ranging from small children to old men and women on Radji Beach. There were twenty-two Australian nurses, some of them badly wounded. There were three officers and several sailors from the *Vyner Brooke*, a dozen soldiers from the previous night's sea battle and about a dozen Royal Navy sailors.

While some of the survivors spent the day foraging on the edge of the jungle for coconuts and pineapples and for material to make stretchers to transport the severely wounded, one party of men was sent to a lighthouse while another party headed towards a second lighthouse a few kilometres away. One of the groups was taken prisoner by Japanese troops.

Viv joined a group led by Bill Sedgeman that headed towards a village a few kilometres inland from the beach.[19] Sedgeman thought a large party of women would elicit sympathy from the local villagers, and perhaps even the Japanese if they encountered them. Walking beside Viv was Clarice Halligan, despite a piece of shrapnel imbedded in her thigh that needed medication and stitches, as well as other nurses Jenny Kerr, Mona Tait, Nancy Harris and Ada Bridge,[20] a country girl from the Hunter Valley of New South Wales, and who in happier times loved to dance. There were also three other women: Alice Rossie, an English nurse who had dodged the massacre at the British Military Hospital in Singapore by boarding the *Vyner Brooke*, Kathleen Hutchings, the wife of a British major, and Mrs Marion Galloway Langdon-Williams, the wife of a Singapore town planner.

They walked for more than half an hour along a narrow trail through the jungle until they neared a village or 'kampong'. Sedgeman told the others he would do all the talking and he approached a trio of old men sitting under a shelter. Using gestures and the little Malay language that he knew, Sedgeman tried his best to explain about the shipwreck and the survivors on the beach; how many of them including some of the nurses were badly wounded, and that they all had urgent need for sustenance. The old men told him the Japanese were now in control of Bangka Island and they should all go to Muntok, where the Japanese could give them food and water.

While Sedgeman was still talking to the men, two elderly women emerged from their huts with food and water for Viv and the other bedraggled nurses, but one of the men, seeing this, put a stop to the generosity. Viv wasn't sure if the villagers were afraid of Japanese reprisals or if they saw the arrival of the Japanese as their salvation from European colonisation.

And so the sad group trudged back to Radji Beach, dejected, demoralised and empty-handed. Their flight to freedom had apparently come to an emphatic halt.

Jimmy Miller had found a fresh water spring behind a nearby headland, but the survivors on Radji Beach realised they were unlikely to receive any help from the local people with food or an escape route. At least they were able to house some of the more seriously wounded in an abandoned fisherman's hut beside the beach.

Sedgeman discussed their dire situation with Miller and Matron Drummond and then called all the survivors together to vote on their next step. He chose a shady spot under the palm trees where the wounded could rest and hear him too.

Viv and the others listened intently as Sedgeman explained in his Welsh lilt that Bangka Island was now under Japanese control and that they were trapped.

As far as he could see it, they could:

1. repair the lifeboats and hope the unpredictable currents would carry them to a place that the Japanese had not yet conquered;
2. move into the jungle and hope they could hide and live off the land with the help of friendly villagers until an escape was possible; or
3. surrender to the Japanese and hope for the best.

The first two options were immediately ruled out because they would involve leaving behind the wounded, the sick and the elderly. Everyone tended to agree that it was surrender or starve.[21]

It was now early afternoon on 15 February. Sedgeman said it would be best to sleep on it and meet again the following morning to make a final decision. He said they should all try to get some rest because the next day would be full of stress and anxiety.

The bonfire was relit, wounds were tended, bandages washed, dressings changed and water carted from the spring. Out in the Bangka Strait, the night sky again flashed demonically with searchlights and cannon blasts as Japanese warships sank the 50-metre Batavian vessel *Pulo Soegi*, which had left Singapore a day after the *Vyner Brooke*.

None of the nurses slept well.

THAT SAME NIGHT, Singapore fell. Realising that the Allied situation there was hopeless, that ammunition and water supplies were almost exhausted and wishing to prevent more civilian and military deaths, General Arthur Percival had started to negotiate a surrender with the Japanese. He maintained that Singapore could have been held if Britain had not sent so many men and so much money to its war efforts in Europe and the Middle East.

The Japanese made Percival march under a white flag to negotiate the surrender at Singapore's Ford Motor Factory, which they had commandeered as their military headquarters.

The Tiger of Malaya, General Yamashita, slammed his fist down hard on the negotiating table and demanded unconditional surrender. Percival, a thin man with buckteeth, looked weak and wan and was completely at the mercy of the Japanese as he tried to negotiate conditions.

In the end he told his troops to stop fighting at 8.30 p.m. Almost 2000 Australians had died in the battle for Malaya and Singapore, with another 2000 wounded.

Despite his instruction to Australian troops to stay at their posts, General Gordon Bennett, commander of Australia's 8th Division, declared it was his duty to flee Singapore, and with two of his staff officers he escaped the city in a commandeered sampan, on the first leg of his journey to Melbourne. General Bennett left 15,000 of his men, among 52,000 Allied troops, to face an uncertain, anxious future as prisoners of war.

'Singapore has fallen and the Malaya Peninsula has been overrun,' Prime Minister Churchill told the British people in a radio broadcast that night.[22]

He assured Australia and New Zealand that 'every effort' would be made to preserve their safety, but he later called the loss of the city 'the worst disaster and largest capitulation in British history'.[23]

Australian Prime Minister John Curtin warned that the fall of Singapore opened the battle for Australia. Japanese commanders were already plotting the imminent bombing of Darwin and Broome.

A FEW HOURS AFTER the surrender of Singapore, a lifeboat arrived on Radji Beach with about twenty-five soldiers and some sailors who had survived the sinking of the *Pulo Soegi*. At least one man in the lifeboat was dead and most were badly wounded, including 32-year-old Yorkshireman Private Cecil Gordon Kinsley,[24] who had been part of Britain's 18th Division. The bombs that had rained down on his ship had also ripped away much of his left upper arm, exposing the bone.

Viv knew some of her nurses and wounded men such as Kinsley would die if they didn't receive proper medical help soon – and in a hospital.

Surrendering to the Japanese was a risk, but what else was there to do? She had heard all the horror stories of their cruelty. When the soldiers, airmen or sailors had come into hospital at Tampoi and Singapore, they had told her with looks of horror that 'the Japs are not taking prisoners'. It didn't matter what branch of the service the Australians were in; the warning was always the same: 'They're not taking prisoners.'

'However when you're young,' Viv recalled, 'and you've got a group of over a hundred people you can't imagine anything happening, and we confidently felt that we would be taken prisoners because of safety in numbers.'[25]

Viv didn't know that Captain Orita Masaru and his men from the 229th Regiment, those same soldiers who had murdered and raped their way through Hong Kong on Christmas Day, had just arrived on Bangka Island as well.

Chapter 14

IN A DIFFERENT TIME, Monday, 16 February 1942, would have been another perfect day in paradise; the beautiful beach, the swaying palms, the bright blue sea.

But there were more than 100 shipwreck survivors on Radji Beach that morning, many badly injured, all of them hungry and afraid. Bill Sedgeman again took a vote on the best course of action. A show of hands agreed that surrender was the safest option.

Sedgeman volunteered to lead a group into Muntok to find the Japanese and explain that there were a large number of shipwreck survivors on a beach who were willing to be made prisoners of war, including many who needed urgent medical attention. He told Irene Drummond that he would ask the Japanese for stretchers to carry the severely wounded, including her nurses. He would also ask for a military escort to give the refugees safe conduct past any hostile patrols.[1]

At 9 a.m., he and two sailors strode off confidently down a jungle track. Viv wondered what would become of her and all the others trapped between the sea and a fierce Japanese military force. On Matron Drummond's advice, Jimmy Miller asked any able British servicemen to start constructing makeshift stretchers in case the Japanese didn't have enough to go around. The nurses began making a large Red Cross flag from salvaged material, just in case there were any doubts if Japanese aircraft flew over again.

Dreading what might happen when the Japanese arrived with Sedgeman, Viv felt depressed and apprehensive.[2] But rather than share her fears with the others, she busied herself fetching water from the spring and tending to the needs of the wounded. Many of the nurses were barely dressed, their clothes having been ruined in the sea or torn apart for bandages. Others wore discarded civilian clothes or shirts given to them by soldiers and sailors. Most still had their Red Cross armbands.

Many of the children, having undergone such a horrific ordeal were still traumatised and, having not eaten for a couple of days, famished. Some of the civilians therefore suggested they should find their own way towards a village or Muntok and throw themselves at the mercy of the Japanese there.[3] Matron Drummond agreed, saying it would save the Japanese time in transporting them to a prison camp and would free up trucks sooner to take the wounded survivors to hospital, which so many of them badly needed. But Irene insisted that all her nurses should stay where they were because their duty was to treat the sick and injured.[4]

An elderly Englishwoman, Mrs Carrie Betteridge,[5] refused to go because she wanted to remain with her badly wounded husband, Tom.[6] He was a successful stockbroker and the Betteridges were leading lights in the social circles of Kuala Lumpur and Singapore. They had been married for the best part of forty years. Carrie was in a state of great disquiet because Tom had taken a hunk of shrapnel in a kidney and would not last long without medical help.

A small group of British servicemen left Radji Beach independently and headed for the Muntok lighthouse,[7] but Jimmy Miller and most of the British soldiers decided to stay with the nurses.

At about 9.30 a.m. most of the survivors watched a group of twenty or so civilians and a couple of sailors whose arm wounds meant they would be useless as stretcher bearers later in the day, leave the beach and head down the same path Bill Sedgeman had taken half an hour earlier. Among the group were Cevia

Warman and her beloved Mischa; Dr Tay; the schoolteacher Louise Beeston; Mrs Langdon-Williams, the town planner's wife; the British nurse Alice Rossie; Kathleen Hutchings, the British major's wife; Myrtle Ward, the wife of a British electrical engineer in Singapore; and an elderly couple from Bright in northern Victoria – John Gallagher Dominguez,[8] a mining engineer for Anglo Oriental Tin, and his wife of forty years, Gerte.[9]

Together they had walked for about twenty minutes towards Muntok when, with the children weary and footsore, they all decided to rest in a jungle clearing beside the path. Approaching from the other direction was Bill Sedgeman, the two sailors, and about fifteen Japanese soldiers of the 1st Battalion, 229th Infantry Regiment, of the 38th Infantry Division. They had just arrived on Bangka Island from their base at Cam Ranh Bay in Vietnam. The soldiers were dressed in khaki shirts and baggy trousers in the style of jodhpurs, and wore caps with a small star. Most had rifles with bayonets attached but at least one was carrying a light machine gun. They were led by the small and smartly dressed Captain Orita Masaru, who had a long sword by his side.[10]

Masaru and the soldiers looked at the dishevelled, distressed group but they took little notice and continued on with Sedgeman in the direction of Radji Beach. The men, women and children eventually made it to Muntok, where they were taken prisoner without incident.

There were now about eighty people resting and waiting on Radji Beach: twenty-two Australian nurses, about twenty uninjured men, mostly sailors from the *Vyner Brooke* as well as British soldiers who had arrived on the lifeboat from the *Pulo Soegi*, and Mr and Mrs Betteridge and about thirty-five other civilian men and women who were wounded, including ten stretcher cases. Under Irene Drummond's direction, the soldiers continued making stretchers using driftwood, belts and planks. When they had put together about a dozen, they moved some of the wounded to the new stretchers, but decided to leave the most serious cases until the Japanese arrived, thinking the Japanese stretchers would be of a much sturdier construction.

Nurse 'Buddy' Elmes[11] was one of the survivors busy treating the wounded. With hazel eyes, her hair worn in a bun, an infectious laugh and a long striding walk, she was a confident, attractive young woman with a quirky sense of humour who used the term of endearment 'old hound' for her friends.[12] Her family adored her and her mother, Dorothy, fretted over her. Dorothy would soon write a letter that began: 'My Darling little Bud, Oh dear, I wish I knew where you are in the world.'[13]

To Stoker Ernest Lloyd,[14] a Manchester sailor who had served on both the *Prince of Wales* and the *Vyner Brooke*, everyone seemed 'pretty cheerful'[15] despite their predicament, and they were optimistic that the Japanese would treat them fairly as prisoners.

Just after 10 a.m., Sedgeman emerged from the jungle and crossed the beach towards them. A small, stern-faced Japanese officer and his soldiers followed behind. When they reached the survivors, Viv watched apprehensively as Sedgeman said to the Japanese officer: 'These are the people I told you about who want to be taken prisoner.'

But Captain Masaru brushed Sedgeman aside.[16] The Japanese officer's face was expressionless as he surveyed the nurses, soldiers, sailors and stretcher cases.

Masaru quickly computed the easiest option to deal with these captives and barked out an order to his sergeant major. As the soldiers cocked their weapons, Viv felt sick. The survivors instinctively drew closer together for mutual protection, and Sedgeman began to protest. Masaru ignored him again, as the soldiers began stabbing bayonets at the survivors, separating the women from the men, just as they had done at the hospital in Hong Kong. The Japanese soldiers searched everyone on the beach and then motioned, with thrusts of the bayonets for emphasis, that the shipwreck survivors must form two lines – one of men and the other of women.[17]

Four soldiers took up sentry posts on the flanks of the two groups, making sure there was no escape. Masaru surveyed all the survivors in silence for so long that, one by one, all but ten of the men broke rank and went back to work on the stretchers, thinking that before long they would be given the command to start toting the wounded to hospital. Then, as Viv waited, hoping they would soon be marched to somewhere where there was hot food and dry shelter, Masaru conferred with one of his soldiers again and finally, by gestures of the bayonets, ordered the ten men who were still standing in line to walk down the beach. Among them were Ernest Lloyd and Able Seaman Jock McClurg, who had been on the *Prince of Wales* before joining the crew of the *Vyner Brooke*. Six soldiers with rifles and a light machine gun followed behind.

The other Japanese soldiers remained guarding Viv and the others.

Lloyd thought his group was being marched into Muntok, but they passed the jungle path that Sedgeman had taken earlier that morning and continued on around the beach to a small bay past a headland of rocks and driftwood. They were about a hundred metres, and out of sight, from the main group.

Here the soldiers lined up their trembling prisoners and motioned for them to stand at the water's edge. The prisoners obeyed.

Lloyd was at one end of the line facing the sea when the man standing next to him, Able Seaman Hamilton, whispered out of the side of his mouth: 'This is where we get it right in the back. I'm going into the water.'

'I'm with you', Lloyd whispered back, and in an instant the line broke. Some men ran along the beach while Lloyd and three others dived into the water. On the beach, out of sight, Viv heard the Japanese open fire. She didn't know it, but they shot the men running along the beach first. Then they turned the guns on to the men in the water.

One bullet scraped Ernest Lloyd across the head, another hit him in the left shoulder, another in the right leg and then one in the left. He lay face down, still and silent, bleeding as he floated out to sea with the tide. The soldiers continued to take pot shots at him to make sure he was dead.[18]

Viv and the nurses froze as the sound of shots exploded in quick succession from beyond the promontory. Eric Germann,

Jimmy Miller and the rest of the men making stretchers looked apprehensively at each other, and then over at the nurses. Someone murmured 'Afraid they're gone', but no one else spoke.

Viv hoped that maybe the blasts were warning shots. With the guns of Masaru's sentries trained on the captives, no one dared move.

Soon the other soldiers reappeared, climbing over the rocks. Masaru now turned his attention to the ten men who had been making the stretchers, and he ordered them to march away, too.

Sedgeman and Jimmy Miller refused, but with bayonets thrust towards them they had no choice. Viv locked eyes with Jimmy as he turned to look at her. A brief boyish grin flashed across his sad face,[19] a half-smile of regret and resignation about what was to come. Then he was gone, hidden among the army and navy uniforms as they tramped towards the beach.

Masaru stood with his thumbs hooked into his sword belt. His legs were spread apart in a confident stance of superiority. He seemed impatient to get this business done so he could get on his way.

As the men set off under guard, Germann and Sedgeman were ordered to lift one of the stretcher cases, a Malayan magistrate named Ernest Watson[20] who, at sixty-eight, was the oldest person on the beach. Watson had been placed under trees at the edge of the jungle with other men and women on stretchers, but he had been sitting up watching the Japanese go about their murderous work.

Germann and Sedgeman did as they were ordered and slowly, reluctantly with bayonets pressed against their backs, they and the other doomed prisoners shuffled dejectedly towards the promontory, all the time looking for a way to escape.

Some thought they could outrun the Japanese bullets. Germann tried another tack. He stopped walking momentarily and called out to Masaru. The procession stopped. From his pocket, Germann pulled a swollen, water-soaked wallet containing his passport and 900 dollars in twenty-dollar bills. He hoped the passport with its gold seal would impress Masaru and that he might be diverted from his cruel course of action.

Masaru studied the passport closely and then threw it on the sand. Some of the twenty-dollar bills had come out of Germann's pocket with the passport and Masaru 'burst into a furious tirade', obviously thinking this condemned prisoner was trying to bribe his way out of a death sentence.

Picking up a piece of driftwood, Masaru swung it at Germann's face. The husky Canadian blocked the blow with an upraised hand and threw the wallet and its contents after the passport, realising money would be no help to him now.

He and Sedgeman picked up Watson and together they struggled down the beach. They struggled even more as they carried the ailing old man, who was in desperate pain, over the rocks and driftwood.

Masaru told them not to bother carrying the magistrate anymore. So Germann and Sedgeman placed Watson gently in a sitting position with his back against a log.

They both shook hands with him and, knowing what was to come, gave Watson a sad goodbye. Then, with the bayonets at their backs, they climbed down the rocks and onto the beach behind the promontory.

Now they were in a small cove. At the water's edge, lying face down, were some of the bodies of the men who had gone before them. Many had slash wounds in their backs, including the English teenager who had helped Germann carry the Australian nurses to the fire. There was a short red bayonet wound under the poor lad's left shoulder blade.

Three soldiers stood near the bodies, wiping their bayonets with rags and polishing them carefully as though anxious to have the cleanest steel possible for their next assignment.[21] A machine gun was at the ready in case anyone tried to run.

Germann, Sedgeman, Jimmy Miller and the others were ordered to stand in a line facing the sea. Two trembling men used their handkerchiefs as blindfolds. No one spoke. Germann looked out over the water and thought the sky and sea seemed especially glorious this morning. *What a stupid way to die*, he thought. *And what a strange ending – here in the morning sun on a strange island, far from anything familiar or any friend.*

At that moment Sedgeman, who was standing on the other end of the line from Germann, dashed for the sea. The machine gun exploded into life as Sedgeman's ended. The brave Welshman, who had helped so many of the nurses escape death only two days earlier, fell to one knee, rose, stumbled again as the gunfire continued before falling down dead at Germann's feet, bleeding from a multitude of wounds. Germann prayed, slowly and with more ardour than he had known existed in him.

On the other side of the headland, Viv and the nurses shuddered at the sound of the gunfire. They had seen so much madness, badness, chaos and carnage over the last few days. Could this really be happening, or was it some sort of terrible hallucination?

Reciting 'The Lord's Prayer', Eric Germann had reached 'deliver us from evil' when a bayonet sliced into his back, exiting out through his chest. His whole body went numb, and he realised he was no longer standing but instead lying face down on the beach, his head in the gently lapping waves. His mouth was open and full of sand and water. All around him, men were being butchered. He heard the sounds of the man next to him vomiting and thrashing about 'as though his body were flopping up and down on the sand'.[22] Bayonets ripped through more bodies. A shot cracked, followed by a deathly silence. Then, as the blood gushed from Germann's body, he felt another body writhe against him. BANG! Another shot. His body tensed all over as he waited for a bullet to crash into his skull.[23]

VIV TREMBLED AT THE SOUND of more shots from behind the headland and, all around, the group of nurses hung their heads at the realisation of their fate. Japanese soldiers stood guard over them, smirking. There was hardly a sound from any of the captives. Five minutes passed. Then the execution squad reappeared, climbing over the rocks of the promontory before sauntering back to where the nurses and the badly wounded lay. As they approached they were laughing among themselves. These men were from the same force that had murdered and raped their way through Hong Kong just a few weeks before.

'Bully,' gasped Jenny Kerr, who was standing behind Viv, 'they've murdered them all.'

Viv felt helpless and devastated, not just for her own life and that of her friends with her on this beach, but also for those dear young men Jimmy Miller and Bill Sedgeman, who had fought so hard to save the lives of all those aboard the *Vyner Brooke*, and who had done such a sterling job getting them to what they thought was the safety of Bangka Island. Those brave men had risked their lives to save the nurses and now those lives had been forfeited.

Lainie Balfour-Ogilvy whispered to the others that they should all just run – run for their lives. They could scatter, bolt in different directions and at least some of them might escape. The strong swimmers could dive into the water, dodge the bullets and swim to another beach or another part of the jungle to get away. However, Matron Drummond reminded her girls that there were many badly wounded people, including their nursing colleagues, lying in stretchers behind them, and their duty was to always help the sick and the injured. Abandoning their patients went against everything they stood for.

So, huddled together under the merciless gaze of their Japanese captors, the nurses prepared themselves mentally for the horrific reality of what they were about to face.

Indifferent to the suffering of their forlorn captives, the young Japanese soldiers who had killed the men behind the headland now marched to a spot in front of the nurses and knelt down. They began reloading their rifles and using rags to clean the blood from their bayonets. Another soldier set up a light machine gun underneath the palm trees about 20 metres from the beach.[24]

'It's true then,' Nancy Harris mumbled. 'They aren't taking prisoners.'

Viv and her desperate friends readied themselves to fend off their tormentors as best they could.[25] Everything became a blur. Eventually, Viv heard Masaru snap an order and his soldiers formed a semicircle around the nurses.

They were about 10 metres from the water's edge. Viv tried to comprehend the end of her young life and of those all around her. Everything became chaotic and jumbled. Were the soldiers tearing at the nurses' clothes? Were her friends being beaten and sexually assaulted? The savagery of what was unfolding made Viv numb. The soldiers made the nurses turn to face the sea and form a line. Old Mrs Betteridge was weeping in the middle. The soldiers kept prodding the sharp tips of their bayonets into the quaking backs of the women, making them walk falteringly towards the water that was gently lapping at their feet amid the unfathomable violence on Radji Beach.

Viv tried to shut out the awful horror of this living nightmare. She thought she heard Jean Stewart cry out: 'Girls, take it, don't squeal.'[26] At the far right of the line Irene Drummond was also quietly telling her girls to be brave.

Viv's mind was in a whirl, and she wasn't sure what she heard or what she thought she heard. She knew she was standing on the far left of the line with Jenny Kerr and feisty Alma Beard, and her brain registered Alma saying: 'Bully, there are two things I've always hated in my life: the Japanese and the sea. And today I've ended up with both.'[27]

Viv was looking out across the water. Somewhere out there lay Australia and home. *How can something as obscene as this be happening in a place that is so beautiful?* she wondered. *What right do these men have to do all that they are doing to these marvellous young lives?*

Some of the women were praying aloud, intoning 'Our Father, who art in heaven …' and 'Hail Mary, full of grace …'

A sense of calm came over Viv. She was thinking that at least it would be lovely to again see her father, George, in heaven and to prepare a place for when her mother and brother, John, joined them there one day.

Then she thought of the shock and grief her mother would feel back home, not knowing what had become of her. She saw her mother's shining blue eyes and, in her mind, they seemed to tell Viv that they would see each other again and they would share carefree days as they had growing up in the Australian bush.

Viv thought she heard Matron Drummond, who was a few paces behind, give one last pep talk to the nurses: 'Chin up, girls. I'm proud of you and I love you all.'[28] Viv turned to the others along the line and smiled one last goodbye at them. Some of her friends returned her smile. Some had an unbreakable inner strength. But some had already decided they were not prepared to leave this world just yet, and when they reached the water's edge they turned and ran as fast as they could. But they were cut down.[29]

Irene Drummond was a few metres short of the water as the other women shuffled into it. One of the soldiers shot Irene in the back and she slammed head-first into the water. Her glasses flew off her head and as she instinctively groped for them, a second bullet tore through her. She did not move again.[30]

The machine gunner then cut loose, spraying the women in the water, those standing stoically, those screaming in fear, those supporting the wounded who could not move without help.

All along the line Viv saw those beautiful women, full of heart and kindness, being cut down, flopping into the sea as bullets blasted them from behind. Some fell limp, face first; others folded and crumpled. There were cries of anguish and terror all about.

Viv was waist deep in the water and preparing herself to step through the gates of heaven and see dear old Dad again. Such was her trance-like state that she could hardly hear the rifles and the machine gun barking.

Then Viv felt something like the 'kick of a mule'[31] hit her in the back and she too fell face forward into the water. Everything turned to black. The Japanese bullet had torn through the flimsy grey fabric of her dress and ripped through her body. Her lifeforce gushed out of her in a red stream.

The blood of all her marvellous friends, those magnificent nurses – kind, beautiful, caring women – mixed with her blood in the water that was gently lapping on the golden shore of Radji Beach.

Chapter 15

A S VIV FLOATED AMONG the blood and the bodies of her friends and prepared to expel the last breath of her short life, the Japanese soldiers went about killing anything that moved in the water. With Captain Masaru supervising, the soldiers plunged their bayonets through any of the nurses who had survived the gunshots. But Viv floated a few metres out to sea away from the bodies of her friends. As far as Masaru was concerned, she was as good as dead.

The Japanese bullet had entered Viv's back on the lower left side and exited her stomach about 5 centimetres above her fabric belt. In a remarkable understatement she later said: 'I was very surprised to find myself still alive.'[1]

> I was young and naïve, I thought that when people were shot they'd had it. I was utterly amazed a few seconds later to find that I was still alive, and then I became frightened and I thought, *Oh, God, I can't go through that again.* I just lay there and, because I had swallowed a whole lot of salt water, and was starting to become violently ill, I thought, *Oh, they'll see my shoulders moving, they'll see my shoulders moving* and I stopped, and I just laid there.[2]

And so Viv lay in the water, face down as she drifted out to sea. The salt water in her stomach made her vomit now and then, so she held her head tilted slightly to one side. Ever so carefully she sucked air into her lungs, as quietly and slowly as she could, in case bubbles in the water or the slightest hint of movement betrayed her. She was stunned rather than elated to still be alive and wondered whether she was hallucinating. The Japanese left her body to drift away as shark bait.

Viv didn't know it, but the Japanese soldiers killed everyone else on the beach, mostly with their bayonets. Some of the nurses who had tried to run had been shot down or had been bayoneted or beaten to death with rifle butts. Then Masaru and his men went about slaughtering all the wounded on stretchers, before going to the nearby fisherman's hut to kill all the badly wounded who were resting there. When the killing spree was done, the Japanese soldiers disappeared into the jungle to cause mayhem elsewhere.

Time seemed to stand still as Viv drifted in and out of consciousness. Eventually, the gentle, rhythmic waves carried her to the shore, where the beach was littered with what remained of her friends.

The sun on her back was warm, but she still felt an icy fear and the cold spread through her body. Her medical training told her it was shock setting in. She thought about finding a nice, warm place where she could curl up and die. But then she began to regain her senses and became deathly afraid. Being shot was an experience she did not want to repeat.

She remained face down on the sand and let the tide run over her again and again and again. The bullet wound was excruciatingly painful, but she gritted her teeth and stayed motionless, listening to the waves, the screeching of the birds and the wind whispering through the palms.

Viv wasn't sure how long she'd been in the water, but the sun had gone past its peak and she figured it was early afternoon. She finally plucked up enough courage to sit up and look around.[3] To her relief the Japanese had all gone, but she knew she could not linger in case they came back. She wondered where all the bodies had gone. Perhaps her mind was playing tricks because soon others would find the bodies of Viv's friends and the other shipwreck survivors strewn like litter across the sand and rocks of Radji Beach.

Carefully, gingerly, Viv placed a hand on her lower back and felt around the hole where the bullet had entered. She found where the piece of hot lead had exited through her stomach, just to the left of her navel. The bleeding had stopped, and the wound had been washed by hours of immersion in salt water. Although her legs felt weak, she had the strength to stand and walk, and she guessed that the bullet had gone clean through her body without damaging any vital organs.

Holding on to her wounded side, Viv took a few halting, painful steps along the sand and started walking in the direction of the jungle. Each step was agony but she saw each one as life-saving.

All I could think of was getting up into the jungle out of the breeze, so I went up this little track about 10 or 20 yards then into the jungle and just lay down. Whether I slept or was unconscious I'll never know. I woke up at one stage and it was pitch dark, the next time it was daylight and I was hot and sweaty, thirsty and very sorry for myself.[4]

Sixty-five Australian nurses had left Singapore on the *Vyner Brooke* just four days earlier. Thirty-three were now dead.

The twenty-one nurses killed on Radji Beach were:

Elaine 'Lainie' Lenore Balfour-Ogilvy, 30
Alma May Beard, 29
Ada Joyce Bridge, 34
Florence Rebecca Casson, 38
Mary Elizabeth Cuthbertson, 31
Irene Melville Drummond, 36
Dorothy Gwendoline Howard 'Buddy' Elmes, 28
Lorna Florence Fairweather, 28
Peggy Everett Farmaner, 27
Clarice Isobel Halligan, 37

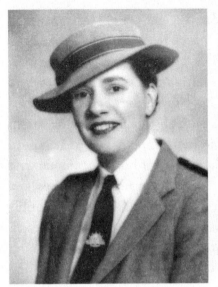

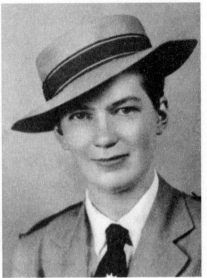

Beth Cuthbertson was badly injured during the bombing of the Vyner Brooke. *Australian War Memorial P04031.001*

As Dorothy 'Buddy' Elmes faced the Japanese on Radji Beach, her mother was preparing to write a letter which began 'My Darling little Bud, Oh dear, I wish I knew where you are in the world'. *Australian War Memorial P01180.001*

Nancy Harris, 29

Minnie Ivy Hodgson, 33

Ellen Louisa Keats, 26

Janet 'Jenny' Kerr, 31

Mary Eleanor McGlade, 39

Kathleen Margaret Neuss, 30

Florence Aubin Salmon, 26

Esther Sarah Jean Stewart, 35

Mona Margaret Anderson Tait, 27

Rosetta Joan Wight, 33

Bessie Wilmott, 28

AS VIV SLEPT INSIDE HER jungle hideout, others were seeing the full extent of the horror on Radji Beach with wide-eyed astonishment.

Captain Masaru and his band of soldiers were ruthless, but they were not totally efficient. While Viv had been floating face down feigning death among her murdered friends, Eric Germann had also been playing dead among other victims beyond the headland on Radji Beach.

After having a bayonet rammed through his powerful body and listening to the death throes of his companions being bayoneted and shot, he had been conscious enough to know that he might soon die from blood loss. But the more time passed as he lay in the water playing dead among the bodies of his companions who weren't playing, the more alive he felt. He heard footsteps and laughter, but did not move, except for an almost imperceptible twist of his head with each wave so he could look along the beach. He waited in the water as stiff and still as the corpses all around, and just as well. Two soldiers had appeared on the rocks and surveyed the cove just to be sure there were no survivors. One of them waved a small flag, as though signalling by semaphore to the other soldiers who were about to murder the nurses.[5] How long Germann waited it was impossible to know, but finally he tested his legs for life and found that they still worked.

He sprang up, spinning his head this way and that to scan the beach once more. It was empty but for the dead. To his surprise one of the men was sitting upright, his sightless eyes looking out over the sea.

Germann ran up the slope and into the jungle. Thorny undergrowth cut his bare feet but the worst pain was the dull throb from his chest and back. Blood oozed from a wound on his lower-right chest and another wound on his back, opposite the wound in front. Just like the bullet that tore through Viv, the Japanese bayonet had gone straight through Germann, somehow missing all the vital organs.

He waited, lying there all day and all night, fighting mosquitoes and ants. The next morning, three survivors from other shipwrecks surveyed the carnage on Radji Beach. Germann emerged from his hideout to tell them that he was a member of a party of nurses, civilians and servicemen who had been murdered.

One of the shipwreck survivors, Corporal Robert Seddon of the Royal Marines, had floated at sea in a life jacket after his ship,

HMS *Yin Ping*, was sunk. He had drifted in towards Radji Beach and saw the horror unfold, undetected by Masaru and his men.

Seddon had seen three groups on the beach, then two or three men and women run to the water in attempts to swim away. One of the men was shot but kept swimming[6] while some of the other men trying to escape were bayoneted and shot. Seddon had floated in the sea playing dead for hours. The next day, he found the bodies of fifteen nurses, fifteen British service personnel and five merchant seamen nearby.[7]

Leading Seaman Dick Wilding told Germann he had reached the shore in a damaged lifeboat after the massacre. He had been on the HMS *Li Wo*, which the Japanese had bombed. Wilding had been ready to collapse when he heard a moaning from the fringe of trees above. He'd forced himself up the slope and found a man lying on his belly on the grass groaning as a cloud of flies buzzed around him. Wilding rolled the man onto his side and saw he'd been lying on spilled intestines. He didn't open his eyes but he'd managed to gasp the word 'Japs' before he died.[8] The dead man was apparently one of the servicemen who had left Radji Beach heading for the Muntok lighthouse on the morning of the massacre.

Before Germann had come out of the jungle, Wilding and Seddon had found a lifeboat on Radji Beach and a dozen bodies – 'all women, except two'. Some were barely dressed, Wilding said, possibly in civilian clothing, while some were in nurses' uniforms and others were naked. Flying from sticks on the beach was a nurse's uniform bearing a Red Cross.

They found another Englishman still alive, but with only minutes to live.[9] The scene 'was too gruesome to go around and accurately count',[10] but Wilding looked closely at two of the female bodies and saw that one had been shot and one had been killed by a sword. Further along the beach the shocked pair found about twenty more bodies, mostly British servicemen, who had also been shot and bayoneted.[11]

On the pile of rocks and driftwood, still leaning against the log where he had been placed, was the old magistrate, Ernest Watson.

His skull had been bashed in. Flies buzzed around the mess that had been his head.

The bodies of most of the nurses were widely scattered along the water's edge, and Germann presumed that some had floated away when the tide went out. Four bodies lay huddled in one group and three in another. Flies were everywhere. The stretchers were where they had been left and on them lay patients staring sightlessly at the sky. Two stretchers were empty: one had been the old magistrate's and the other had been for the wounded soldier Kinsley. What had become of Kinsley?[12]

At the fisherman's hut near the beach they found one man who fell forward, right onto his face, as they entered. They sat him up. 'Japs been here?' they asked. He mumbled, dribbling and managed to point back along the beach to where the bodies of the nurses lay. As he sat upright the man's intestines spilled out of a gash in his belly but somehow he masked his shocking pain. Beyond where he sat dying were the bodies of three sailors, fly-blown and stinking, sprawled across fishing nets.

THE DAY AFTER SHE WAS SHOT, Viv woke inside her jungle hideout, dazed and confused. Her bullet wound was throbbing and she felt famished and parched. The humid air weighed down on her like a heavy shroud and fear clawed at her very being.

Nervously, she poked her head out from the palm fronds around her hiding place and looked about for danger. She was near the track to Muntok and she knew that a freshwater stream was nearby.

But her relief quickly turned to panic when she saw a metallic glint from a bayonet. Despite her pain she scurried deep within the protection of a fern tree. Then she heard Japanese voices. Nearby. Every muscle inside her tensed and the throbbing in her side grew worse. She sucked in a breath and held it as from behind a veil of leaves she saw the same soldiers who had murdered her friends come walking down the track right beside her hiding place.

She thought her heart would burst and was sure that the Japanese could hear it pounding. She prayed they couldn't. The soldiers were so close she could almost touch them, and she hoped beyond hope that they wouldn't see light reflecting from her pupils.

She began to shake uncontrollably, but the last soldier in the patrol walked by without noticing her. On they went, down to the beach where they'd snuffed out so many lives.

THE MURDERS ON RADJI BEACH had not satiated the bloodlust of some of the Japanese soldiers who showed so little regard for humanity or rank. Eric Germann would later explain that the Japanese soldier in World War II 'seemed to possess the personality of a Dr Jekyll and Mr Hyde. He could be gentleman or beast with equal naturalness and facility.'[13]

Germann and his companions were desperate for food. They met some Malay fishermen who gave them water but had no food to spare. Everywhere they went, villagers refused to assist them because they feared Japanese reprisals.

And so, despite everything that had happened to him and the viciousness he had seen and experienced, Germann convinced himself that not all the Japanese were heartless killers. He eventually surrendered in Muntok to Japanese soldiers who received him with little concern and pointed to the local cinema, where a thousand or so prisoners were already being housed, including Cevia Warman, little Mischa and the other women, children and old men who had walked away from Radji Beach on the morning of 16 February.

How odd, Germann thought, that these same people had met the murderers being guided by Sedgeman to Radji Beach, and yet they were spared while all the others were killed. 'Not only did the fate of a prisoner vary according to the individual Japanese who found him,' Germann mused, 'but also according to the particular moment the Japanese found him.'[14]

Imprisoned at Muntok, Germann met another survivor from the massacre on Radji Beach: Stoker Ernest Lloyd. Lloyd's head wound from the first round of killings beyond the headland had rendered him unconscious, but he'd still managed to breathe as he drifted away, while the Japanese took pot shots at him. Then, when the coast was clear, he'd returned to the beach. From there he'd crawled into the jungle, where he collapsed and lay for three long days. After he had recovered, he went down to the beach again and came to the spot where he had originally landed.

> There I saw the Australian nurses. All were dead. I recognised two or three. I counted twelve or fifteen nurses and about twenty-five men dead. Two or three of the women had practically all their clothes torn from them. They were in the most horrible positions – some kneeling – some doubled up. Some had bayonet wounds as well as bullet holes. I saw the chief officer [Sedgeman] dead and his clothes covered with blood. The nurses were scattered. Some had fifty yards between them. I reckoned they had been dealt with individually.[15]

Lloyd spent four days at the scene of the carnage in a terrible physical and mental state. With his wounds festering and weak from a loss of blood, he could hardly walk. He hid in the jungle and was nearly dead from his wounds when he met Chinese labourers, who strung him on a pole and carried him into Muntok to be handed over to the Japanese.

Lloyd's captors chose not to finish him off. He was luckier than so many of the prisoners, and luck played such a big part in the treatment of Japan's captives. The day after the slaughter of the nurses, Japanese patrol boats captured the 13-metre launch *Mary Rose* in the Bangka Strait and escorted it into Muntok's harbour.

On board was the high-ranking diplomat and public servant Vivian Bowden,[16] who held the title of Australia's Official Representative in Singapore, effectively Australia's ambassador to the island city. Bowden had lived in Japan at different times and had been Australia's Trade Commissioner in Tokyo and Shanghai. The launch had left Singapore two days after the *Vyner Brooke*, with General Percival insisting that Bowden and his two senior assistants flee the city and return to Australia.

Bowden was locked up in the Muntok cinema with about a thousand other prisoners, including some of the Australian nurses. He protested loudly to the Japanese about his diplomatic status being ignored and remonstrated when one of the soldiers tried to steal his watch.

The soldiers beat him almost senseless and then dragged him outside. There this distinguished, elderly white-haired gentleman was forced to dig his own shallow grave before the Japanese shot him.

THE REAPPEARANCE OF Captain Masaru and his men unnerved Viv for hours. She was thirsty, hungry and afraid, but she dared not even peek out from behind the palm fronds that she now saw as life preservers.

Finally, she willed herself out of her hiding spot and, crawled along the ground on her hands and knees in search of the freshwater stream.

When she finally reached the stream, she knelt beside it and bent forward. She was about to dip her cupped hands into the water for the drink she'd been craving ever since the Japanese bullet tore through her body. But before she could taste its cool sweetness, her heart froze.

She almost fainted when she heard a male voice from the undergrowth. 'Where have you been, Nurse?'[17]

Viv wheeled around, her eyes wide.

Chapter 16

SLACK-JAWED, VIV STARED at what might have been a ghost. How was British soldier Cecil Gordon Kinsley, who had been slashed and tossed aside like rubbish by the Japanese, still alive and still talking?

Kinsley had arrived on a lifeboat on Radji Beach with most of his left upper arm torn off down to the bone. He had been one of the stretcher cases lying under the trees while the nurses were shot, and now here he was in Viv's jungle hideout, propped up on one elbow, legs splayed, wearing his British Army khaki shirt and shorts. They were covered in his blood, as was the field dressing on his upper arm.

'I saw what they did to you girls,' Kinsley muttered, with little life left in his voice or in his wasted body. 'Then they came back to put the bayonet into us wounded.'[1]

A Japanese soldier had rammed his bayonet through Kinsley twice as all the injured men and women around him were stabbed too. But after their murderous spree, and having left the dead nurses strewn across Radji Beach, the Japanese had gone back down the track towards Muntok without checking that all their victims were actually dead.

Kinsley was made tough. Despite his horrific wounds, he'd managed to walk, stumble and crawl to a small, empty fisherman's hut where he'd spent the night. He'd left at first light to drag himself to the stream near Radji Beach for water. But when he'd heard the Japanese returning, he'd crawled into the jungle and hid.

Kinsley could see Viv was badly wounded too. But she was more interested in his welfare than her own. She knelt beside him, unbuttoned his shirt and gently removed the bloody bandage from his arm. She surveyed the two bayonet wounds in his belly. All of the poor man's gashes showed evidence of infection. He needed immediate surgery and intensive care, but there was none here in the jungle. Viv had to improvise as best she could. She told Kinsley to lie as quietly as he could, despite his pain, in case Japanese patrols were near, while she went back to the beach to search for medicines and bandages.

With a look of terror on his face, Kinsley told her to be careful because there were soldiers everywhere and they would think nothing of coming back to finish the work they had started. After reassuring Kinsley, Viv carefully climbed out from her hiding spot and stumbled down the bush track in her bare feet, having left her shoes behind when she dived from the *Vyner Brooke*. Along the way, she suffered a multitude of cuts from twigs and spiny grasses.

When she reached the edge of the jungle, Viv lay flat and carefully scanned the beach. Once she was certain there were no Japanese nearby, she emerged onto the sand.

There was a body in the water. Viv suspected it was one of the murdered nurses but on closer inspection she saw it was a young Asian woman, most likely from another shipwreck, her bloated face suggesting she'd been in the water for days.[2] The young woman's hair trailed behind her like a long black veil.

Viv had no time to feel sad. She retrieved an army water bottle half-buried in the sand and picked up two life jackets that would make good pillows. She filled the water bottle from the stream, and on the edge of the jungle collected a large bundle of coconut fibre from beneath the palm trees that would do in lieu of bandages.

When Viv returned from her mercy dash, Kinsley breathed a sigh of relief. Viv placed one of the life jackets under his head then began shaping the coconut fibre into long strips. After gently washing and cleaning Kinsley's angry wounds, she began bandaging them with the fibre strips, using vines torn from the jungle undergrowth to hold them in place.

To help take Kinsley's mind off the pain, Viv asked him about his life. He told Viv about Elsie, his wife of eight years, and about their home in Hull, and how he had been an insurance agent before enlisting.[3] She told him about Kapunda and Broken Hill and Adelaide and Melbourne. She told him about William Shegog, the mounted policeman, and how the Bullwinkels had come from Germany. Viv also told Kinsley about how her baby brother, John, a good lad, was flying Spitfires in England.

What a strange war this was, Kinsley said. Here he was an Englishman dying in the Far East and her brother, an Australian, was flying in England.

By the time Viv finished ministering to Kinsley's wounds she was utterly exhausted. She lay down with her head on a life jacket, and looked across at her patient. He was unconscious.

AS VIV FOUGHT TO KEEP Kinsley and herself alive in the jungle, Japan stepped up its relentless invasion of the South-West Pacific, and its forces finally reached the Australian mainland on 19 February 1942. The US, still reeling from Pearl Harbor just two months earlier, was unable to curtail the Japanese as they swarmed south.

In two separate raids within an hour and a half of each other, 242 Japanese aircraft bombed Darwin, an outpost on the roof of Australia with a population of just 6000. The city's strategic position had seen rapid construction of airfields and naval bases, but its defences were inadequate and crews manning anti-aircraft guns had little training because of ammunition shortages.

As the sun rose over the Timor Sea on 19 February, 188 Japanese aircraft – Zero fighters, dive-bombers and torpedo-bombers – were readied on four aircraft carriers that had been instrumental in the attack on Pearl Harbor. At airfields on the Japanese-held islands of Celebes and Ambon another fifty-four heavy bombers revved their engines as ground crews prepared an assault unlike anything Australia had ever seen.

Just before 10 a.m., Darwin's air-raid sirens began to scream, and for the next thirty minutes fire rained from the sky. Three warships and six merchant vessels were sunk and at least twenty-one wharf labourers died. The hospital ship AHS *Manunda* was strafed with shrapnel and set ablaze with the loss of twelve lives. The American destroyer USS *Peary* went down with eighty-eight men.

Ninety minutes later, while rescue crews worked feverishly, fifty-four Japanese heavy bombers appeared 5500 metres above the scene of destruction and unloaded hundreds of tonnes of mayhem. In the end, more than 200 people were killed, eleven ships were sunk and thirty aircraft destroyed.

Fear gripped Australia in the hours after the carnage. Prime Minister John Curtin told his countrymen that the enemy now thundered at Australia's 'very gates'. 'Everything we cherish,' Curtin said, 'is in immediate peril. We must face this test with fortitude and fight grimly and unflinchingly. Darwin has been bombed, but not conquered.'[4]

News of Japanese atrocities – beheadings, mass executions, rapes – had spread far and wide in the days after they had overrun Singapore, and not everyone was convinced that Australia could hold off the invaders. After Darwin was savaged, fear took hold. Shirley Ingram, a Perth schoolgirl at the time, recalled how her mother, a young war widow with three small children, had nightmares about Japanese soldiers capturing her family. She would have preferred they be dead than fall into the enemy's cruel hands. 'I vividly recall huge searchlights scanning the night skies,' Shirley said. 'My greatest concern was after overhearing Mother inform our next-door neighbour over the back fence that "if the Japs come, I will kill the girls".'[5]

WHEN KINSLEY WOKE FROM his deep sleep, he and Viv discussed their limited options. Both had survived the most brutal murder attempts by the Japanese and did not want to give them another chance.

'We were both adamant that we weren't going to give ourselves up,' Viv explained later, '... that we'd rather die out free.'[6] All of

Viv's experience told her that the Japanese didn't take prisoners and she had an aching hole in her left side to prove it.

Tempers quickly frayed and the frightened, desperate pair argued over the best hiding spot. Viv wanted to move deeper into the thick jungle; Kinsley wanted to return to the fisherman's hut, which had a roof as protection against tropical downpours. Viv argued that the hut would be the first place the Japanese would search and that since both had been badly wounded, they needed to be close enough to the stream so they wouldn't use up what little energy they had to obtain water.

Kinsley protested but Viv knew she was right and threatened to leave him, though she had no intention of doing so.

They propped each other up as they tottered cautiously down the track and further into the dense undergrowth, constantly on the lookout for Japanese soldiers and snakes. Eventually, they found another hiding place and fell asleep surrounded by dense undergrowth.

The next morning, Kinsley's condition had worsened. Viv suspected that he could not survive long but she was determined to give him the best chance she could. It had been at least four days since either of them had eaten, and the only thing Viv could see to make any sort of meal were coconuts. But she had nothing with which to break them open. Despite the fact that Viv and Sedgeman – poor Bill – had been rebuffed when they'd sought help a few days earlier, Viv decided to approach the first village chief she could find and beg for help. The risk of being betrayed by the villagers to the Japanese was one Viv would have to take. It was either that or starve. And so she made Kinsley comfortable and left him semi-conscious in the jungle.

With bloodied feet, a bullet hole in her side, a pounding heart and fear in her blue eyes, the tall Australian nurse dressed in a tattered grey dress smudged with oil and blood, set off limping down the jungle track in search of food. Viv knew their lives were on the line, so for mile after mile she fought against the blazing tropical sun and her burning desire to lie down. She arrived on the verge of collapse at the same village she had visited with

Sedgeman a few days earlier, but this time her circumstances were even more dire.

Warily, as Viv tried to keep her balance despite her fatigue, she approached a small group of the women around their cooking fires. They were the same women she had met a few days earlier. They eyed her with equal apprehension as she used broken English and the few Malay words she knew to explain that she wanted to see the village headman.

The women sent a young girl to find him and stared blankly as Viv stood in front of them, balancing on a stick to stay upright. The headman arrived and Viv did her best to explain that she needed food for herself and a very sick companion.

The old man shook his head, saying he could not help and that Viv should surrender to the Japanese. She didn't tell the headman that she had tried that once before and it had ended very badly.

The old man walked away, telling Viv curtly over his shoulder, 'You give up to Japan, man get food.'[7]

Crestfallen, Viv spun around extending her arms with hands stretched out to the impassive women.

'Please,' she spluttered, 'please, just a little food.'[8]

They looked away from her to their cooking pots and Viv realised that after cheating death on Radji Beach she and Kinsley now faced a slow death by starvation in the jungle. She still had her pride, though, so clutching at her painful wound, she walked out of the village trying to hold her head high.

She had just rounded a bend in the track when her blood ran cold. There was a rustling in the palm fronds near her. Japanese were everywhere. Viv knew that. Her heart was beating uncontrollably. She froze, transfixed by the rustling leaves. Then her terror was released like a lanced boil. Two smiling women from the village stepped out from the bushes. Quickly and quietly they placed two parcels wrapped with banana leaves on the ground, before disappearing like shadows into the sea of green. The parcels contained cooked fish, boiled rice and big chunks of pineapple.

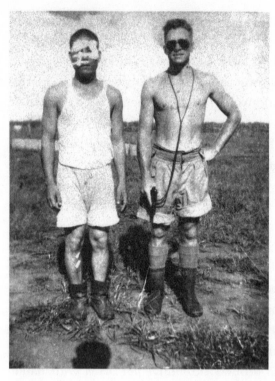

Zero pilot Hajime Toyoshima (left, with Australian Sgt Les Powell), was captured after crashing on Melville Island following the Japanese attack on Darwin. *Australian War Memorial P00022.001*

FOLLOWING THE JAPANESE RAID on Darwin, pilot Hajime Toyoshima[9] crash-landed his A6M Zero fighter on Melville Island later on 19 February. He had run out of fuel due to bullet damage to the tanks of his aircraft, sustained when attacking an aerodrome on nearby Bathurst Island.

Toyoshima tried to escape the scene, but Matthias Ulungura,[10] a young Indigenous man from the Tiwi Islands, crept up on the disoriented fighter pilot with a hatchet, and pressing the handle into Toyoshima's back as though it was the barrel of a gun, pulled Toyoshima's pistol from his holster and took him prisoner.

Ulungura took his prize catch to RAAF guards stationed on Bathurst Island. Toyoshima was eventually moved to the new prisoner-of-war camp in Cowra, west of Sydney. Cowra was near the home of nurse Jenny Kerr, who had just been murdered beside Viv on Radji Beach.

WITH HER PRECIOUS FOOD parcels under one arm, Viv had renewed vigour as she staggered back to Kinsley. Together they ate a little of the food then and there. It was the most delicious meal Viv could remember. Then Viv divided the rest of the food into small portions, which she figured could sustain the pair for the next four days.

But with the Japanese now in control of Bangka Island how long could the generosity of the villagers last? How long before the Japanese found these two lucky victims and finished them off? Viv thought her wound was on the improve but how many more days could Kinsley stay alive without proper medical care? His body was a mass of wounds and he had the washed-out face of a dead man.

Viv was also plagued by questions of why she alone among the nurses had survived. It made her feel depressed at times, but she eventually concluded that her height had saved her. Because she was the tallest nurse on Radji Beach the bullet had hit her lower back, while the rest of the women were shot through their hearts, lungs or livers. Spending so long in salt water had killed any infection. She forced herself to overcome the heavy dose of survivor guilt.

In the late afternoons as darkness approached and Kinsley slept fitfully in their hiding place, Viv would creep down to the beach to bathe and check her wound. While the bullet hole was ringed with a large purple bruise, there was no evidence of gangrene, and even the pain was beginning to recede.

Both she and Kinsley had jangling nerves from fatigue, post-traumatic stress and fear. At one stage, Viv exploded with anger because Kinsley kept calling her 'Nurse' rather than 'Sister', though she soon apologised to her stricken companion.[11]

After the food ran out, Viv trudged back to the village, this time in a tropical rainstorm. Once more, the old headman refused to help, and once again, to her great joy, two women appeared on her return journey with more parcels of food. But she knew this couldn't continue indefinitely, and Kinsley was becoming weaker by the day. He was in great physical pain.

Being in far better shape than her companion, Viv knew that it was up to her whether they lived or died. Surrender or starve. The Japanese might kill them but they might not. And if they didn't get help soon Kinsley would surely die.

Viv broached the subject with her companion, but he told her he did not want to risk being bayoneted again. He said they had both been spared for a reason and they should take their freedom one day at a time.[12]

Although her father had been staunchly Anglican, Viv was not overly religious, having attended church only occasionally. She figured God would be too busy with thousands dying every day in this horrific war to listen to her complaints or pleas. But they had now been hiding in the jungle for ten days, and with all avenues to her blocked, Viv felt a need to speak to her Creator. With Kinsley asleep again, she knelt in prayer and whispered:

> Lord, I haven't really prayed to you before, but you know I believe in you. I don't understand why you spared me when all the other girls used to go to church regularly. You must have your reasons. I'm sorry to worry you because there must be a lot of others asking for your help right now. I don't want a miracle, all I want is your guidance. I want you to help me know what to do. You see, there's Kinsley. I think he's going to die. When that happens, I will be on my own and Lord, you know how much I fear being alone. I couldn't bear that, I can't be on my own. Tell me what I should do, please show me the way.[13]

Viv did not hear the voice of God, only the screech of a seabird. But she remembered a saying she had heard many times, that God helps those who help themselves.

Chapter 17

ENERGISED AFTER HER PRAYERS, Viv felt she had
found the way to salvation. She woke Kinsley from his fitful
sleep and told him that if they didn't do something soon he would
be dead and she would be close behind. They could not survive in
hiding.

She said she was going to take a chance and see if the Japanese
would take them prisoners. Surely not all of them were murderers.
If the Japanese really weren't taking prisoners, then even a quick
death at their hands would be a relief compared with slow
starvation.

Kinsley, a forlorn figure with tangled hair and a scraggly
beard over hollow cheeks, reluctantly agreed. His legs were now
so wasted they looked like they'd been swallowed by his army
shorts, which were now a couple of sizes too big for him.

'If it comes to the worst,' Kinsley said weakly, 'I hope the Japs
do a better job of it this time.'[1] He asked if they could stay in their
hideout for another day. Tomorrow would be 26 February 1942,
his thirty-third birthday, he told Viv, and if it was to be his last
birthday, he wanted to spend it as a free man.

Viv thought that was a splendid idea. In the morning, she rose
to organise Kinsley's birthday lunch. While he was still asleep,
she set off through the light mist and made her way to the place
where the kindly village women were now risking death from
the Japanese to hide food parcels at regular intervals. Viv returned
with a small leaf-wrapped parcel. She moulded a small amount of

the rice into an approximation of a cupcake and stuck a twig in it to represent a candle. Then she gently woke Kinsley.

As his eyes fluttered open she presented him with the gift. 'Happy birthday,' she said.

They chatted again about their lives, and then it was down to business. Viv re-dressed Kinsley's wounds with fresh coconut fibre, then used sand and water to scrub his shirt to obscure the bayonet holes as much as possible. She did the same to her uniform to hide the bullet holes front and back. If the Japanese suspected they were witnesses to a massacre they might never live long enough to talk about it.

IT WAS NOW TWO WEEKS since news had reached Australia about the fall of Singapore. In Adelaide, Eva Bullwinkel was frantic. She sat down to write Viv another letter, hoping that the very act of writing it might bring her beloved daughter some much-needed luck.

My Darling Girl
The suspense of the last couple of weeks has been dreadful, not knowing how you are – where you are and what has been happening to you.

I have rung Mrs. Drummond several times but they have not received any word from Matron Drummond at all. Mrs Drummond seems to think some of the nurses are still on Singapore Island. There is only one comfort, the Japanese have, from all accounts, respected the Red Cross in Malaya and my only hope is that the nurses will be well treated. Even if you have left Singapore the dangers are so great that one feels in constant fear of what may happen.

Oh Viv dear, if only you were back in Australia. Every day I have been hoping for a cable from you … I am going to the Red Cross to see if they can find out where you are.

I have not heard from John for some time so I cannot give you any news of him.

Darling I cannot write more in this letter. If you ever receive it you will understand.

... I do hope and pray I will receive some news of you very soon – good news.

With fondest love to your dear self and may God guard and protect you, is my constant prayer.

Your loving mother.[2]

VIV COULD FEEL NOTHING but compassion and admiration for the shell of Private Kinsley as he staggered to his feet to face the might of the Japanese empire once more. 'Do I pass inspection, Sister?' he muttered as he supported his emaciated, patched–up frame with a stout stick.

Viv didn't say so but she knew that both she and Kinsley had seen better days. Just standing was an effort for him, and now he was about to undertake a jungle trek of several kilometres to face men who had blown him up and twice run him through with a bayonet.

Viv's bare feet were cut to ribbons and her legs covered in scratches. She had washed her grey dress, but blood and oil were difficult stains to remove, even when scrubbed with sand. She used a water bottle slung over her shoulder to hide the bullet wound in her dress.

She later wrote:

Saturday 28th February 1942 – Finally made up our minds. We both decided to go and get it over with rather than starve back on the beach. Commenced our last walk of freedom.[3]

As the sun rose over the jungle, Viv and Kinsley set off from their hideout and down the track towards Muntok. They placed a supporting arm around each other's waist to stay upright. Kinsley used his stout stick to help, taking one halting step at a time with a brief pause between them.

Viv was worried by Kinsley's poor condition and suggested she hide him in the jungle while she went ahead to find the Japanese.

But gasping, he told her that he did not want to die alone. So together, they tramped and staggered and stumbled on, slowly, methodically, through the heat and humidity and along the rough track, Kinsley leaning heavily on Viv on one side and his stick on the other.

They stopped at the village where the women had secretly given them food and the old chief was now helpful when they told him they were surrendering to the Japanese. He gave them something to eat and showed them the track to Muntok.

They pressed on. Viv's feet were caked in blood and she was exhausted from supporting Kinsley's weight. They were alarmed to hear footsteps behind them but when they wheeled around it was only a small Sumatran man in his thirties. He waved to them and called out in perfect English, 'Good morning to you.' He asked them where they were going and Viv told him they were going to surrender to the Japanese.

He said that was the safest option for them because in Muntok there were prison camps and many women wearing grey uniforms and Red Cross armbands. A wave of relief washed over Viv as she realised that many of the other nurses, her dear friends, were still alive.

Viv and Kinsley lurched on until the early afternoon, when they realised that the whining sound behind them was an approaching motor vehicle. The driver was blowing the horn furiously.[4] Automatically, they stepped to one side to let the vehicle pass when Viv realised that the only people driving cars in this area would be Japanese.

Viv held the water bottle tightly to her side to hide the bullet wound in her dress as an old open tourer car came to a halt with a grinding of gears. A Japanese soldier was at the wheel and beside him a naval officer.

The officer spoke sharply in Japanese and the driver jumped out of his seat and jogged across to the two westerners, who looked to be at death's door. He pointed a revolver at them[5] and then searched them for weapons. He then climbed back behind the steering wheel and turned to them. 'Get in,' he said in faltering English.

Viv was taken by surprise.

'Quick,' the driver snapped.

It took some effort to help Kinsley into the back seat. Then Viv climbed in behind him. With more grinding of gears, the tourer started moving and spluttered off down the track towards Muntok.

After the exertions of the day, it was a relief to be sitting in the open-top car with a cool breeze blowing. Despite their apprehensions about what the Japanese might do to them, they began to relax a little. Viv eased her aching muscles by stretching out her long legs. Her feet bumped something big under the front seat: a large bunch of bananas. Leaning forward, she asked the driver if he would seek permission from the officer for her and Kinsley to share a banana, as they were famished.

When asked, the officer grunted, and Viv and Kinsley each wolfed down half a banana.

THE JETTY AT MUNTOK seemed to stretch on forever out into the Bangka Strait. Six hundred metres long, it extended from the huge Customs House. Along with a white cement lighthouse, it dominated the port town of 10,000.

Viv and Kinsley looked all around them as the old car rattled on down the narrow streets of the main residential area before stopping in front of a large bungalow. On the bungalow's wide verandah, which ran the entire length of the building, were several Japanese men clad only in G-string underwear.

As the officer dismounted and entered the building, the driver barked 'Out!' Viv had to virtually carry Kinsley from the vehicle. Then the soldier led them up the wooden steps to the almost naked Japanese men. Viv's heart was beating fast as the soldier told them to sit at a cane table.

As the men spoke in Japanese they shot glances at Viv, causing her to sweat as though she was in a sauna. Were any of them the killers she and Kinsley had met on Radji Beach? Then, as if Viv was in a strange dream, six Japanese men wearing exquisite kimonos came from inside the building out onto the verandah.

They stopped in front of the two prisoners, and the most senior of the group summoned the driver of the tourer, who marched over and bowed his head to the men. The leader spoke quickly in Japanese to the driver, who then turned to Viv and barked in broken English, 'Colonel wishes to know how many British soldiers in Singapore?'[6]

'I don't know,' Viv said honestly. 'I'm a nursing sister and know nothing of military matters.'

The soldier then asked Kinsley the same question, and he told them truthfully that he had arrived on the last convoy into Singapore and had been in the fighting for only a few days before being evacuated. He had no idea how many British soldiers were there.

The colonel asked Kinsley if he was prepared to work in prison, and he said yes. Viv said she too would work, providing it was tending to the sick in hospital.

The men in kimonos went back inside. Soon a soldier appeared with a tray of biscuits and hot tea and set it down in front of Viv. This was a lot more hospitable than getting shot or stabbed.

Viv and Kinsley wolfed down their unexpected afternoon tea and then one of the men in kimonos came back onto the verandah and approached Viv with a rolled-up bandage. He sat beside her and pointed to his ankle. He was testing to see if she really was a nurse. She bandaged it carefully to his satisfaction and he then went back inside.

Then one of the near-naked soldiers at the end of the verandah approached Viv in a far more menacing way. He pointed to her neck and demanded the rising-sun badge – the official insignia of the Australian Army – from her collar.

She looked him straight in the eye. 'No,' she said.

He was not prepared to take no for an answer, though, and became boisterous and threatening.

Kinsley implored Viv to hand over the little piece of metal. Sensing the danger after they had come so far, Viv reluctantly gave it to the man.

The soldier studied the badge closely, turning it over and over and holding up the little trophy to show his laughing comrades. Then he closed his fist over it and turned to leave.

From somewhere deep within, Viv forgot about the murders on Radji Beach and threw herself in front of the startled thief. 'That is mine,' she shouted, 'and I want it back.'[7]

If looks could kill Viv would have died on the spot then and there, but before the soldier could strike her, the colonel shouted orders from the doorway of the bungalow, and reluctantly the soldier gave back the badge. His savage glare suggested he would get even if he could.

VIV AND KINSLEY WERE PARTED a few hours later when the driver of the tourer reappeared and told the wounded soldier to follow him. Kinsley could barely move so, again hiding her bullet wound with the water bottle, Viv helped him to the back seat of the car.

His sad eyes reflected constant pain and there was no strength left in his broken body. He was ready for the end, but he whispered: 'I would never have made it this far if it hadn't been for you, Sister. I used to look at you and wonder what with everything that happened to you where you got your strength from to go on ... You made me determined to be like you.'[8]

The two held hands, bonded by the incommunicable experience of war, the spilling of their own blood, and their desperate fight to stay alive.

'Kinsley,' Viv whispered, 'I want you to know that I admire you very much and I feel a great pride in having had you as a companion.'

'Goodbye, Sister, and may God bless you,' Kinsley murmured so quietly that Viv strained to hear him.[9]

The old tourer trundled off down the dirt road and Kinsley's head flopped about as he no longer had the strength to hold it still. Viv was now utterly alone among the same people who had tried to murder her.

As the car disappeared into the distance Viv heard a woman's voice. 'Don't be afraid, Sister, the Japanese are really very kind people.' Startled, Viv turned to see a woman of medium height in her early fifties, with short dark hair and a slight figure swathed in fine European fashion. She was Vichy French, a supporter of the Nazi invaders in her homeland and thus an ally of the Japanese.

But Viv was more interested in the old tourer, which was now returning to the bungalow. Another Japanese soldier trotted out from the bungalow and gestured for Viv to get in the car. She climbed in, covering the bullet hole in her dress by bowing to the soldiers – a practice she hated – and then the car drove off in the same direction Kinsley had gone.

The driver pushed the old car hard down the narrow streets, hitting the horn and gesturing to pedestrians to get out of his way. It had been a wearying day of physical and mental fatigue and in the afternoon sun, Viv started to fall asleep. The tourer rounded a bend, swerved, bucked and swung to the opposite side of the road before jolting to a stop that hurt Viv's neck.

The driver had just dodged a column of marching men. Gaunt and haggard, the men were wearing a variety of tattered, filthy rags that had once been military uniforms. It was a sad procession, but at least Viv knew for sure that the Japanese were taking prisoners.

The car travelled on. Viv's fatigue, the afternoon sun and the gentle swaying of the tourer lulled her into a half-slumber again. Another abrupt stop shook Viv awake once more. As her eyes opened, the first thing she saw was a careworn European woman with a Red Cross armband filling a bowl with water from a tap.

The car had stopped in front of a high wall. Soon the driver was ushering Viv through an arched doorway. Inside was a large open area surrounded by dilapidated huts. A young man wearing what remained of a British Army captain's uniform rushed out from a long hut with a red, rusting iron roof.

He held out his hand. 'Welcome to the Coolie Lines, Sister,' he said in a well-modulated English accent. 'It is indeed a pleasure to see you.'

She took his hand in hers, and he asked her to follow him to the large shed where he would record her details.

While they were walking there, Viv was explaining how she came ashore and with whom, when a familiar woman's voice cried out. 'It's Bully!'

The sound of Viv's nickname stopped her in her tracks and a feeling of elation ran through her veins.

'Hey, Bully, over here.' Viv stumbled on her torn feet in the direction of the voice. Behind a gate she saw thin, sunburned faces gawking at her. They belonged to women dressed in sarongs and army or navy shorts – khaki and white – and singlets given to them by some of the male prisoners.

The gate flew open and suddenly Australian Army nursing sisters ran to embrace Viv. As she was enveloped in hugs and kisses, they all cried with joy. They all looked very different, but she realised they were all from the 2/10th.

'Come on, Bully, the rest of the girls are over at the Coolie Lines.' Viv recognised that voice. It was Betty Jeffrey, who had been so kind to her in Malacca.

And so Viv was reunited with thirty-one of her dear friends in the grounds of this dilapidated old prison, the Muntok jail and the adjacent camp for Chinese labourers. The nurses showered her with affection and inundated her with queries about her ordeal in the water.

Viv's boss in Singapore, Jean Ashton, stopped her in her tracks with one question. 'But Bully,' Jean asked, 'where are all the others?'[10]

Everyone fell silent.

Chapter 18

THE MUNTOK JAIL WAS a concrete quadrangle with an iron roof, and the Coolie Lines were mostly large huts and sheds that had housed the Chinese labourers employed to load goods on the Muntok jetty.

After the hell of the previous two weeks, Viv found it a wonderful relief to finally be among familiar, reassuring faces.

'Viv is a tall, slim girl with very fair straight hair cut short, and blue eyes,' Betty Jeffrey noted in her diary. 'She is not an excitable person at any time and she quietly walked in through the door of the jail clasping an army type water bottle which was slung over her shoulder to her side. We immediately saw why she did this; it was hiding a bullet hole in her uniform. We took her into our dormitory and as we all gathered round her she told us what had happened.'[1]

All the nurses had heard rumours that had filtered down from the Japanese guards about the massacre of shipwreck survivors at Radji Beach. But they dared not believe them. Viv had made up her mind not to say anything about the murdered nurses because she feared that if the secret was exposed she would be instantly killed. So, at first, Viv denied any knowledge of the killings or the nurses' whereabouts, even when the women kept tossing her names, the names of their friends.

'For the first half dozen I said, "No, I don't know",' Viv recalled later. But in the end she could no longer keep the truth from her comrades, and as the tears gushed from her eyes she spluttered, 'Yes, I do know what happened to them.'[2]

The thirty-one other nurses around Viv were 'absolutely appalled'[3] as they listened in stunned silence to the horror story. Two of the male prisoners who were there listening to Viv's tale were Army Intelligence officers, and they cautioned everyone not to talk about it, because the Japanese would not want a living witness to a war crime. Any gossip about the murders, they said, would quickly lead to Viv's death.[4]

'After we heard this story,' Betty Jeffrey recalled, 'we decided then and there never to mention it again ... The subject was strictly forbidden.'[5] Instead, Viv would concoct a different story of shipwreck and survival to satisfy the curiosity of her captors.

VIV WAS UTTERLY EXHAUSTED and severely traumatised by her ordeal. The group agreed that she could not be treated in the hospital, where the Japanese might discover her bullet wound, so Wilma Oram found a spot for her on the concrete floor of the sleeping quarters and shared with Viv her mosquito net and food.[6]

It had been a gruelling day physically and emotionally and Viv's head had hardly touched the cold surface when she was fast asleep. When she finally awoke and looked around her new home, Viv wondered how long she could survive there. The dormitory for the Australian nurses was a dilapidated shed with a concrete floor that sloped from the edge to the centre, where a long sewer drain ran the entire length of the building. The drain was just a gutter with no protection, nor privacy, and was used by both the Japanese and the nurses. Night and day the stench enveloped everyone and everything.

Forty female prisoners slept on the hard floor, which was open to the elements. Betty told Viv that she had been able to scrounge a mattress for a while on which five of the nurses slept together, but she had given it up for some English nurses who had spent six days in the sea after their ship was bombed and had arrived at Muntok badly shocked and sunburned.[7]

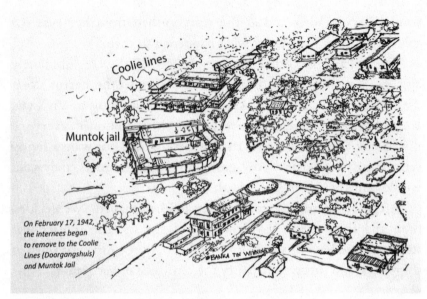

Coolie lines

Muntok jail

On February 17, 1942, the internees began to remove to the Coolie Lines (Doorgangshuis) and Muntok Jail

The Muntok jail compound and Coolie Lines. *Muntok Tinwinning Museum*

There was just one tap in Viv's dormitory that only produced a drip into a large concrete trough, and there was a constant queue for a little bath water which the nurses would splash on themselves. There was no soap and only one towel. There were no sheets, no blankets, no combs, and very little food. Someone found an old toothbrush in a drain, and after cleaning it, shared it with five other nurses. An old milk tin became a food plate; a rusted shoehorn was used as a spoon.

The Muntok jail housed about 600 people, most of them from the seventy or so boats that the Japanese had bombed in the Bangka Strait over the course of a week. There were servicemen and women, civilian men, women and children and many nuns. Most had arrived with just the clothes on their backs. All but one of the nurses had lost their shoes on the *Vyner Brooke* so thirty-one of them were barefoot. Those who could sew converted clothing that Allied servicemen and Chinese labourers had left behind into shorts and tops, or made dresses out of curtains or blackout material. Many kept their uniforms folded to use only on special occasions.

Food was mostly boiled rice, which was often burnt and often filthy. It was served every morning at ten o'clock and the nurses collected some to eat then and some to eat later in the day as their dinner. Viv shared a plate and spoon with Wilma until she was able to find her own rubbish that could be converted into cutlery, and eventually someone found a set of dainty Chinese bowls that they could all share.

Among the prisoners were three women doctors – two British, Drs Smith and McDowell, and one German, the imperious and haughty Annamaria Eleanor Goldberg, who had survived her battles with the sea and with Veronica Clancy and Blanche Hempsted to make it into Muntok jail fighting fit. The Australians did not like or trust her.

The nurses had busied themselves on arrival, clearing one dormitory to use as a hospital for the large number of wounded inmates. However, due to the injuries and exposure that the Australian nurses had experienced, only half of them were considered fit enough to work in the hospital, and those who did work could only do so in short shifts. It was to the hospital that Private Kinsley had been taken by the Japanese guards when he and Viv first arrived in Muntok.

Viv had only been in the prison camp for a few days when she was woken from her sleep by Wilma Oram. Wilma told her that a Chinese man was looking for her as she was wanted at the hospital urgently. Viv leapt from her concrete bed and rushed over. There, a British nurse led her halfway down a central aisle before stopping beside the stricken figure of the brave young soldier who had endured so much alongside Viv for two weeks in the jungle.

Viv sat on the edge of a wooden platform on which Kinsley, his untidy beard saturated with sweat, was resting with eyes closed, his breathing raspy and laboured.

She lowered her face to his. Kinsley's eyes opened weakly. Viv spoke gently to him. She carefully took his hand in hers and lightly squeezed it.

A wave of emptiness washed over Viv. Here was this brave, adventurous man who only a couple of years earlier had been a happy insurance agent living in the north of England. Now he was in this filthy stinking hellhole thousands of miles from his wife and loved ones drawing his last few tortured breaths with infected lungs.

'Thank you,' Kinsley gasped between splutters. 'Thank you for everything, Sister.' Kinsley squeezed Viv's hand just a little, using all the strength he had left.

'No thank *you*, Kinsley,' Viv said.

Kinsley's dull eyes smiled weakly.

Viv had seen many young men die senseless, needless deaths over the last few months but Kinsley's final fight for life affected her deeply.[8] Together they had fought with everything they had left against the insanity of warfare, two human beings who had tried to maintain their spirit of life and their pride in their humanity.

Viv remembered the words of Florence Nightingale bringing comfort to the servicemen in Crimea: 'No soldier should die alone upon a foreign soil.'[9]

Viv promised Kinsley she would write to his wife, Elsie, back in Hull and tell her of his bravery.[10]

This brought a faint smile to Kinsley's face. Then, after a few minutes of silence, he told Viv that she best be going because she probably had more important things to do. But Viv sat with Kinsley, holding his hand until he fell into a deep sleep.

Viv stood up to leave. She nodded to a man in the next bed who looked familiar. It was Stoker Ernest Lloyd.[11]

WHILE THE SURVIVING NURSES all swore not to speak about the massacre again, many told Viv about their own death-defying adventures after the sinking of the *Vyner Brooke*. Some had suffered bloodied chins from the chafing life jackets, while others had deep burns to the hands from using ropes to descend the sinking vessel. Some had multiple lacerations and shrapnel wounds inflicted by the bombs and bullets.

Veronica Clancy had used her uniform as a sail to guide her raft into Muntok and arrived at the Customs House there to be taken prisoner with 'complete nonchalance, strolling in dressed in her corsets and a man's overcoat'.

'It must have been a sight, for Veronica is a big girl,' Betty Jeffrey wrote.[12]

When Viv had arrived at the prison, Betty's hands were heavily bandaged. She had burned them raw sliding down a rope from the sinking ship and they had become badly infected, so much so that the other nurses had to feed and clean her for weeks.

Betty told Viv that when Captain Borton, who was also in the Muntok prison camp, had steered the *Vyner Brooke* into hiding at one of the picturesque tropical islands, she had looked out over the railing and imagined how lovely it would be to have a nice, long swim in the beautiful blue water. She didn't realise how long that swim would become.

Betty and Iole Harper eventually spent three days in the water, fighting against 'those vile currents'[13] in the Bangka Strait, and then fighting their way up and down salty rivers and creeks in crocodile-infested mangrove swamps on Bangka Island. At one stage they discussed the possibility of swimming to Australia. They had not met before the sinking of the ship and had been swimming together for twenty-eight hours before they thought to introduce themselves, after which they realised they had many mutual friends.

Betty and Iole had both suffered severe cuts and scratches. Malay fishermen gave them food and water, and the pair were eventually convinced to give themselves up to Japanese troops.[14]

Now all the nurses had become accustomed to sleeping together on the cold hard floor amid swarms of mosquitoes and with the more sadistic of the Japanese guards walking in and out of the dormitory all night to ensure none of the prisoners slept well. The guards hit the women on the shins with their bayonets, and turned on all the lights, only switching them off when the babies and small children of the civilian mothers began to cry.

A FEW DAYS AFTER VIV ARRIVED, on 2 March at 3 a.m., the Japanese guards woke the camp with flashing torches. Shouting commands, they used bayonets to prod the inmates out of the huts and into the compound.

Viv tensed all over, expecting the worst, but the talk among the nurses was that they were moving camp across the Bangka Strait to Palembang, the largest city in southern Sumatra. The nurses grabbed the few possessions they had, mostly just their uniforms and an eating utensil, and lined up in the humid darkness.

Each of them was given a small lump of rice for breakfast and another small amount 'looking quite revolting'[15] wrapped in a banana leaf to sustain them on their journey. They were then herded like cattle onto a fleet of open trucks fitted with wooden rails for livestock.

Trucks overflowing with Allied prisoners, including mothers with babies and small children, rumbled out of the camp as the first orange rays of the sun began to creep over the horizon. The convoy lurched through the streets of Muntok, prisoners swaying from side to side with the motion of the vehicles as they bumped over the rough roads. At last the trucks arrived at the Muntok jetty, which seemed to point across the blue-green water of the strait like a long, slender finger. The prisoners were told to get out and head to the end of the pier and wait.

The two ships assigned to take them across the Bangka Strait were twin-deck riverboats, 'dirty, old tramp things,' Betty Jeffrey called them.[16] The nurses sat waiting on the jetty's rough timber floor, though it made a welcome change from the concrete of Muntok prison. Launches ferried twenty of the heat-stressed prisoners at a time out to the anchored riverboats, with men taken to one overcrowded vessel and women and children to the other.

As the barges set off under a stunning sunrise complete with a double rainbow, Viv, sitting on a large pile of wood, enjoyed the fresh sea air after days of sleeping beside the open sewage drain in her dormitory. It was a thirty-kilometre journey across the Bangka Strait, and as she stared out to sea, Viv thought of her mother and brother who, not knowing her fate, must have been anguished to hear of the slaughter in Singapore.

At least there was the occasional laugh to take Viv's mind off the turmoil. Two of the prisoners were the wealthy Mary Brown and her 26-year-old daughter Shelagh, pillars of colonial high society in Singapore. Mary was an enormous woman who battled with the single narrow toilet cubicle on the ferry that was perched over the side of the ship above the propellers and was guarded by a Japanese soldier with a bayonet, just in case of who knows what. Several of the Australian nurses had to help Mrs Brown squeeze into the cubicle backwards, and then engage in a fierce tug-of-war to extract her.

By the time Viv's boat entered the Musi River for the final 100-kilometre leg of the journey to Palembang, the conditions had become hot and sticky and there was no protection from the sun. Most of the nurses were hatless. Then a tropical downpour drenched them. Japanese guards brought out some old and dirty tarpaulins just as the downpour was ending, and as the hot sun emerged from behind the clouds, the canvas just made the humidity worse.

Hot, dirty and sweaty, they sailed through the mangroves and past the isolated villages of Sumatra, with the male prisoners on the second ferry close behind. Gradually the grassy fields gave way to numerous houses on both riverbanks and there were increasing numbers of other river ferries and many small boats propelled by locals using paddles. At about 5 p.m., as the two riverboats full of prisoners neared Palembang, Viv saw burnt-out buildings and two ships half-sunk in the water.

The boats docked at the ferry station in Palembang, then a city of more than 150,000 people. One of the major export centres of the Dutch East Indies, it had been captured by the Japanese three weeks earlier.

Viv and the other prisoners were kept on the barges while a handful of Japanese, stripped to the waist, supervised the unloading of both ships by teams of Malay labourers. When the cargo was finally unloaded, Japanese soldiers, with bayonets, rushed onto both vessels and began pushing the captives towards a thin rickety plank that served as the gangway to disembark. Mary Brown needed help with that too.

Then, for two hours, Viv and the others sat dismayed on the wharf in the hot afternoon sun with their small bundles of possessions. Eventually, more cattle trucks arrived to take them to their new prison, an abandoned school at Bukit Besar, about 10 kilometres west of the dock.

The prisoners had to stand inside the cattle trucks, holding on tightly to the sides as the vehicles rocked and swayed on the bumpy roads. To humiliate them further, Japanese soldiers had assembled a crowd of locals to line their path and forced them to jeer at the captives as they went by. As Viv's truck approached the reluctant hecklers, the nurses fired back at them with even more vitriol, using the most unladylike language, tongue poking and finger gestures. The crowd was stunned into silence by the fury of the Australian women, and the Japanese became so angry that they began shouting and hitting out at the bewildered crowd.[17] The trucks gathered speed for the last part of the journey and Viv feared she would be toppled out at every bend.

Finally, they arrived at an old, disused school. Dutch servicemen were there to welcome them with hot tea, a hot meal of stew made from potatoes and spinach and whatever else could be scrounged. The back of the truck quickly emptied as Viv and the others scrambled out and rushed into the school building to eat their fill.

After this most welcome dinner, a British officer split the prisoners into groups of forty, assigning each a classroom where they could sleep in rows on bare floorboards as Japanese guards watched them. The lights were left on all night and the windows left open so that swarms of mosquitoes covered the prisoners in bites, and the poor mothers among the group worked overtime trying to protect their children.

THE FOLLOWING DAY, 3 March 1942, the Japanese followed up their lightning raid on Darwin with an aerial attack on Broome in Western Australia. Broome was then a small pearling port, but it was an important refuelling depot on the air route between Batavia and the Australian cities, so had become an Allied military base.

That morning, nine Mitsubishi Zero fighters and a reconnaissance plane took off from their base at Kupang in Timor and
at 9.20 a.m. made strafing attacks on the flying boats anchored at
Roebuck Bay in Broome and the nearby RAAF base.

The Japanese pilots spent an hour firing their machine guns,
destroying twenty-two Allied aircraft, including an airborne US
Air Force B-24A Liberator full of wounded personnel. About
twenty people died when it crashed into the sea.

Among the Allied aircraft destroyed at Broome were fifteen
flying boats that had been anchored there, and many Dutch refugees
escaping the Japanese assaults on Sumatra and Java were killed.

Three Japanese fighters also chased a KLM Douglas DC-3
airliner that was approaching Broome carrying refugees from
Bandung on Java. The pilot managed to land on a beach near
the town, but machine-gun bullets killed four people on board.
Diamonds worth £150,000 on the aircraft went missing.

In total, the attack killed at least eighty-eight civilians and
Allied military personnel.

AT BUKIT BESAR, Viv and many of the nurses woke with puffy
faces from the mosquito bites. They were given another small
ration of rice for breakfast and were then visited by the senior
British officer in the prison, 53-year-old Air Commodore Charles
Modin. A decorated World War I pilot, Modin had approached
the Japanese with a request that all thirty-two Australian nurses
be treated as military personnel rather than civilians, and therefore
accorded the status of prisoners of war rather than internees. Under
the Geneva Convention, the Japanese had to feed prisoners of war.
Internees might get a little food if the Japanese felt generous, but
mostly they had to feed themselves as best they could.

The Japanese had refused the POW status and had also refused
appeals for Red Cross support. They told Modin that all the women
and children would be moved to a separate camp later that day.

Viv and two of the senior Australian nurses, Nesta James and
Jean Ashton, had something they wanted Modin to know before

they were shipped out, just in case they were not seen alive again. They told him about the murders at Radji Beach. Viv gave the startled officer the names of all those who had been killed. She feared it might be her last chance to tell the story.

In the early afternoon, the guards ordered all the prisoners out of the school and lined them up, men, women and children three abreast. They were all marched along a rough road and Viv, whose bare feet became more bloodied and swollen with every step, concentrated not on the pain but on the happy memories of Sunday picnics with her mother, father and brother in Broken Hill under the shady gum trees beside the Darling River.

After a tramp of several kilometres that left Viv limping badly, it was getting dark as the prisoners reached a row of fourteen freestanding brick houses built by the Dutch and arranged in an L-shape in an area called the Big Hill.[18] The houses had steps leading to a verandah and space underneath them to allow cooling air to circulate.

Viv and the other 2/13th nurses occupied one house and the nurses of the 2/10th and 2/4th occupied another, with two houses occupied by Dutch internees separating them. Local male prisoners occasionally supplied the women with a little bread and cheese over the fence separating the properties.

These new prison houses were large and in good repair and had electricity. Viv guessed that the previous inhabitants had fled Palembang in a hurry. There was European food still on the kitchen table and in the cupboards, and in the wardrobes there was clothing that had clearly belonged to European adults and children. In the bathrooms the nurses found the treasure of soap, and in the house occupied by the 2/10th there was the latest model of electric stove.

Jean Ashton, as the acting sister in charge of Viv's house, doled out chores for her nurses, which included building a fireplace and oven in front of the house for cooking. Very early in their stay, Mavis Hanna said she still had ten Singapore dollars and volunteered to buy food at a local store. Dutch women also called in to help the prisoners with a few toothbrushes, loaves of bread and bunches of bananas. They came later with soup, a meal of rice and beans, and hot tea. It was the most food any of the nurses had seen since they left Singapore, just three weeks but, seemingly, a lifetime ago.

The camp at Bukit Besar was paradise compared with the filth of the Muntok jail and Viv and Wilma Oram became one of many district nursing teams assigned to visit the sick in camp at regular intervals.

None of the nurses ever forgot that they were the prisoners of a brutal military force. One nurse was bathing in her prison house when she saw a Japanese guard in the doorway ogling her. She froze with fear as he took his time looking over her before leaving with a laugh.[19]

The women were ever vigilant to protect themselves against sexual assault and were always careful to make sure they were never completely alone when guards wanted to take them on work assignments. A few days later, a Japanese non-commissioned officer and an English female interpreter who had lived in Malaya for many years and been with the nurses on the *Vyner Brooke* visited the nurses and told them they had to move out immediately as the camp commander was converting their houses into an officers' club. The order was that the nurses would be accommodated in the two houses between the properties they currently occupied.

The Japanese commanded the nurses to ensure the houses were spotless, because beds, couches and other furniture would soon be delivered. The interpreter told the nurses they were to provide entertainment for the officers as 'geisha girls'[20] or 'comfort women'. If they did not comply, they would receive no more food.

Viv and the others looked at each other aghast. The 'officers' club' would be a makeshift brothel, and the nurses were being ordered to provide their Japanese captors with sex.

Chapter 19

VIV AND HER COMRADES had an unbreakable pact when it came to the most personal and harrowing incidents of war and prison life. In later years, with the horrors of those days long behind, they rarely spoke of the massacre on Radji Beach and if they did so they repeated a version that Viv gave publicly in which the nurses nobly walked into the water without fear or panic.

The nurses also closed ranks over the Japanese demands to use some of them as sex workers, though it was later revealed that the Japanese had identified those they wanted to work at the 'club' – Jessie Blanch, Win Davis, Jess Doyle,[1] Pearl 'Mitz' Mittelheuser and Nesta James, all small, dark and pretty as well as 'medically clean and free of disease'.[2]

Viv and the others did as they were ordered as far as leaving their houses and moving into the newly vacated properties between them. They formed a human chain during a thunderstorm to move the few sticks of furniture, the fly wire, curtains, light cords, floor coverings and the precious electric stove. They had to ensure the officers' club was clean and stocked with beds and couches for the 'comfort' and 'entertainment' of the men. But that's as far as they said they were willing to go.

Wednesday, 18 March, was to be the club's opening night.[3] Viv and the others felt sick about the Japanese officers' expectations. Iole Harper said the club, which had even more rooms in some nearby houses set up for entertainment, should have been named 'Lavender Street' after the red-light district in Singapore.[4]

According to their recollections of the events, Jessie Blanch, Win Davis and Nesta James were initially ordered to attend a meeting with six Japanese officers, where they were told to sign a document agreeing to entertain the officers of their own free will.

Jessie refused to sign, infuriating the Japanese officer who had presented her with the document.

> I yelled at him, and he yelled at me, we argued about this, and I said I wouldn't sign. He said 'if you don't sign, you'll starve to death. We're going to starve all of the sisters'. And I said, 'As far as I'm concerned, I'm not signing it. I'll die first'.[5]

One of the officers presented Win Davis with the same document. He looked her in the eye and said, 'No sign, you die.' But Win and Nesta James also refused to sign. All three women said they felt sick about it, knowing that all the prisoners would suffer because of their stance.[6] And the whole camp at Bukit Besar was indeed denied food for the next four days, putting enormous pressure on the meagre stocks the prisoners had stored, though some of the Dutch locals came to the fence of the prison and gave the nurses a little Australian flour.

The nurses later said that eventually they realised they had no choice but to go to the club on opening night. However, they decided that they would somehow try to trick and frustrate the Japanese into leaving them alone. The reality, though, as shown on Radji Beach, was that the Australian nurses were at the mercy of a cruel and merciless invading force who would not hesitate to destroy them. The nurses had no power, no protection and no bargaining chips. As Jessie Simons later admitted:

> It is hard to express our feeling of horror and helplessness under these most trying conditions. Certainly, we did not want even to arrange furniture for the club, but we knew what had happened to the other girls on the beach, and we wanted to get home someday.[7]

The women came together as a group to discuss their best form of defence. Betty Jeffrey recalled the discussion.

> One sister said she wasn't going to be a plaything to all and sundry in the Japanese Imperial Army. If the worst came to the worst she was going to concentrate on one man, preferably the doctor. Another girl thought it might be a good idea to teach them to play cards. Somebody else suggested we should all swear never to mention it or tell any tales about anyone if and when we were released.[8]

Viv recalled that on the morning of the announced opening of the officers' club, 18 March, two Englishmen and the English female interpreter visited the nurses and said the Japanese were demanding six women to attend the club that night, and that they were to make the officers happy.

The two Englishmen said they would be running the bar in both the houses that constituted the club and that they would ensure the women were never left alone with the Japanese. What good the Englishmen could do in this situation they did not relate, and everyone knew they could do nothing. But the Englishmen told the nurses that if the women did not go to the club as instructed the Japanese would start executing prisoners.[9]

The nurses would later say that they met at 4 p.m. that day and decided their strength lay in numbers. While they would tell the Japanese that some of the nurses – the younger and more petite ones such as Pat Gunther – were sick and needed others to care for them, twenty-two of the women, Viv included, would go to the club together, ensuring they looked as unattractive as possible.

Viv and Wilma wore their uniforms because the loosely hanging garments hid the curves of their bodies. They rubbed dirt on their faces and put twigs and leaves in their hair. Viv went barefoot while Wilma and some of the other nurses slipped on borrowed men's army boots. Altogether there were more than twenty women who arrived at the officers' club at 8 p.m.

The six officers were already there and, according to Jessie

Simons, were startled by the invasion of all these 'gaunt harpies'.[10] 'Our numbers made the [officers'] romantic ideas a little difficult to put into practice,' she wrote, 'and we densely refused to comprehend their poor English.'[11]

The nurses had agreed as a group to not accept liquor from the Japanese, and Viv told an amusing story that when one of their captors enquired what the nurses would like to drink, they replied 'milk'. When told there was no milk, only liquor, the usually fiery Blanche Hempsted, replied in a sweetly innocent voice that 'Australian girls were nice and did not drink alcohol'. Some of the nurses had a hard time keeping a straight face at that line.[12]

Despite the gravity of their plight Jessie Simons nearly burst out laughing as she caught Blanche's eye.[13] The English waiter was giving the nurses soft drinks, biscuits and salted peanuts, and the nurses, in turn, were thinking of ways to give the Japanese the slip.

A hypodermic syringe and drugs lay on a table. Jessie Simons wanted to steal them to use as pain killers for the injured nurses

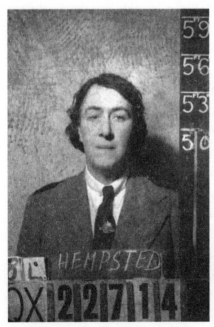 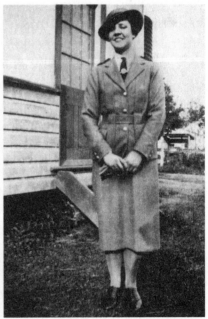

Queensland nurse Blanche Hempsted was always ready for a fight. *Australian War Memorial P02783.019*

Win Davis refused to 'entertain' Japanese officers. *Australian War Memorial P02783.019* but knew it would have been a death sentence if she'd been caught.[14] And so the nurses continued to play along, pretending not to understand a word the officers were saying.

Then, without warning, the six officers rose to their feet and the one who could speak English best ordered six of the women to go to the house next door. According to Viv, half the sisters stood up and immediately left the room for the adjoining house, with Blanche Hempsted falling into a coughing fit as though she had tuberculosis. Val Smith, from North Queensland, was a chain smoker and she also broke into a hacking cough.

Eileen 'Shorty' Short,[15] a resolute veteran nurse from country Queensland, kept the Japanese officer who had attached himself to her walking up and down the road in front of the club, ostensibly for him to sober up. She said she kept him walking until, exhausted, he finally let her go home.[16] The officer with his arm around Mavis Hannah was so drunk that she said she pushed him over and dashed home.[17]

Viv claimed that all the girls escaped the night unmolested, and other accounts by nurses who were there recalled the incidents in a similar way. They were amusing stories and Viv and her comrades often used humour when talking about the most harrowing times of their captivity, no doubt as a coping mechanism to deal with the much grimmer reality of what they'd endured.[18]

The truth is, the Japanese were not known for their sense of humour in World War II, and would rarely have taken no for an answer, especially from skylarking women. But in later years the nurses all spoke of how they banded together to prevent the abuse, and that while other interned women succumbed to the Japanese threats of starvation, the Australian nurses did not.

After this escape from the officers' club, the nurses said later that they talked into the night about what to do if they faced reprisals the next morning. Betty Jeffrey said the week after the opening of the club was 'too awful' to write about, and that the nurses did not sleep well for weeks. She said the mental strain of that time 'was far worse than being bombed and shipwrecked'.[19]

Jessie Simons recalled sadly that:

I think all the girls would agree that this club experience was the most repulsive and unpleasant in our whole imprisonment. I know it stands out grimly in our memories. For two weeks after this we were under enormous tension and became mentally worn with expectation. Any sound, at night especially, set our hearts pounding.[20]

A delegation was formed including Viv, Nesta James, Jean Ashton and Wilma Oram, to complain to the Dutch Red Cross representative, Dr Jean McDowell, about the coercion. Dr McDowell was a handsome, distinguished British woman with greying hair[21] who was trying her utmost to keep everyone at the camp alive.

The Japanese had a record of ignoring any requests from the Red Cross but, according to the nurses, Dr McDowell informed Air Commodore Modin and the Japanese commanders in Palembang. Viv said that, after this, the nurses were left alone. The Australian nurses would later claim that there were apparently other prisoners chosen as comfort women.

This however may have hidden a darker truth.

More than fifty years after the incident at the officers' club, author Susanna de Vries interviewed the elderly Longreach-born nurse Sylvia Muir, who was then suffering from breast cancer. She wrote:

Sylvia claimed that at a secret meeting held in the Japanese officers' club, four older nurses agreed to replace the younger ones and become comfort women to spare the rest of the group from being starved to death. The other nurses swore on the Bible that the names of 'the four' would never be revealed, to spare pain to them and to their relatives, and no one ever broke this promise.[22]

THE NURSES AGAIN HAD their rations cut in the immediate aftermath of the club's closure. The locals offered to sell the nurses chickens, eggs and fruit but would not accept

Singapore money which, at the time, was all that the nurses had. So the nurses split into pairs to see what they could scrounge. Jessie Simons and Mavis Hannah dug up a large tapioca root. Then a friendly local man who spoke good English gave them ten guilders to buy some food.

The man also had a radio, and he risked his life using it. He would creep to the barbed-wire fence near the women's homes at night to give them the latest developments on the war,[23] and he had welcome news from Australia: the *Empire Star*, which had left Singapore just before the *Vyner Brooke*, had made it safely home with more than fifty of their colleagues. Despite their own predicament, the nurses were overjoyed, though Jessie Simons was a little miffed that the gramophone and records she had given to one of the girls on the *Empire Star* was back home while she remained at the mercy of the Japanese on Sumatra.[24]

The nurses broke open a storeroom at the back of the house they were sharing and found an RAAF greatcoat and some magazines, including a copy of *The Australian Women's Weekly* from a year before. It featured the article by Tilly Shelton Smith about the good times the nurses were enjoying in Malacca. The photos showed the nurses in smart, starched uniforms, including shiny shoes and stockings and capes. They were all smiling and talking about how much they loved playing tennis and swimming and enjoying life in the tropics. Some of the women pictured in the photos were now dead. The others felt like they were halfway there.[25]

It was around this same time that Lieutenant Arthur Mann arrived in Fremantle with a terrible tale to tell of how he had survived the sinking of the *Vyner Brooke*. He described how dozens of nurses had been cast into the sea but said he did not know of their fate. Mann told reporters in Perth that he had floated on a piece of timber before finding a raft, and he had eventually made it to the swampy Sumatran coast.

There, he and two other men walked barefoot through swamp and jungle before finding an upturned sampan in a creek. They paddled the boat towards Bangka Strait, found a ship's lifeboat with survivors from another vessel and eventually made their way to an RAF unit still on Java.

Lieutenant Mann had received medical attention at Serang and Batavia,[26] and together with twenty Dutch soldiers they eventually reached Cilacap, on the south of Java. Three weeks after the sinking of the *Vyner Brooke* they boarded the SS *Verspyck* for Australia.

Mann said that during the night after the *Vyner Brooke* was bombed he was floating in the sea when he was passed by a small raft just 5 feet, 3 inches (about 1.6 metres) long. Twelve Australian nurses were desperately clinging to it. He hoped they had made it to Bangka Island.[27]

When she heard this news, Eva Bullwinkel in Adelaide was beside herself with anxiety, and as the Japanese continued their surge towards Australia, she fretted over her daughter's fate.

While Viv and the nurses were at the Big Hill camp, Private Kinsley, who had stayed in the Muntok hospital, died from his wounds.[28]

Chapter 20

VIV WOKE UNEASILY to the sound of shouting and running feet. It was 6 a.m. on April Fool's Day, 1 April 1942. At the time, Jessie Simons was feeding a baby, the son of the Englishwoman who seemed more interested in convincing the nurses to become geishas than looking after her child. Two Japanese guards with bayonets on the end of their rifles burst into the nurses' houses and screamed something at them they couldn't understand but which they knew would not be good.

The Japanese were moving the women again. They began to confiscate knives and scissors, so those nurses who had these invaluable utensils had secreted them as best they could in their miserably small collections of clothes and personal belongings. They were all heartbroken at the thought of leaving their precious stove.

Viv snatched up her small bundle of possessions, put on a pair of clogs that a Dutch woman had given her and shuffled outside. The Japanese herded the prisoners into two lines before marching them about 800 metres to a *padang*, an open space on top of a nearby hill. After being rushed there, the prisoners – men, women and children with small bags and here and there a battered suitcase – were made to wait for eight hours under a sun that grew redder and fierier as the day dragged on. Some of the babies and children were already crying and as the day progressed many of the nurses, especially those who were hatless, began to complain of splitting headaches. All the time the guards sat laughing in the shade of nearby trees.

Then, in the middle of the afternoon, the Japanese suddenly began to push the prisoners apart – men on one side, women and children on the other.

The families were being separated, and the nurses watched pathetic scenes[1] as the Japanese guards marched the men away to Palembang jail accompanied by the wailing of their distraught wives and children.

Would this broken-hearted group ever see their husbands and fathers again?

Viv thought the exercise was calculated torture designed to cause the civilians maximum pain.

Another half-hour under that brutal sun followed before the women and children were marched to another part of Palembang. Rumours spread that they were going to the docks and would be shipped back to a prison camp in Singapore.[2] But after a wearying journey that lasted until late afternoon, the dispirited, sunburned women and children found themselves in front of a row of ten newly built three-room cottages[3] on a street named Irenelaan.

With the arrival of more female prisoners and nurses from Muntok, many seriously ill with dysentery, the Irenelaan camp would eventually accommodate more than 400 Australian, English and Dutch women and children.

Each house had two bedrooms, a lounge-dining area, a bathroom and a small kitchen to the rear. It had an electric light but no power; taps but no water. There was no furniture, no stove and no cooking pots.

The homes had been built to accommodate three people each, but Viv had to share her house with twenty-two others – the rest of the 2/13th nurses, the women from the 2/4th, and five civilian women and three children.

The Japanese squeezed the nurses from the 2/10th and seven more civilians into the adjoining house, the occupants there numbering twenty-four. Another house, further along, had to accommodate thirty-six people.[4]

Most of the women slept on tiled floors, which were cooling after a day in the hot tropical sun, but Nesta James, at barely

150 centimetres, made her bed in a discarded child's cot,[5] and Jenny Greer slept on a table.[6] Pat Gunther wrote that the accommodation was so crowded that after Perth's Mickey Syer[7] trod on her face one night, 'I decided to move, and join Beryl Woodbridge on the porch'.[8]

One of the guards had told the nurses they would only be in the house for a night. Having all bedded down in rows like sardines, and battling swarms of mosquitoes and the flashing torches of the watchful guards, they woke the next morning to see a barbed-wire fence being erected. Their one-night stay at Irenelaan would eventually stretch to seventeen torturous months.

The Japanese used the hillside behind the camp for training, and at the sound of the soldiers going through their bayonet drills Viv would think of all her friends being run through with Japanese steel and would shake in horror. Sometimes the troops ran from house to house in camouflage gear making blood-curdling screams as they practised attacking towns.[9] Viv hoped that the Japanese officer who had ordered the massacre on Radji Beach had moved on and that no one from that morning would recognise the tall and lanky Australian nurse.

THE WOMEN MOVED QUICKLY to make the most of their bad situation. They made a cooking fire by removing a back door and smashing it to bits for wood, then borrowed a match from a guard to light it. They cooked in a Mobil Oil tin that had been half-full of oil and spider webs. They ate boiled rice with the flavour of oil and drank tea with a similar taste for weeks, eventually using all the hut doors for fuel as well as several photograph albums retrieved from a fire heap in the backyard of the huts. They also burned most of Nesta's cot. Later they used some of the retrieved photos to make playing cards for games of bridge.[10] They also found an enormous old black cooking pot that they named Matilda.

The severe overcrowding overloaded the septic system, which had been designed for just fifty people. Pipes burst and threatened to cause an epidemic by sending raw sewage into the two stormwater drains, which seemed to have been constructed with the idea of defying gravity by running uphill. For a long time, the camp was awash with faeces and barefoot women struggled during the clean-up.

The huts became so crowded that some of the nurses were forced to sleep on the floor between the latrines. When there was occasionally some clean water they had to shower briefly under a bucket of water in cubicles without doors, in full view of the leering Japanese guards.[11] The lack of water to clean themselves quickly became a major hygiene issue.

The nurses had an emergency discussion, nominating Nesta James as their spokesperson to deal with the Japanese and making her assistants 'Mitz' Mittelheuser, house captain for the 2/10th, and Jean Ashton, house captain for Viv's hut.

Committees were organised to deal with the heavy workload of keeping everyone alive. Emptying the septic tank was the most pressing issue, but there were groups assigned to clear blocked drains, and to look after housekeeping, cooking, rationing the food supplies and procuring additional sustenance, since the rations were meagre and often putrid. There was a light entertainment committee to lift spirits, and a district nursing committee. Dr McDowell opened a dressing station in a garage.

On Sundays, almost everyone attended church services. Roman Catholics met for prayers in the quarters allotted to a group of Dutch nuns.[12] One garage, known as 'The Shed', where fifteen women lived, became on Sundays a Protestant chapel run by Englishwoman Margaret Dryburgh.[13] Miss Dryburgh, as everyone called her out of respect, had been a missionary schoolteacher in China and Malaya before being interned. She became a vital source of spiritual and musical sustenance for her fellow prisoners and was cited by those in the camps 'as a beacon of hope during their long ordeal'.[14]

Like Miss Dryburgh, Flo Trotter was a devout Christian and she met regularly for prayers with other nurses of deep faith, including Sylvia Muir, Mitz Mittelheuser, Joyce Tweddell, Mickey Syer and the convent-raised Brisbane nurse Chris Oxley.[15]

Children also had regular school classes in the camp, in both English and Dutch. One of the missionary women had a volume of the complete works of William Shakespeare. Each day she would read passages from it to the children and gave them lessons in spelling and writing. The children used the charcoal at the end of sticks in lieu of pencils, and they wrote in the clear margins of pages torn from a Dutch telephone book.

The Japanese ordered the children to work alongside the adults, and among the tasks was tilling the vegetable gardens. Every prisoner hated the work because all the food they grew was sent to the Japanese and if any of the plants died the children were savagely beaten.

The Japanese provided rations daily: sacks of rice and usually rotten vegetables – bad cabbages and bad carrots – thrown from a truck to the roadway. Sometimes there would be *kangkong*, better known as 'swamp spinach', which grew in the gutters and sewers.[16]

Every now and then the guards would throw a piece of wild pig from a truck, only for it to be immediately surrounded by hungry camp dogs. The prisoners were not allowed to chase the dogs away. Instead, a Japanese guard would cut a small piece of wild pork for each house, placing his dirty boot on the meat to steady it as he hacked away. Betty Jeffrey remembered that the piece given for the twenty-four people in her house would not cover the palm of her hand, so there was always great excitement if one of the women found a tiny piece of pork in her stew.[17]

Each prisoner received just a cigarette tin of rice per person per day. Luxuries such as an egg often had to be split five ways. It was particularly hard on the children, who went to sleep and woke up with gnawing hunger in their bellies.

As they came closer and closer to starvation, the prisoners became more accustomed to eating rotten food. Jessie Simons remembered breaking into a dish 'the one egg that was the week's protein and nearly fainting from the odour – it had a ripe abscess … However, after mixing the offender with rice and curry before baking it in a tin over hot coals, I got the mess down and kept it down – with an effort'.[18]

Wilma Oram learned to stomach eggs that had a partly formed embryo in them.[19]

Jessie Blanch remembered when, late in her captivity, the Japanese included some corn in the prisoners' weekly ration. 'I had some in a little basket tied up on the rafter for my next meal. I looked up when I woke and here's a rat in it. So, I grabbed him and went off to sell him to the Eurasians. I said "He's a lovely fat, good healthy rat!" And he popped out of my bag, and I lost [the equivalent of] $2.50. They were going to pay me $2.50 for a rat.'[20] As their hunger bit hard, some prisoners gladly ate snake.

Before long the nurses kept their eyes out for the Chinese funeral processions that passed the prison camp. Cymbals, tins and rattles shaken by mourners were all part of the funeral rituals, as was leaving food on the graves for the spirits to use in the afterlife. The nurses were pleasantly surprised when, after one funeral passed, some young lads shared the cemetery food with them. Perhaps they thought the nurses would be dead soon as well.[21]

Viv and the others didn't see soap for months at Irenelaan. When they were finally thrown some with their rations, it was divided among them carefully and treated as preciously as gold. Once the women had washed their few belongings with it, the soap was gone.[22]

EARLY IN THEIR TIME AT Irenelaan Viv and Wilma Oram were doing their rounds as part of their district-nursing duties when they heard the startling screams of a teenage girl seated beside a camp fire. A middle-aged woman was standing over the girl pouring boiling water from a kettle onto a cloth and then applying it to the youngster's head.

Viv rushed to the rescue. The woman identified herself as the youngster's grandmother, Violet Kenneison.[23] She said that flies had laid maggots in the girl's scalp and she was killing them with an old remedy. Viv tried to convince her that boiling water was not the best way to treat the problem, but the grandmother remonstrated and told Viv to mind her own business. With her

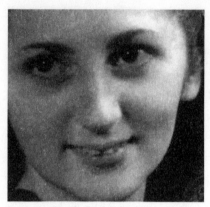

Teenager 'Little Bet', Edie Kenneison, became Viv's close friend in the prison camp.

jaw set firmly and her blue eyes blazing, Viv took the girl by the arm and led her away to safety.

The girl told Viv that her name was Betty Kenneison[24] and that she was fourteen. She said she remembered seeing Viv weeks earlier walking into the grounds of Muntok jail while supporting a badly wounded English soldier. She remembered all the other nurses being overjoyed to see her as they all shouted 'Bully'.[25] Viv called her new friend 'Little Bet'. Viv's intervention proved a blessing for the young girl who later reported that the maggots were actually cleaning up the pus in her scalp.[26]

'Little Bet' Kenneison was born at Batu Caves in Kuala Lumpur, Malaya, where her English grandfather Ernest Kenneison[27] ran a construction company. When the Japanese invaded Malaya, he and his second wife – Bet's step-grandmother Violet – took the girl to Singapore in the hope of travelling to safety back in England.

With Singapore ablaze, they'd boarded HMS *Giang Bee*, a Chinese-owned coastal steamer requisitioned and used as a patrol vessel, on the same day that Viv climbed onto the *Vyner Brooke*.

The next day, as Japanese bombers attacked, Betty held her grandfather's hand while panicking passengers pushed them towards the railing. In the chaotic rush after a bomb blast tore off a section of the ship's bridge, Betty became separated from her grandfather. She never saw Ernest Kenneison again.[28] More than 200 others went down with the ship.

Betty was thrown into the water and with her grandmother was plucked out of the sea by men on a lifeboat. Other survivors were pushed away from the crammed boat as they threatened to capsize it in their panic. Betty was haunted by her grandfather's death and the cries and screams of others as the current carried them away to their deaths. Fifty-six survivors from the *Giang Bee* drifted for two days until 15 February, when they washed up at Djaboes, a bay on Bangka Island's north-west coast. Malayans gave them food and clothes before the Japanese came and took them as prisoners, carting them to Muntok jail in cattle trucks.

Violet blamed Betty for her grandfather's death and constantly reminded the girl that she had been instructed to look after him and never let him out of her sight. She had failed to do that, and Betty was perpetually sad as a result.

At Muntok jail, Betty had waited at the front gate every day, praying that her grandfather had somehow survived the shipwreck. She hoped to see him walk down the street. She never did see him, but one day she'd watched Viv and Kinsley stagger into the prison, and she found her hero. Betty came to idolise Viv, later remarking that despite the struggles all the prisoners had to deal with in the camp, Viv was always 'very caring and made me her responsibility'.[29]

Viv's broad smile and infectious laugh comforted and reassured Betty in such a violent, chaotic world. But often the horror of their lives under Japanese control made the traumatised teenager despondent. On one starry night, Betty and Viv were walking around the perimeter of the camp when Viv rested her hand lightly on Betty's shoulders and told her not to look down at the ground but look up at the shining stars. Imagine you are just like those stars, sparkling and free, Viv told the girl. Freedom is everywhere, Viv said – in the wildflowers and birds, in the heavens, and especially in the imagination. The Japanese could not control the thoughts of their prisoners. Viv told Betty she could leave the Japanese prison camp behind any time she chose and escape into her beautiful mind.[30]

Chapter 21

IN THE FIRST FEW MONTHS of internment, the nurses were doing all they could to remind themselves of home and their loved ones. They even organised an 'Ashes' cricket Test between English and Australian prisoners, the nurses fancying their chances against their traditional sporting enemy. Viv was a natural athlete while Jess Doyle and Iole Harper were from famous cricketing families – Jess's clan had produced Test players Charles, Dave, Ned and Jack Gregory, while Iole's were well-known cricketers in Western Australia.

The match didn't come off, though, and Betty Jeffrey wrote, 'I'm sorry, for I'll never get another opportunity to play cricket for Australia.'[1]

Soon that was the least of Betty's worries. As the war dragged on the nurses became too weary for sports or any other leisure activity, spending much of their time foraging for food and trying to cook what little they had into something edible.

Mavis Hannah and Jessie Simons earned Dutch guilders from other prisoners by making and selling grass hats and bags. Mavis also borrowed a sewing machine from one of the Dutch internees and used it to make new clothes from old garments.

Win Davis used the machine to make seven pairs of black shorts from a nun's habit that was given to her, and she and Pat Gunther made hats from the woven-reed bags in which fish were delivered to the camp, adding pieces of coloured material to give them the feel of Australian summer fashion. Pat also drew remarkable sketches of camp life. Val Smith repaired sandals using nails salvaged from old furniture that was being broken up for firewood, and Iole Harper worked as a washerwoman and nursemaid for a Dutch family. Cecilia Delforce chopped wood, and Beryl Woodbridge made rag dolls for the camp's many children. Flo Trotter and Betty Jeffrey set themselves up as hairdressers, while most of the others either did laundry or cleaning in the Dutch civilian area of the camp. Viv made some money by crushing soybeans, which, when flavoured with vanilla essence, made a palatable drink. Viv and Wilma also elected to sort bananas before they were distributed to the internees.

'Viv and I had no money to buy bananas,' Wilma remembered later, 'so we stuffed in as many as we could while we were cutting them ... There were ways and means of looking after yourself!'[2]

Then the Japanese banned the local people from trading in food with the prisoners.

Disease became more common and food scarcer.

A group of Englishwomen were looking after little Mischa Warman, now an orphan, after his mother, Cevia, succumbed to the disease and dismay of life under Japanese captivity.[3]

Many of the Japanese guards were routinely cruel, their sadism stoked largely by the shame and resentment they felt at being ordered to watch over women and children when other troops were being lauded for their courage in combat.

One morning, Viv and the others watched horrified as the guards dragged a frail old local man, semi-conscious, to the centre of the camp and tied him to a post with barbed wire. He had been caught trying to sell a few duck eggs to the prisoners. The old man had already been badly beaten, his mouth and face cut and swollen and his head lolling to one side. Before leaving, the guards told the women that they were not to give him food or water or they would suffer the same fate.

All day the cruel sun tortured the old man. Blood caked on his head and his throat became parched. The nurses heard his ravings when he began to hallucinate. The old man's pleas for water echoed through an awful night until he finally fell silent.

At noon the next day a middle-aged British woman went to the man with a cup of water only to be knocked to the ground by a guard wielding his sheathed sword like a club.

The blow to the side of her head opened up a deep cut and caused a scream of anguish. As the guard lifted his sword to strike the woman again, Jean Ashton rushed at him. 'Stop!' she cried. Viv and the others had followed her and now the guard sneered at them all as he smashed the sword into the woman's head once more. Satisfied with his work, he strode away as the nurses lifted the stricken, bloodied woman to her feet.[4]

The next morning, prison roll call, or 'tenko', was held at the usual time on the *padang* in front of the post on which the old man hung, clearly dead, held up only by the barbed wire. All the women had to bow to the guards as the roll call was taken. Either that or face a beating or hours hatless under the sun as punishment. This was the reality of prison life under Japanese rule.

As the women and children gazed forlornly at the pathetic little body tethered to the punishment post, Japanese guards approached behind their new camp commandant, Captain Miachi, a dapper officer with a Clarke Gable haircut and neat moustache. Pat Gunther remembered him as being 'quite a handsome man and incredibly conceited'.[5]

Miachi told them that if the prisoners had any complaints – apart from being forced to watch an old man murdered in the most obscene way – they should speak to Dr McDowell, who would then report their concerns to him.

For a long time, the women were not allowed to have papers or do any writing. Day and night, guards would wander into their sleeping quarters with fixed bayonets to search them. Any personal papers were burned. Still, many of the nurses, including Viv, recorded their thoughts. Viv wrote hers in a discarded Dutch diary, and Betty Jeffrey wrote hers in a child's exercise book and hid it in a pillow.

Mistreatment and malnourishment affected everyone, especially the civilian internees and their children, who were not used to living in a regimented fashion in such close proximity to strangers.

Sometimes the nurses' meagre possessions were stolen. Everyone's nerves were stretched to breaking point.

There was constant turmoil inside the huts with so many people crammed in. 'Life is not easy next door, there are some rather odd types living with our girls, and they are hard to get on with, especially at ration time,' Betty wrote of the situation in Viv's hut.[6]

Jean Ashton recorded one of the fights in the hut she shared with Viv and twenty-one other women: 'Final blitz – Mrs Close and ... Raymont have a fight in the bathroom about 7 a.m. We others all still in bed. We rush out to help – Miss McMurray from the back room joins in fray by standing behind Mrs Close and hitting Sr Gladys Hughes on [the] head with a piece of wood'.[7]

JOHN CURTIN HAD ONCE been a terrier for the Brunswick Australian rules club in Melbourne, but the Australian prime minister had never enjoyed good health. The stress of faction fighting in the Labor Party had taken its toll on him long before the Japanese began ravaging Asia and the South Pacific. Curtin suffered from stress-related illnesses and depression, which he masked early in his career with heavy drinking. He was a chain smoker, too, until wartime shortages of tobacco hit even him.

And yet for all his vices and insecurities, this sad, sickly bespectacled man became Australia's tower of strength in 1942. Not long after the bombing of Pearl Harbor and with Australia under obvious threat, Curtin had defied tradition and many of his own colleagues to say that in this time of crisis, Australia now looked to America as its rock, rather than the United Kingdom.[8] He recalled his troops supporting Britain in the Middle East so they could prepare for the defence of Australia.

Following air raids on Tokyo and other Japanese cities by the American pilot Jimmy Doolittle and his raiders, an immense naval war raged in the Coral Sea from 4 to 8 May 1942. Casualties were massive but the Japanese fared the worst, with 966 killed, ninety-two aircraft lost and ten ships destroyed or damaged. It was the first time the Japanese advance had been checked so severely.

But there seemed no end to the Japanese cruelty and the senseless deaths. A few days later at Rabaul, 5000 kilometres west of Viv's prison camp on Sumatra, a group of Australians were caught with a radio and a pistol. Among them was an eleven-year-old boy, Dickie Manson, and his mother, Marjorie. The group were denounced as spies and driven in the back of an open truck to the base of a volcano. Marjorie tied a strip of red material around Dickie's head to cover his eyes. She then held her little boy's hand as a firing squad of six soldiers shot them dead.[9]

ON THE PARADE GROUND one morning, Viv and Wilma were hobbling badly with extreme cases of tinea that had been exacerbated by overflows of the sewerage system. Viv also had painful furuncles – or boils – on her thigh. Jean Ashton took the two nurses back to their hut and said they should be admitted to the hospital in Palembang. But just as they were about to leave to seek permission from Dr McDowell, a large British woman who was sharing the hut with the Australians barged in and confronted the three nurses, saying she wanted more sleeping room.

Jean tried to reason with the woman, only to be brushed aside as the intruder stormed past Viv and Wilma and began hurling the Australian nurses' possessions out onto the floor of the main room while screaming obscenities at them. Wilma leapt to her aching feet and told the woman to cut it out. Blanche Hempsted marched through the door and told the woman to 'belt up or there [will] be a bloody big blue'.[10]

The British woman charged at the Australian group and raked Wilma's face with her fingernails. Two more civilian women arrived and one grabbed Blanche's hair and pulled it. Mina Raymont waded in and was punched in the head before she wrapped her arms around her assailant and wrestled her.

A young woman brandishing a large knife threatened to stab the Australians if they didn't stop. Suddenly there was silence and stillness.

Dr McDowell arrived and demanded an end to hostilities. As a compromise, she asked the nurses to surrender the second

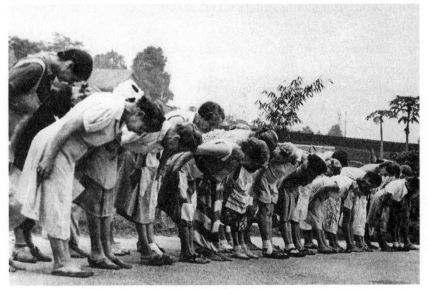

A group of internees bow their heads to their Japanese captors at the morning roll call. *Singapore National Archives*

bedroom to the civilian women and their three children. She also insisted that Viv and Wilma have their miserable feet treated in Palembang.

Captain Miachi approved their transfer the next day. On 25 May 1942, a rickety, old ambulance took the ailing pair over rough and bumpy roads to the Charitas Hospital, a small building staffed by Dutch doctors and nuns. Patients had initially been treated with medicines hidden before the Japanese arrived, but those medicines had gradually run out.

Viv and Wilma were escorted to a tiny ward. That night was the first time since leaving Singapore that the pair had slept in beds, though they were topped only with a thin mattress and pillow.

The next day, the nun in charge of the ward, a Dutch woman named Sister Renelda, told Viv and Wilma that Australian soldiers had previously gotten her into strife. When she had gone about the wards killing bugs, her Australian patients had told her she was using the wrong English word and that the proper noun for bugs was 'buggers'. When the nun later told her priest that she'd been going about the hospital looking for dirty 'buggers' the priest was mortified.[11]

The humour of the Australians could only mask the horrors of war ever so briefly. A month later the Japanese merchant ship *Montevideo Maru* left Rabaul carrying 1054 prisoners, mostly Australians, bound for the Chinese island of Hainan.

On 30 June the ship was spotted by the crew of the submarine USS *Sturgeon* near the northern Philippine coast. Unaware that it was carrying human cargo, the *Sturgeon* fired four torpedoes just before dawn on 1 July. The ship sank eleven minutes later and all 1054 prisoners, most of them locked below deck, drowned.

VIV SPENT TWENTY-FIVE DAYS in the Palembang hospital being treated for tinea but returned to Irenelaan alone as Wilma still needed more care. The doctor who treated Viv told her that, in lieu of medicine, she should rub butter or margarine into the affected parts of her feet. It was ridiculous advice, Viv thought, because she had seen neither butter nor margarine since leaving Singapore and even if there was a skerrick to be had at Irenelaan, the prisoners were so hungry no one would be allowed to rub food on their feet.[12]

When Viv returned to the camp, Betty Kenneison was waiting for her at the gates. She ran to her as the other nurses crowded around. The Japanese had relaxed their iron grip just a little, and Viv found that her hut now contained an old piano, donated by some Dutch women who couldn't play it and needed extra sleeping space in their quarters. At first the women had considered chopping up the piano for firewood, but fourteen Australian nurses had swarmed over the instrument like so many hungry ants, and with many grunts and damaged knees[13] they'd moved it into their place. None of the half-starved nurses were as strong as they had been before captivity, but they knew that music could lift them a little. The always frail[14] but perky Tasmanian Shirley Gardam was a fine pianist.

The nurses also produced a newsletter with a barbed-wire masthead written by hand and passed around. It was called the

Camp Chronicle and was full of stories about Australia and recipes to make their camp food more palatable. There was a noticeable lack of hard news about the Japanese atrocities.

On 5 July 1942, church attendance at The Shed was rewarded with the very first performance of Miss Dryburgh's own composition, 'The Captives' Hymn', an uplifting masterpiece that she sang with the prisoners Shelagh Brown and Dorothy MacLeod, a former teacher at Singapore's Anglo-Chinese school. After its debut, the song was performed by the whole congregation of women and children every Sunday.[15]

RUMOURS BEGAN TO SPREAD that salvation was near for the nurses. Following their halt in the Coral Sea, the Japanese had suffered catastrophic losses in the naval Battle of Midway and setbacks at Milne Bay and on the Solomon Islands. They were in retreat down the Kokoda Track after having failed to reach Port Moresby.

Some of the nurses heard that they would soon be released in a prisoner-swap deal. The rumours grew legs when several Asian inmates of Irenelaan were set free. But the hopes of Viv, the other nurses and most of the internees were quickly dashed, adding to the boiling tensions.

Jean Ashton, dressed in a two-piece summer dress made from an old curtain, was making jam over a fire in front of her hut under the noon-day sun, when two of the civilian women from their earlier fight demanded she stop. With a foul-mouthed tirade they said the smoke was making them suffocate in their tiny bedroom.

The larger of the two women kicked Jean's cooking pot away, sending it rolling across the campground and spilling all the jam. The smaller of the two women hit Jean with a punch to the ribs that knocked off her grass sunhat and sent her sprawling into the spilled jam. With a cackle,[16] the large woman ripped off Jean's bra top and held it aloft as a trophy. Bare-breasted Jean leapt at the big woman and wrestled her, spinning her around and sending her to the ground, winded.

Thinking she had settled the matter, Jean was putting her top back on when the second woman smashed her in the side of the head with a lump of wood.

The always pugnacious Blanche Hempsted led the charge of Australian nurses but before they could take their revenge, Jean McDowell arrived to make peace once more. A Japanese guard also ran to the scene, ready to make war. He pointed his rifle at the nurses, daring them to take another step.

Nesta James defended the Australians to Dr McDowell, emphasising their camaraderie and the fact none would tolerate their colleagues being bullied.[17]

Dr McDowell said that the Japanese would not allow fighting and, regardless of who was at fault, if it happened again everyone knew that the Japanese punishments could be 'excessive'.

Viv and Veronica Clancy helped Jean Ashton back inside while Jessie Simons recovered Jean's top.

The nurses decided that it was best for everyone to surrender the house to the civilians and move all the nurses into accommodation that was already overcrowded. For the first time since internment, the two groups of nurses became one. Thirty-two of them were then confined in a three-bedroom house.

Not long after they became prisoners, the starvation diet caused the nurses to stop menstruating,[18] and over time they began to lose their hair[19] and teeth due to a lack of Vitamin C.

Mina Raymont and Iole Harper had abscessed teeth extracted without anaesthetic. Betty Jeffrey and a friend had to carry a semi-conscious Iole back to the nurses' hut after her ordeal and it took her a long time to recover.[20]

Viv and Wilma were hospitalised again with severe tinea that made it almost impossible for them to walk. Viv's big toenail on the right foot was removed. Gladys Hughes also went to the hospital with an excruciating ear infection. Shorty Short and Shirley Gardam both suffered cuts to their legs that became terribly infected. Veronica Clancy was floored by myocarditis and Betty Jeffrey suffered an attack of appendicitis.

Jessie Blanch had developed a throat infection in the water after the sinking of the *Vyner Brooke*, and while lying 'sick and miserable' on shore recovering from the tribulation, she was kicked by the Japanese soldiers as they walked past.[21]

'When we got salt,' Jessie recalled, 'I never put it on my food. I'd gargle with it to try and stop my throat infection … [it] flared up and it was dreadful.' The throat infection developed into an abscess. One day, it burst and the infection spread, leaving her deaf in her left ear for the rest of her life.[22] She eventually had a heart attack because of overwork in the camp. Win Davis nursed her back to health.[23]

A lack of Vitamin B caused Mavis Hannah to battle beri-beri, which badly damaged her heart and left her unfit for any form of physical exertion.[24]

Viv came down with tonsilitis in November 1942 and recalled that there was a complete lack of modern medicine within Irenelaan. 'We had nothing, literally nothing to care for a patient,' she said. 'No mattresses or linen or anything like that, nothing. We did pound the embers of the fires into a powder which we gave to our patients. That's supposed to be reasonably good for diarrhoea, but our patients all had dysentery by this time.'[25]

Many of the other nurses, including Jessie Simons, came down with dengue fever.

Despite their physical condition the women were routinely slapped across the face by guards and often made to stand all day in the sun hatless as punishment. There was always the constant threat of rape and execution.

Still, they tried to find moments of light in their dark suffering, playing bridge, making mahjong sets from broken tiles and furniture and forming a library from books abandoned by the Dutch when they fled Sumatra. They celebrated each other's birthdays as best they could, and, on 11 November, Jean Ashton helped to organise an Armistice Day commemoration.

The nurses also staged a comical fashion parade with their oddments – clothes by 'Paula of Palembang' – and a series of Saturday night concerts with themes such as 'The Jolly Swagman' and the 'Running of the Melbourne Cup'. The songs had sarcastic lyrics about their captors, their conditions and even some of their fellow prisoners, including Mrs Brown, who was portrayed using enormous padding and a waddling walk.

One of their favourite songs was written by Val Smith and Mina 'Ray' Raymont and sung to the tune of 'The Quartermaster's Store'.

There is rice, rice, mouldy rotten rice
Nothing more, nothing more
There are eggs, eggs, growing little legs
Let's throw them at their shaven heads ...[26]

The shows became so popular that many Dutch and British women squeezed into the crammed house for the performances or, if there was no room at all, peered through windows and doors. Mina Raymont was the driving force behind the shows, which included impressions of the stars of the time. Viv made an excellent Greta Garbo, Wilma Oram played Mae West, Beryl Woodbridge became Shirley Temple and Sylvia Muir was perfect as the glamorous and exotic Dorothy Lamour in a sarong.

Margaret Dryburgh helped the nurses with their songs as did Margery Jennings and Norah Chambers,[27] two women who had been living in Malaya before the war. Norah was a graduate of London's Royal Academy of Music, and both women were the wives of prisoners of war.

Back home in Adelaide, Eva Bullwinkel had no idea what had happened to Viv and continued to write to her on spec, but the letters and cards were all returned. Then Eva was sent word that her son, Flight Sergeant John Bullwinkel, had suffered a badly broken leg 'during a parachute descent following action against the enemy in the Middle East'.[28] He was so badly injured that eventually he would be discharged as 'medically unfit for further service'.[29] John's best mate, Tom Worley, had been killed six months earlier when the Wellington bomber on which he was flying stalled and crashed in Oxfordshire.[30]

AS THE NURSES' FIRST Christmas in captivity approached, Chris Oxley and Jenny Greer found a shrub that made a passable Yuletide tree. They decorated it as best they could, and Chris even brewed some potent chilli wine in secret.

Christmas drew near with a storm on its tail, which Viv considered a gift. Torrential rain had become a blessing for the nurses because rain meant a decent wash in a hellhole where clean water was always scarce.

At one point Betty Jeffrey was moved to write, 'We haven't sighted soap for months and are a fine colour! When it rains we still dash out and stand under the nearest piece of leaking roof, the only decent wash we get.'[31]

Late one day, just before Christmas, the married women gathered with their children behind the barbed wire at the camp perimeter to catch a glimpse of the men from Palembang's male camp being marched from a work site, where they were being used as slave labour. For most of the civilian prisoners the sad procession was their only chance to see loved ones since their separation from Bukit Besar's Big Hill eight months earlier.

The path the men trod was almost 400 metres from the women's compound and the men were but faint outlines in the distance. Many of the women and children were ravaged by dengue fever and malaria but they ignored their distress to quietly wave to the men as tears ran down their faces. For Wilma Oram this was 'proof that, no matter what savagery their captors inflicted on them, civilisation would prevail for the vast majority in the camps'.[32]

One woman, defying the Japanese guards, began to sing the Christmas carol 'O Come, All Ye Faithful', and soon the whole group was singing as the Japanese soldiers hurried the men along with the points of their bayonets.[33]

Chapter 22

THE TROPICAL STORM arrived as something of a gift at the Irenelaan Camp to usher in Christmas Day 1942. Wild winds battered the huts but the driving rain soaked the prisoners, who were glad for the wash.

After they had dried themselves, Viv sat next to Blanche Hempsted at a Christmas morning service at The Shed with other Protestants, listening to readings from the scriptures and singing hymns and carols.

The two nurses were captivated not so much by the nativity stories but by the performance of Sally Oldham, a small, middle-aged Manchester missionary also known as 'Florrie'. She seized upon the Christmas celebration as a time for confession, rising before the assembled women to cast her eyes heavenward and declare it had been thirty years since the Lord had saved her from sin.

'I wonder what the bloody hell she did,' Blanche said to Viv loud enough for others around her to hear.[1]

'Shoosh, Blanche, you're in church,' Viv whispered.

'Come on Bully, I know that. I just wish she could get to the point,' Blanche replied.

Veronica Clancy was another 'fascinated' by Sally's sin and wanting all the salacious details.[2]

With her eyes closed, Sally, who had preached for many years in China, crossed her arms over her breasts and told how the Lord had led her from evil into a life of self-righteous enlightenment.

She then launched into the hymn 'Jerusalem' and the congregation joined her.

In a loud voice that could be heard over the singing, a flummoxed Blanche asked, 'Yeah, but what the bloody hell did she *do*?'

Viv burst out laughing but when some of the congregation turned their heads in annoyance, she and Blanche joined the singing with gusto.[3]

The nurses had saved some tea leaves for Christmas, as well as rice, which they ground to make cakes and biscuits.[4]

The male inmates at the other camp had agreed to reduce their rations so the women could have a decent Christmas meal. Through some humane guards they managed to send the women a little beef with a sack full of potatoes and some tiny onions.[5] The nurses even made a plum pudding of sorts from brown rice, ground peanuts, cinnamon and local palm sugar known as 'gula jawa'.

Later they gathered around the piano to sing carols and songs of home.

The Japanese also brought in typed messages of Christmas greetings from England, America and Australia for the inmates of those countries. The Australian message came from the prime minister and read: 'Australia sends greetings. Keep smiling. Curtin.'[6]

In the late afternoon the Dutch women invited the Australians to their celebration. They had a tree and had decorated it for the children in whatever colourful tinsel and trinkets they could scrounge. Under the tree were small gifts for all the youngsters – handmade toys and dolls.

As the sun began to set, Viv watched as a procession of children carrying candles to light their way as they approached the tree. They were singing 'Away in a Manger'.[7] Thinking of her own mother back in Adelaide pining for her children, Viv could hardly hold back the tears.

THERE WAS NO CHAMPAGNE, but Chris Oxley's chilli wine was a big hit at the Christmas party and there was plenty left over for New Year's Eve six days later, as the nurses tried to forget the horrors of 1942.

Perhaps 1943 would see the end of the war. That was the collective prayer of the women who 'let down their hair' as the Japanese guards left them in peace for a short while. The keys on the battered old piano were hammered like never before.

Blanche Hempsted had an acid tongue but even the chilli wine was a bit too hot for her taste. She had offered some to Viv and Wilma in a cigarette tin, but they'd declined. Viv didn't like the sound of it and Wilma was teetotal. Just as well. When Blanche took a sip from the tin her face became a mask of horror. Several drops of purple liquid dribbled down her chin. 'It's like pouring petrol down your throat,' Blanche said, 'and setting it alight.'

Blanche walked away singing at the top of her lubricated voice, 'There were eggs, eggs, nearly growing legs in the Quartermaster's Store.'[8]

Poor little Blanche. Viv thought often of Blanche working to a state of exhaustion at the hospital in Singapore and then crying herself to sleep thinking of the boys who had died that day.[9]

As midnight approached, Jean Ashton gave a short speech in which she encouraged the nurses to think of the wonderful time they would have when they finally reached home. She ended her speech with a shout of 'Happy New Year!' Blanche drank the last of the chilli wine from her cigarette tin and the nurses linked arms to sing 'Auld Lang Syne', kicking up their feet with optimism.

It did not take long for that optimism to be crushed.

ON 16 FEBRUARY 1943, the nurses held a quiet, secret commemoration service for the sisters murdered on Radji Beach and those who had died in the water in the hours preceding. Later that morning, the piercing whistle was the signal for Viv and the others to line up and be counted by their house captains.

On the parade ground the children were feeling the heat and humidity while their frightened mothers tried to quieten them in case the unpredictable guards became angry. Viv watched cautiously as one of the soldiers leaned on his rifle with a look of scorn. He scanned the rows of prisoners and gave a low growl of contempt. Ominously, he marched over to a woman in the front line of the Dutch contingent. His nose was almost touching hers, then, before she knew what hit her, the guard slammed the butt of his rifle into her face. The woman was knocked backwards, sending women behind her toppling, before she hit the ground unconscious, blood gushing from a mouth full of broken teeth. The guard then turned to his right and smashed his rifle butt into another unsuspecting woman. She went down just as awfully as the first, out cold with blood all over her face. The prisoners had learned a little Japanese and knew the guard had screamed in his language something about 'scarlet lips' and the nurses knew he meant lipstick. Any who still wore that little connection with the world they had left behind quickly wiped it off with the back of their hands.

Viv made her way back to her hut on feet still plagued by tinea and asked Blanche to help her cart water to clean up Wilma, who had come down with dysentery and was getting sicker by the day. Even during the storms around Christmas, Viv had gone out in the driving rain and thick mud to get water, even though it worsened her tinea. No task was too daunting for her if it meant saving the life of a friend.

Wilma explained later, 'You see, you did need a friend when these things happened, because they would happen without warning.'[10]

As Viv and Blanche were leaving for the well, a kindly Englishwoman Mrs Blake rushed over to the Australians' hut to tell Jean Ashton that the camp commandant wanted to see her immediately. Jean dare not delay.

Viv had no time to wait for Jean to return because Wilma was desperately ill. She and Blanche took a large pole with a bucket secured in the middle and trod carefully down a winding, slippery jungle track to the camp's well. They lowered the bucket more than six metres to hit water and then, with their weary, malnourished arms, hauled it to the surface.

On the way back, the weight of the water quickly evaporated their strength and the pole holding the bucket cut into their bony shoulders. Viv was afraid that her infected feet would defeat her, but as they neared the end of their tough journey they found Jean Ashton waiting. Viv and Blanche put down their pole and bucket and flopped onto the ground, and Jean handed them some precious gifts – small cards about 7 centimetres high and 12 centimetres wide. They were prisoner-of-war service cards. The Japanese had finally agreed to pleas from the Red Cross that their prisoners be allowed to write a short, heavily censored letter to their loved ones.

As Viv and Blanche carried the water for Wilma to their hut, it suddenly seemed much lighter.

VIV SAT DOWN TO COMPOSE her first letter home in a year. She was as much in the dark about Eva and John as they were about her. She was careful not to offend her jailers in case the letter card was torn to shreds, and was even more careful to paint a picture of happiness to assuage Eva's fears, even if it meant stretching the truth as far as she could.

> Women's Internment Camp
> Palembang. Sumatra.
> 18.3.43
> Dear Mother,
> Sorry to cause you so much worry but don't. I have not
> and never will regret leaving home. My roving spirit has
> been somewhat checked. I am very well in fact I'm close
> on 11 stone [70 kg] I'm sure. I have let my hair grow and
> am now sporting a nob if you please. We do a little nursing
> about the camp but the sick cases go to the hospital. We
> find suntops and shorts the ideal uniform. Have learned to
> play contract bridge you should learn to play it is by far the
> superior game and we have a very keen school of players.
> How is John my love to him and ask Zelda and Con to tell
> all friends that I am well and often think of everyone give
> them all my love. I hope it will be possible to hear from
> you soon. Many happy returns of last month mum I hope
> you are well and keep smiling and don't worry over me.

Once again love to all in Melbourne, Perth, Adelaide and Broken Hill.

Lots of love. Viv.

On the same day that Viv penned her sunny note, Flight Lieutenant Bill Newton and his two-man crew on a Douglas Boston bomber attacked Japanese ammunition dumps and fuel stores at Salamaua on the north-eastern coastline of New Guinea. Two days earlier, Newton's heroics in the same area had earned him the Victoria Cross. Newton was a handsome, dashing young man who looked like movie star Errol Flynn. Before the war he'd been a star fast bowler in Melbourne and friends with Keith Miller, another swashbuckling wartime pilot who went on to become one of Australia's most celebrated cricketers.[11]

The Japanese responded to the Australians' attack on Salamaua with cannon fire. Newton's plane burst into flames and he ditched it about 900 metres offshore. The navigator[12] was killed on impact but Newton and his wireless operator, Flight Sergeant John Lyon, survived, and they swam ashore to hide in the jungle.

The two Australians were eventually captured by a Japanese patrol. Lyon was bayoneted to death, but Newton was taken back to Salamaua where, on 29 March 1943, the naval officer who had captured him used a Samurai sword to behead him.[13]

Three weeks later, on the morning of 18 April, sixteen American Lockheed Lightning fighter aircraft intercepted a fleet of Japanese warplanes acting as an escort for Admiral Isoroku Yamamoto, the man who oversaw the attack on Pearl Harbor and the Battle of Midway. Yamamoto was killed by two .50-calibre machine-gun bullets, and the Mitsubishi 'Betty Bomber' on which he was travelling crashed into the jungle on Bougainville.

Then, on 14 May, just before dawn off Queensland's Moreton Island, the Australian Hospital Ship *Centaur*, ablaze with lights shining brightly on the vivid Red Cross markings along its white hull, was hit by two Japanese torpedoes. Thirty-year-old nursing sister Lieutenant Ellen Savage[14] was the only one of twelve army nurses to survive. Of the 322 souls on board the *Centaur*, only sixty-four were rescued.[15] Among the dead was young doctor Clem Manson, who had welcomed Viv and the other nurses to beautiful, exotic Singapore just a year and a half earlier.

At the same time, the Japanese army were forcing about 60,000 Allied prisoners of war – including 13,000 Australians – to build a railway linking Thailand and Burma. Their methods again involved cruelty, murder and starvation. About 2800 Australians died.[16]

AT IRENELAAN, Viv and the other prisoners found ways to take their minds off their predicament. There were the concerts, the library, card games and, until the Japanese banned them because they were too popular, a program of informal lectures on Thursday nights. Miss Dryburgh had spoken on the subject 'Northumberland Legends', and Shirley Gardam told everyone about the delights of her home state, Tasmania. Iole Harper spoke about the joys and heartbreaks of 'Life on a Sheep Farm'.

Eileen Short told Viv that she wished she could lecture the people at home about what was really happening in the prison camps under Japanese control. Shorty had grown up at Maryborough in country Queensland and could chop wood like a champion axeman as she provided firewood for the women. Dressed in sun top and shorts, she almost always had in the corner of her mouth a cigarette made from dried leaves found in the camp wrapped in half pages from a Bible.

Shorty told Viv that she ached for the day when a big suntanned Aussie soldier came striding through the front gates of Irenelaan, the muscles in his thighs twitching as he arrived to tell them they were all free. 'I just love those short shorts they wear, don't you, Bully?'[17] Shorty rolled her eyes in such an exaggerated way that Viv burst out laughing.

As it turned out, it would be the women, and not sun-bronzed Aussie men, who would soon pass through the gates of Irenelaan.

IN SEPTEMBER 1943, the women received a note from some of the male prisoners in the nearby camp. It was hidden in a chunk of firewood, about the only way the two camps could communicate.

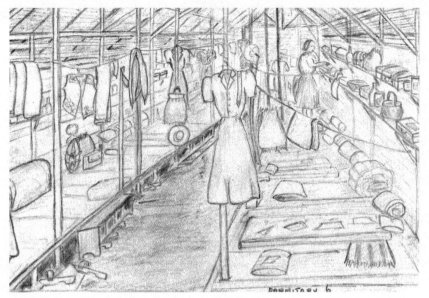

Pat Gunther sold drawings such as this in exchange for Dutch money to buy food at Palembang. This sketch is of the interior of the nurses hut. *Australian War Memorial ART29438*

'We are leaving tomorrow,' the note read. 'We think you will be moved too. Prepare for journey.'[18] The men had spent nine months carving their prison camp out of the jungle, and the women thought it was typical of their illogical captors to move them again.

The note gave some of the women hope that the war was over and that their internment was about to end. Others reasoned that the Allied forces were threatening Sumatra. But just about everyone was happy to leave Irenelaan, thinking that there could be no place worse.

The women were given permission to take anything movable, so Viv and the others busied themselves loading the old Japanese lorries with everything they could think of, including scraps of wire, old tins that could be used as cooking pots, bricks to build fireplaces, nails and stools and chairs that could be used for firewood. The piano had to stay but the lorries still looked like overloaded junk shops.[19]

If the women thought they would see some new and interesting sights after seventeen months of confinement at Irenelaan their hopes were dashed. The old lorries lumbered to a halt after just fifteen minutes at what would be forever called 'the Men's Camp'.

Immediately, the women knew that their change of circumstances was 'a bad bargain'.[20] The Men's Camp was situated in a low-lying, damp, unhealthy area that looked like a rubbish dump. Believing that the camp was being taken over for use by Japanese soldiers, the male prisoners had left it worse than a pigsty and stripped it bare of anything of any possible use to human beings.

Fully enclosed with barbed wire, the Men's Camp was about 100 metres long and 60 metres wide at one end, narrowing to 30 metres at the other. In the centre of the compound was an open space or *padang*. On each of the camp's four sides was a long barracks made of bamboo with open sides and a thatched roof of palm leaves. Each building consisted of two huts divided by a mud path. There were bamboo platforms on each side with a shelf above for the prisoners' belongings. There were sixty women to a hut and the bed space was just 50 centimetres wide by 168 centimetres long. Bugs, rats, lice and mosquitoes were constant companions for the prisoners.[21]

There were two communal bathrooms: one for the Dutch, and one for the British and Australians. Once again, fresh water was a problem but one of the women cut a hole in the bathroom roof to let the rain in. Lavatories were just one long cement drain with no privacy.

The roofs of the huts either leaked or blew off in heavy rain. On one stormy night, a short circuit started a fire in a beam and the roof was aflame until guards brought it under control. The roof of the kitchen was always catching fire.[22]

The Japanese had taken over the hospital in Palembang for their own use, and the Dutch nuns had been sent to the Men's Camp to establish a hospital there in one of the barracks, after asking the prisoners to squeeze in even tighter.

In addition to Dr Jean McDowell there were several other doctors, including Dr Goldberg, who had proved so difficult for the nurses on the raft after the sinking of the *Vyner Brooke*. The Australian nurses noted that while they were starving, she always seemed to have a good supply of money and always looked well fed, when even one of the camp's musical conductors, the esteemed Norah Chambers, had to sift rat droppings from rice to find enough for a small meal.[23]

Jean Ashton rostered ten nurses to help the nuns in the hospital, while the others, including Viv, were to tend to the rest of the camp. Some of the nurses found a large quantity of empty rice sacks and stuffed them with grass for the hospital patients to use as beds and pillows. They fashioned a cigarette tin into a lamp for the hospital, improvised a wick and filled it with red palm oil.

CHRISTMAS 1943 ARRIVED, and while they no longer had the work parties of male prisoners to serenade with carols, the women still concocted the best Christmas dinner they could from peanuts, bananas, a few onions and greens from the garden and a few scraps of meat.

Two days after Christmas, Miss Dryburgh gave the nurses one of the great gifts of their shattered lives when she announced what had been Norah Chambers' brainwave – a 'Vocal Orchestra' to give a prison-camp concert unlike anything any one of them had ever experienced.

The orchestra would do its best to replicate musical instruments with human voices. So, at 4.30 p.m. sharp on 27 December, after weeks of secret rehearsals, Norah led the thirty musicians to a sheltered area in the centre of the camp. Each carried paper in one hand and, as they were all too weak to stand throughout the whole performance, a little stool in the other.[24]

The audience sat in rows around them. Many of the prisoners had put on their best dresses while some had curled their children's hair in an effort to smarten them up for the concert.[25]

Three Australian nurses, Mickey Syer, Flo Trotter and Betty Jeffrey, were part of the orchestra, along with Shelagh Brown and Dorothy MacLeod, who had been part of the trio to first sing Miss Dryburgh's 'The Captives' Hymn'.[26] Also in the choir were some Dutch nuns, and British nurse Olga Neubronner, who had never really recovered from her miscarriage after the sinking of the *Vyner Brooke*.

Margaret Dryburgh, bespectacled and with her greying hair tied back, introduced the concert and requested that the audience close their eyes and imagine themselves in a better place. Then the Vocal Orchestra launched into Dvorak's 'Largo' from his *New World Symphony*.

Norah Chambers slowly raised her arms, paused momentarily and then with a sweeping movement stroked the air. A soft distant note, barely audible, rose and fell. Viv and the rest of the audience strained to hear it. The volume increased and the music carried them all away from the bonds of prison, at least in their imagination. Some said later they had never heard anything so beautiful before.[27]

Viv, sitting with her eyes closed, was swept up by the heavenly voices of her friends, who only a few hours before were downhearted prisoners of a brutal regime. The misery of camp life seemed to melt away as the orchestra and audience together soared with elation.[28]

Several guards arrived but rather than call a halt they stayed to listen to one of Mendelssohn's *Songs Without Words*, a Brahms waltz, 'Londonderry Air', Debussy's 'Reverie' and a Beethoven minuet.[29]

The program went without a hitch and concluded with 'Auld Lang Syne'.

That night, everyone forgot about the rats and the filth.[30]

By popular demand, the entire concert was repeated on New Year's Day and again at occasional intervals. More and more Japanese came to the concerts but although some roundly applauded the efforts of the prisoners they made no attempt to preserve the waning strength of the women with extra food or medical attention.[31]

Sadly the orchestra eventually had to disband. Just months later, more than half of the women who had made such soul-stirring music were dead.

Chapter 23

CAPTAIN KAZUO SEKI, a small hard-faced man with a malevolent stare and one permanently bloodshot eye,[1] assumed command of the Men's Camp on 1 April 1944. Seki was a product of a brutal Japanese military system that regarded prisoners as refuse.

He immediately insisted on a roll call of all his captives, so several hundred women and children formed a long snaking line on the *padang*. One by one they appeared before him, bowing politely – lest they receive a rifle butt in the face – before their names and ages were recorded. Jessie Simons thought it was interesting that some of the women were still sensitive about making their ages public, and a few had remained the same age after more than two years of captivity.[2]

Seki gave the prisoners a long speech, translated by interpreters into English, Dutch and Malay, in which he told them of Japan's glorious victories in the war. However, the nurses were sceptical of the captain's claims after he warned them that the camp may soon be bombed by Allied planes targeting the nearby Pladjoe oil refinery. In case the bombs started falling, the prisoners were organised into evacuation groups that would be housed in a nearby rubber plantation.

Following Seki's arrival, there was even less to eat. All the women were weighed and food was allocated on the basis of a collective average of how much was needed to keep all of the painfully thin prisoners alive.

The women were given injections to prevent typhoid, dysentery and cholera, but the Japanese seemed unconcerned that the prisoners were wasting away from hunger.

Food became even more scarce with the arrival of Malays and other locals in the service of the Japanese. The numbers in the camp swelled to more than 600 and overcrowding worsened.

The nurses would watch the Japanese unpack Red Cross parcels, help themselves to whatever they fancied, and then bring the leftovers to the camp some days later. Flo Trotter recalled that by the time the Red Cross gifts were divided among the whole camp 'each person got about one inch of chocolate ... a spoonful of coffee essence, a spoonful of butter, an inch of cheese, half a cup of powdered milk, a half-tin of jam, one small tin of meat and one of salmon for fifteen of us, a small packet of soup powder for three and twenty cigarettes.' It was still wonderful to taste real food, even in such tiny amounts, though. Those who didn't smoke were able to trade cigarettes for an egg, often rotten, or some gula jawa.[3]

Seki ordered the prisoners to cultivate large areas outside the camp and even the camp's *padang*, which had become like concrete due to the traffic of hundreds of feet. The digging was done with five-kilogram hoes called *chungkals* that many of the women had trouble lifting. The work went from 5 a.m. to 6 p.m., except for a break of about three hours during the hottest part of the day. The ground was so hard that the impact of the steel hoes on the earth jarred the women's bones all the way down to their toes. They planted sweet potatoes and tapioca and had to carry water all day from a pump about 500 metres down a steep hill. The captives were not allowed to keep any more than a litre of water a day for themselves, so every time the guards weren't looking they spat in water intended for the Japanese.[4]

SOME OF THE MOTHERS perished not long after their arrival at the new camp. Most had been forgoing their meagre rice ration, giving it instead to their hungry children. Once the women were hospitalised, the nurses had to force-feed them but most still succumbed to starvation.[5]

Mrs Frances Anderson, whose husband had been imprisoned at Changi in Singapore, had been a large, very keen golfer with a booming voice when the Japanese arrived at Penang. She had become desperately thin and frail on the camp's starvation diet and had died just before Seki took over. Sally Oldham, the little missionary from Manchester, died a few weeks later.

For nurses such as Viv, their days at the Men's Camp became the most morbid and depressing of the war, even considering the horrors they had already seen. Not only did they provide comfort for the dying but, after having endured so much together, they then had to prepare the bodies of their friends for burial and use a makeshift stretcher to help carry them to the cemetery just outside the camp.

Often in poor health themselves and constantly hungry, Viv and the other nurses had to dig the graves with the heavy *chungkals* in stifling humidity. Then they bowed their heads and listened as a nun prayed for the soul of the person going into the ground. Viv and the others would then have to carry the empty stretchers back to the camp, knowing that they would tread the same steps again before too long.[6]

Sometimes the Japanese would provide a truck to carry the dead to the cemetery, but not often. 'No woman died on her own,' Viv recalled later, 'but then, if the guards were not in the mood to bring in the coffin and the lorry to bury them, we would have to look after their corpses at night, fighting off the rats.'[7]

Even when requests were made for extra food for sick children, the Japanese would reply that there was plenty of room for them in the graveyard.[8]

Soon there were funerals every day. Two of the women in the camp made wooden crosses on which Norah Chambers would engrave with a hot-wire poker the names and dates of death.[9]

Viv recalled a time when she was mentally and physically spent after a day of death and despair. Sitting on the hospital's dirt floor in the dim light of the makeshift palm-oil lamp, she was watching over two very sick women laid out on bamboo platforms. One, a middle-aged woman, was dying. The other, a younger woman, was unconscious but might last another day. Viv took an old milk tin full of water, dipped a piece of cloth into it and wiped the brows of her two fading patients. She sat down on the floor again, contemplating her own mortality, but before long she detected a movement on the matting between the two women. At first she was puzzled by what she saw in the dim light, but when she realised what it was she almost vomited. A horde of lice were jumping off the older woman and scurrying to the younger one. Viv checked the older woman's pulse and heartbeat. The woman was dead. The lice had left the corpse in search of a new host.

Viv tried hard to cry in an effort to exorcise the gut-wrenching misery, but she was so sad that not even tears could comfort her. She had reached the lowest point of her life.[10]

FACE-SLAPPING AND PERVERSION by the guards continued unabated. They would watch and laugh as the women were forced to go to the toilet in front of them. Wilma Oram said that Seki 'let his guards do just what they liked to the women', and that one guard with the nickname Fatty 'derived pleasure from voyeurism and he was also one of the cruellest guards'.[11] Nesta James frequently saw women punched and slapped, and 'women with their teeth hanging out and faces blackened'.[12] Pat Blake had long slept with an iron bar near her bed because she never knew what might happen during the night.

Betty Kenneison knew all about that. Rags now covered her emaciated body and in place of shoes her feet were wrapped in leaves secured by jungle vines.[13] She had grown a pumpkin and tied it to her leg at night for safekeeping until it was ripe, but she had woken one morning to find the pumpkin gone.

At different times all the prisoners had to fight large camp rats for leftovers, but for a while a saviour arrived in the form of a beloved cat the nurses called 'Hitam', meaning 'black'. Hitam became a favourite of all the inmates, especially the children, as he waged war on the rodents before lolling on his back so the infatuated children could rub his belly. When some of the guards realised how attached the children had become to their precious pet, they kicked the cat to death.[14]

BY THE MIDDLE OF 1944, there were about 20,000 prisoners of war under guard on the Australian mainland. Among them were more than 2000 Japanese, more than 14,000 Italians, most of them from battles in North Africa, and about 1600 Germans, including those captured from the raider *Kormoran* after the sinking of HMAS *Sydney*.

The prisoners were well treated in accordance with the Geneva Convention, but at the Cowra prison camp, west of Sydney, there was constant angst among more than 1000 Japanese prisoners there who regarded their captivity as a source of shame. Despite being given adequate food, shelter, cigarette rations and even baseball bats for their leisure activities, the Japanese constantly plotted their escape.

Rumours of a move to a new prison camp at Hay, 400 kilometres to the south-west, ignited an already volatile situation.

At about 2 a.m. on 5 August Hajime Toyoshima, the fighter pilot captured on Melville Island after the bombing raid on Darwin, sounded a bugle.

Three huge gangs of prisoners, armed with knives, baseball bats, and clubs studded with nails. shouted 'Banzai', and began breaking through the camp's barbed-wire fences.

Privates Benjamin Gower Hardy and Ralph Jones began firing their No. 2 Vickers machine gun into the swarm of escapees but they were quickly overwhelmed and hacked to death.

Eventually 359 POWs escaped, although many took the opportunity of freedom to commit suicide soon after, apparently as a way to assuage their guilt at being captured.

Some of the escapees were shot dead by local civilians or soldiers, the luckier ones merely surrendered to farmers or police and went back to their prison.

All the survivors were recaptured within ten days of the breakout.

In the end the death toll stood at four Australian soldiers and 231 Japanese, including the bugler Hajime Toyoshima.[15]

ON THE NIGHT OF 11 AUGUST 1944, Viv was gently administering a damp cloth to the brow of a sick woman when a loud bang made her jump with shock. It sounded like a distant explosion. Several other bangs soon followed. Then there was an ear-piercing shriek, a sound Viv hadn't heard since the air-raid sirens in Singapore. At the sound of another explosion in the nearby jungle, Viv threw herself over her patient.

Allied aircraft were bombing the oil refinery as Seki had predicted, and a few of the bombs were missing the mark. Over the noise of the exploding bombs, the cheering from hundreds of women and children drowned out the frantic shouting of the guards. Viv sensed that deliverance was near. The bombing raid gave everyone hope, and it was the first morale booster the nurses had experienced since their capture.

Furious, Seki issued an order confining prisoners to their barracks during air raids. A few nights later, though, Mina Raymont and Val Smith were unable to curb their curiosity and watched with delight as the Japanese ran around the camp in frantic confusion, unsure of what to do under bombardment. A sergeant and a guard hauled Mina and Val before the commandant. One of the guards, a fiend the women called 'Rasputin', had seen a hole in the wall of their hut. The hole had been there before they entered the camp, but Mina and Val were accused of making it.[16]

Seki ignored pleas for mercy from the nurses, who told him that Mina not only had malaria but had developed a heart condition. He sentenced the two Australians to stand in the blistering heat all day without hats for as long as he deemed appropriate. 'Rasputin' slapped their faces hard, too, so their skin was red and swollen before the sunburn took effect.[17]

During the hottest part of the day, Mina's eyes turned up to the sky and she keeled over. Ignoring the guards waving their bayonets, Dr Goldberg and the nurses picked up their unconscious friend and carried her to the hospital. The other sisters took turns to stand beside Val Smith, and when she finally wilted at sunset, they carried her into the barracks and treated her for sunstroke.

Less than a week later, on 17 August, the nurses were playing bridge to mark Wilma Oram's twenty-eighth birthday when a wave of euphoria gripped them again. For the first time since their imprisonment, mail from home had arrived, and the Japanese, sensing they might need friends if this war continued to go badly for them, decided to share the good cheer.

For the first time in two and a half years, Viv heard from Eva, who, realising messages would be heavily scrutinised by the enemy, wished Viv a happy birthday and a merry Christmas and thanked her for her letter card.[18]

To Viv, the message was precious beyond words, and she and the other nurses celebrated the first evidence that their loved ones at home knew of their internment on Sumatra and of their survival after the *Vyner Brooke* catastrophe. Sadly, some of the loved ones back home still did not know what had happened to many of the nurses, including those who had perished beside Viv on Radji Beach.

While the letters from home were a fillip for all the nurses, only five of the thirty-two captives, including Viv, now weighed more than 50 kilograms, and they were getting thinner every day.

IN OCTOBER 1944, with thousands of Javanese prisoners being taken to Sumatra, Viv and her fellow internees were told to move again,[19] this time back across the Bangka Strait to Muntok. The resettlement of all the prisoners, to a camp a little further inland than the Coolie Lines, would stretch into November.[20]

Amid the flurry of activity before their departure, Viv and Wilma were flat out making stretchers to transport the many seriously ill patients. Then there was the desperate search for food to sustain them all on the journey as well as the gathering up of their personal belongings.

They were to travel on a series of dilapidated vessels that included at least one that was regarded as unseaworthy.

The ships crossed the Musi River and docked adjacent to Kertapati railway station where 240 Indonesian and Indo-Dutch internees plus some Dutch nuns were waiting.

The nurses were ordered to load everyone's luggage from the railway onto the ships, a move designed to humiliate them in front of the other prisoners. For several hours, Viv and the others struggled with the luggage of more than 250 people as the guards yelled at them and hit them on their legs with their sheathed swords.

When the women had finally finished loading the luggage, they were marched at the end of bayonets to load hundreds of sacks of rice from the locomotive up the gangways and onto the ships. Viv staggered under her load and Wilma was bent almost in two, but they did their best to block pain from their minds as, robot-like, they worked on and on into the night until finally, at 3 a.m., they collapsed in a weary heap on the deck of their barge.

After travelling 100 kilometres down the Musi River, Viv's barge arrived at Sungsang, where the nurses boarded an antiquated triple-decker ferry to join other vessels in crossing the Bangka Strait.

The boat carrying the hospital staff to Muntok was struck by a violent tropical storm that almost overturned the vessel.[21]

At Muntok, the prisoners were loaded onto a convoy of trucks and taken to their new camp on the outskirts of town. The health of the women was in freefall, but the accommodation was far more comfortable than the Men's Camp they had left behind at Palembang. There were six large huts, each capable of accommodating 140 people. They would have much more bed space, and because their hut was built on a rise, Viv and the others even had the benefit of a little sea breeze.[22] There were nine wells and the grounds were covered in gravel, which meant Viv and the other prisoners would no longer have to tramp through mud every time it rained. The Japanese had, however, disregarded normal health procedures and built the toilet pits and communal bathrooms alongside the kitchens.

The camp would eventually contain 700 prisoners and internees, of whom 150 were children.[23] Male prisoners from Palembang were now occupying Muntok's old Coolie Lines, and Captain Seki was in charge of both camps.

By the end of November many of the women were laid low with what was termed 'Bangka Fever', a mosquito-borne sickness that caused savage headaches, raging temperatures, skin eruptions and then unconsciousness, which in some cases led to death. John Gallagher Dominguez, the elderly mining engineer from Bright in Victoria, and Gerte his wife of forty years, died at separate camps at Muntok without being able to say goodbye. Mrs Mary Brown, the large English woman, was by now reduced to skin and bone and died on 17 January 1945.

Betty Jeffrey, Shirley Gardam, Mickey Syer, Jenny Greer and Mitz Mittelheuser had been taken to the camp's new hospital, which had a main ward capable of holding nineteen patients on one long platform made from rubber-tree branches lashed together.

There were four doctors responsible for the health of more than 700 inmates, and drugs were almost non-existent. At one stage, thirty-one out of the thirty-two Australian nurses had malaria, and although the Japanese now and then provided a few quinine tablets, the only treatment for most of the cases was to have the patient chew a bit of bark, said to have anti-malarial properties.[24] Many of the nurses also had different forms of beri-beri. Mavis Hannah and Jessie Simons complained that the beri-beri swelled their legs, while for others it accelerated heart rates and caused confusion and numbness in the limbs.

MINA RAYMONT HAD NEVER fully recovered from being forced to stand in the sun as punishment. And by the time the prisoners arrived back in Muntok, she had been seriously ill for quite a while. Her condition deteriorated quickly in the new camp, and she had little resistance left to fight cerebral malaria, the severe neurological complication of the infection. As her brain went haywire, she was gripped by seizures and abnormal behaviour.

Viv watched her friend dissolve physically and mentally and thought back tearfully to all the concerts and singalongs Mina had organised to boost morale, and how, when Mina and Wilma

Oram were rostered on night shift together, they would arrive at the hospital arm in arm and singing.[25] Viv remembered how, when her softly spoken, ever-smiling friend could no longer work in the garden to earn money for food, she sewed little handkerchiefs from scraps of material and traded them for food with Dutch civilians.

Viv and Wilma spent as much time at Mina's bedside as they could, as did Mina's great pal Val Smith. Lying on the hospital platform, Mina would slip in and out of consciousness as her swollen, infected brain induced agony and hallucinations. At times her high-pitched ranting and screaming continued for hours, making all in the camp wince. Mavis Hannah despaired that the illness had turned lovely, sweet Mina into a 'raving lunatic'.[26]

Her colleagues prayed for a fast, merciful end. So did Dr Goldberg, who found the screams confronting. 'Can't you shut her up?' she asked Viv one day.

'She can't stop,' Viv shot back. 'She doesn't even know she's doing it.'

'Well, I'll stop her if you won't,' Goldberg said, brushing Viv aside to deliver a vicious slap to Mina's face.

Viv and Wilma leapt to their feet. 'Don't ever do that again,'[27] Viv said menacingly.

The doctor left the room hurriedly as Mina's friends stood in front of her, defiant.

Mavis Hannah begged Captain Seki to give Mina anti-malarial medication, which the Japanese had withheld from the Red Cross parcels. Seki laughed and smacked Mavis across the face. His guard then hit her with his rifle.[28]

Lieutenant Wilhelmina Rosalie Raymont, of the 2/4th Casualty Clearing Station, died on 8 February 1945 at the age of thirty-three.

Val Smith was not with her friend when she died, and in her depressed, enervated state was plagued by feelings of guilt that she had deserted her pal when she was needed the most. For a long time, none of the nurses' assurances that Mina would not have known could relieve Val's depression.[29]

The camp cemetery was outside the barbed wire in a hillside clearing surrounded by thick jungle and gorgeous flowers. Here and there were Chinese and Malay markers, many fallen down, but in the few weeks since the internees had arrived, more and more wooden crosses were dotting the hillside and the track to the cemetery was becoming worn by constant traffic.

On the hot, humid morning after Mina died, the stronger of the nurses used their heavy *chungkal* hoes to dig her grave. Val Smith and others dressed Mina for burial and some of the other nurses pieced together some pieces of packing cases to make a coffin.

Viv and other nurses who had not lost their uniforms in the sinking of the *Vyner Brooke* retrieved these precious, carefully folded garments from their storage places and dressed as well as they could. Despite some of the clothing being torn and oil stained or, in Viv's case, having a bullet hole straight through it, they wanted to give Mina a proper military funeral.

The camp fell silent as three nurses either side of the coffin carried Mina up the hill to the old Chinese cemetery, with the rest of the nurses in the uniform of the Australian Army Nursing Service[30] following slowly, solemnly behind.

As they reached the prison gates the guards snapped to attention and removed their caps,[31] something they had never done before.

Mina was the first of the nurses in the Japanese camp to perish, but disease and sickness had a grip on all of them now. Soon Lieutenant Vivian Bullwinkel would be fighting for her own life again.

Chapter 24

BY FEBRUARY 1945 MANY of the surviving nurses weighed just 38 kilograms, and some were down to 32 kilos. Betty Jeffrey was so thin she could bend her elbow and span both her wrist and her upper arm with her finger and thumb.[1] The prisoners were able to scrounge a little goat meat from time to time, or some turtle eggs and turtle soup. But not enough. And disease was so prevalent that most did not have the strength to hold it off.

Sometimes, there were three funerals a day in the nurses' own circle of acquaintance. One woman saw four of her five children die within a week from the effects of malnutrition.[2]

The Japanese frequently made the comment 'plenty of room in the cemetery' when complaints were made about the lack of food and hygiene, but Jessie Simons would lament that even the cemetery was becoming overcrowded.[3]

On 20 February the once-bubbly Melbourne nurse Rene Singleton[4] died from dry beri-beri, the disease consuming her flesh from within as her body sought sustenance. Emaciated, almost beyond recognition save for her deep blue eyes, Rene was always hungry in camp. On the day she died she kept asking for 'more breakfast please'.[5] Viv lamented the loss of a woman who had done so much to help lift the spirits of all the others when they needed it. Rene died unaware that the two brothers she idolised, Douglas and Ken, had been killed within ten days of each other during heavy fighting in North Africa almost two years earlier.

Margaret Dryburgh delivered the eulogy at Rene's graveside, not far from Mina Raymont's plot. The coffins now were just pieces of ill-fitting wood pieced together with a few nails. They were filled with the body and as many flowers as the women could pick because the scraps of timber rarely fitted together and without the flowers covering the gaps in the wood, the body could be seen moving about on its way to the cemetery.

Completed coffins were stored at the back of the hut that Miss Dryburgh used as a church, and they cast an ominous shadow over the camp.

By early 1945, there were no more of Miss Dryburgh's concerts or charades or singalongs; the voices of the women were all too weak and there was no energy for enjoyment. A lack of rain meant the wells were dry and the tiny creek beside the camp was filthy. Olga Neubronner, the British nurse who survived the sinking of the *Vyner Brooke* and a miscarriage after reaching land, died on 2 March.

'The mud and heat and mosquitoes of Palembang are preferable to this,' Betty Jeffrey wrote. 'We are told [Bangka] Island is known as Dead Man's Island.'[6] Several of the civilian internees were so weak that they collapsed in the latrines and fell through the slats.

Feisty, hardworking Blanche Hempsted died on 19 March, a victim of malnutrition and beri-beri. She told a friend sitting with her that she was sorry for all the trouble her sickness had caused for the others, and she apologised for taking so long to die.[7]

CAPTAIN SEKI TOLD THE prisoners they would be moving yet again, but Viv knew that many of the prisoners would be too frail to survive another arduous journey. From the description of the new camp, located across the Bangka Strait and near the city of Lubuklinggau (formerly Loeboek Linggau) in the southern Sumatran jungle, it seemed to Viv an ideal place for the Japanese to kill all their prisoners in secret, and bury the evidence in the jungle.

On 4 April Viv was feeding what remained of Shirley Gardam from a small bowl of rice. Shirley could hardly speak but she told Viv a little about the beauty around her home in Tasmania. Suddenly she raised her head, let out a sharp cry, then fell back. Shirley, who played the piano so beautifully, had died unaware that her mother had passed away three years earlier. She had a passion for flowers, and the other nurses covered her body and her coffin with as many petals as they could before lowering her into the ground beside the other nurses.

By now the women were so weak it took twenty of them to carry a coffin to the cemetery. Three poles were placed under the coffin and eighteen people lifted the poles. One person led, holding her hands behind to steady the coffin and keep an eye on the track. The end of the coffin was supported by the twentieth person, to avoid any risk of it slipping.

Pat Gunther recalled:

> The funeral services were carried out most correctly by the missionaries and nuns, while we ragged remnants of humanity stood with bowed heads. The burials took place any time after 3 p.m. The usual 'Sumatra' – a noisy electric storm – frequently blew up as we finished filling in the graves.[8]

In the few months they had been back on Bangka Island, a hundred of the 700 internees had died. Margaret Dryburgh no longer had the voice to perform the eulogies.

On 8 April, four days after Shirley's death, about 200 women were packed in trucks and set out on the two-day journey to the new prison in Sumatra. Half of the Australian nurses, including Viv, went with them in the first convoy.

The trucks roared to the long pier at Muntok at breakneck speed, sending the frail women flying all about as they hung on for what was left of their dear lives. Viv and other nurses had to then tote stretchers carrying sick women for the length of what seemed an endless jetty as Japanese crews manning the new anti-aircraft guns at Muntok watched their struggles dispassionately.

When they reached the end of the jetty, the nurses gently placed their stretcher cases down and walked back to pick up more patients. While they were doing this, one of the stretcher cases died and the nurses had to dig a shallow grave for her in the foul-smelling mud under the wharf. When the rest of the stretcher cases were delivered to the end of the pier, the guards loaded all the prisoners onto a coastal steamer for the next leg of the journey.

It took the best part of a day to make the crossing, during which time eight of the sick died and were buried at sea.[9] Their bodies were simply rolled over the side, a task the Japanese would not help the women do. Since they had no weights to sink the bodies in the water, the dead floated along beside the ship for a while in a ghoulish procession.[10]

After anchoring overnight at the mouth of the Musi River, the 'lumbering old tub'[11] moved upstream at first light and docked at Palembang just before noon. The prisoners were then transferred to a waiting train, with stretcher cases in the cattle trucks and the others crammed into carriages thick with black coal dust. The engine had not arrived, and the Japanese made the prisoners wait all day and into the night in stifling conditions. Dysentery was so bad that the women and children had to use a ditch beside the train tracks to relieve themselves in full view of the curious locals.[12]

The train was still parked as the mosquitoes arrived after dark. Finally the engine appeared and with a jolt and a hiss of escaping steam they began to move. As the train gathered speed, Viv, exhausted, tried to stay awake to see where they were going. The train sped through thick forest, past the 3000-metre volcano Mount Dempo, over an upper tributary of the Musi and then through a series of hillside tunnels.

Thirty-four hours after leaving Bangka Island, Viv and the others reached the end of the line. The trip was just too much for many of the patients, including the marvellous Miss Dryburgh, who died in her new prison camp on 21 April. Mrs Evelyn Madden, whose husband had died in her arms after the sinking of the *Vyner Brooke*, and who had constantly circulated rumours about the imminent release of the prisoners, died the following day, still unrescued. Miss Dryburgh's musical offsider Margery Jennings succumbed two weeks later.

HAVING SUFFERED ONE crushing setback after another, the Japanese forces now resorted to kamikaze attacks on the unstoppable American navy, their pilots deliberately turning their aircraft into missiles and flying them into United States warships. These suicide missions, sometimes carried out by teenagers, had intensified as the Allies loomed over the Japanese island of Okinawa.

American firebombs rained down on Japanese cities for a year, laying waste to a large part of the nation and killing as many as 900,000 civilians. In one bombing raid in March 1945, American aircraft dropped massive loads of cluster bombs onto the densely populated wooden homes of Tokyo using highly flammable napalm. A fifth of Tokyo was left a smouldering wreck with more than 100,000 confirmed dead, many of them burned alive. And still the Japanese warlords drove their people on, insisting they fight to the last man. In North Borneo, almost 2500 Australian prisoners of war, victims of beatings, starvation and disease, would die on a series of forced marches from the Sandakan POW camp to the town of Ranau 250 kilometres away.

For Viv and her fellow prisoners in the Sumatran jungle, the fight for survival was harder than ever. At dawn, the day after their arrival at their remote outpost, the prisoners were taken on trucks down a narrow dirt road for 25 kilometres to an abandoned rubber plantation at a place called Belalau.[13]

In what they regarded as their most primitive camp yet, most of the Australians were confined to a series of poorly built huts with leaky thatched roofs and dirt floors on a hill overlooking a shallow creek. There were no bathrooms, so the women would have to bathe in the creek in full view of the guards. There were no doors on the toilet boxes, either, though mercifully they had been placed downstream from where water was taken for the kitchen.

The inmates supplemented their meagre rice ration with grass and ferns from the creekbank. Occasionally they were tossed scraps of deer, bear and, once, some monkey. Each of the nurses had received two pieces of monkey the size of dice.[14] There were banana and pawpaw trees outside the camp, but the prisoners were beaten if they tried to take any.[15]

By May 1945,[16] most of the nurses had made out a will, largely in part to stop the guards from confiscating their possessions after death, since the Japanese at least had an appreciation for formal legal documents.

The nurses were unaware of all the Japanese setbacks or that, on 30 April, Adolf Hitler and his wife had killed themselves in a Berlin bunker with the Russian Red Army on their doorstep. Nor did they know that, on the following day, the new Reich Chancellor Joseph Goebbels and his wife murdered their six children before committing suicide, hastening an end to the war in Europe.

While the wheels were falling off the war machines of Germany and Japan, more and more of the prisoners were also falling at the finish line. In the camp hospital at Belalau, women lay on long benches with no means to isolate those with contagious diseases. Unhygienic conditions that appalled the nurses had to be accepted now as inevitable.

Some of the women sold the few possessions they had left in a bid to buy food. The deeply religious Chris Oxley sold four back teeth on a gold bridge to stay alive.[17] Young women, aged well beyond their years by their privations, lay haggard and emaciated in the last stages of exhaustion.

One of the most pathetic cases in the hospital was a poor Dutch woman who had become mentally ill from all her terrible experiences. Long before she was interned with the Australians, her husband, dying of starvation in solitary confinement, had been unmercifully beaten by the Japanese. The guards said they would take the woman to see him. She thought he had recovered, but the shock of seeing her husband's starved, battered, naked body lying in a crude coffin was too much to bear.[18]

Little Betty Kenneison was admitted to the primitive camp hospital on a day heavy with humidity and growling thunder. She was semi-conscious and desperately ill with fever and dysentery. Viv bathed the teenager's wasted body but knew that, without drugs, her little friend would almost certainly die too. Over the next few days, Viv carefully nursed Betty and shared some of her meagre food. While Betty was fighting her illness, the woman to the right of her died, and with her tired eyes Betty watched as the body was picked up and placed in a flimsy coffin. As the coffin was being lifted a plank came loose at its base and the dead woman's head flopped out. Betty was not afraid, though. She had seen worse things in the camps.[19] A nun gently tucked the woman's head back into the coffin and held the crude box together as best she could.

While Betty was still in the hospital, another of the nurses, New Zealand–born Gladys Hughes, who was always coming up with new cooking ideas to make the camp muck more palatable,[20] perished on 31 May 1945. Her friends suspected that her heart simply gave out because she despaired at ever being released.

Betty eventually left the hospital but the conditions for the prisoners were so toxic, Viv feared that she would soon have a relapse. As it turned out, it was Viv whose health collapsed.

WILMA ORAM WANTED Betty to see Viv one last time before Viv died. It was June 1945 and Viv had been battling beri-beri and malaria for weeks, which had left her on the edge of the abyss.

Knowing how close Betty and Viv were, Wilma sought out the teenager and told her Viv had been in and out of hospital and her chances of survival were slim. Five of the nurses in the camp had already passed away and it looked like Viv would be number six. Wilma had given Viv Epsom salts supplied by Chris Oxley but was desperate to secure some limes for her friend, thinking that the Vitamin C might save her.[21] There were no limes in the camp and even if there were, no one had any money to pay for them now.

Betty promised she would do everything to help her friend. Having just recovered from her own close call with illness, she ran off on her skinny legs in search of a woman trader in the camp known as 'The Half-Baked Banker', who exchanged jewellery, money and promissory notes for food and other goods.[22] Betty had a gold bangle on her arm and she knew that it was real currency. Her mother had given her two bangles before the war, but Betty had already sold one for food. She had carefully disguised the remaining bangle with tar and mud to hide its value from both the prisoners and guards.

Betty pleaded the case in the Banker's hut but was turned away as limes were nowhere to be found. The Japanese had recruited Javanese guards at Belalau, and now Betty thought she might have some success with one of them.

Hidden behind a hut close by the perimeter Betty took off the bangle and cleaned and polished it so that it looked its best. She waited for a guard who had shown mercy to the prisoners and who she believed might actually trade food for the bangle rather than steal it from her.

She was right. A deal was done. The guard took the bangle and brought back twelve limes that Betty delivered to a grateful Wilma as Viv slipped in and out of consciousness. Using the precious limes to revive Viv, Wilma and the other sisters cared for their friend until she slowly began to pull through.

Smiling widely despite her exhaustion, Viv told her teenage saviour: 'Little Bet, you helped save my life.'[23]

Viv wanted to preserve Betty's life too. Betty later explained:

When [Viv] found out that I was detailed on the burial squad she went to Mrs Hinch [the British spokesperson for the prisoners]. The Japanese in the end wouldn't let us go out and bury our dead. They had special days, so they piled up the dead bodies perhaps for a couple of weeks. The whole place stunk of death, and so when I went to pick up the dead bodies the decayed flesh just left the torso and the bones. Viv, as sick as she was, said, 'No, you're not going on that squad', and Mrs Hinch listened to her and I was detailed to another squad.[24]

Thanks largely to her youth, Viv recovered more quickly than most of the patients, but when she picked up a mirror and began to comb the hair on the left side of her head, the hair came away with the comb. Before the war she would have cried hysterically, but now she was just glad to still be breathing.

JOHN CURTIN DID NOT LIVE to see the end of the war in the Pacific, but he did live long enough to see Hitler's fantasy of a thousand-year Reich of German rule in Europe end in ruins. Curtin was just sixty when he died in Canberra on 5 July 1945 from a stress-related heart attack, as Australia's 7th Division began its last operation to liberate Borneo from the Japanese.

Ten days later, on 15 July 1945, Win Davis, one of the youngest of the nurses and much loved by all, died despite Pat Gunther scrounging potatoes and eggs to feed her.[25] 'Win had so much to live for,' Betty Jeffrey said, 'she wanted so badly to have six sons.'[26]

American forces hastened the Japanese capitulation when they virtually obliterated the Japanese city of Hiroshima with an atomic blast on 6 August, the first time a nuclear bomb had been used in warfare.

The following day, Russia declared war on Japan and went on to take much of the territory in China that the Japanese had swept through a decade earlier. Among the soldiers failing miserably to hold off the Red Army was one Major Orita Masaru, the man who had ordered the massacre of the nurses on Radji Beach.

As the Japanese military collapsed, Rene Singleton's best friend, Dot Freeman,[27] died suddenly in hospital on 8 August.[28] Dot had been fading for days and while chatting softly with Flo Trotter over a cup of tea suddenly curled into the foetal position, closed her eyes and breathed her last.

The next day a second American nuclear bomb was dropped on the city of Nagasaki.

Seventy thousand people were killed instantly and 70,000 more injured. The killing was indiscriminate. Husband and wife, old man and baby, pacifist and warmonger were all consumed by a 3000-degree wave of energy.

At least eight prisoners of war working as slave labour in the city, including one Englishman and seven Dutchmen, were killed, but all twenty-four Australian prisoners somehow survived in their camp 1700 metres from the epicentre of the Nagasaki blast.

With other Japanese cities under threat of further apocalyptic fires, Emperor Hirohito issued a radio broadcast announcing the surrender of Japan on 15 August 1945.

The news had still not reached Belalau three days later when one of the most popular of the Australian nurses, Pearl 'Mitz' Mittelheuser, died covered in an old dry sack used to keep her warm against the malarial chills.[29] Her best friend Sylvia Muir was with her when she died, but Sylvia was so dehydrated that she couldn't cry, only wail. Of the sixty-five sisters who left Singapore on the *Vyner Brooke* there were now only twenty-four alive and many of them were in hospital. Pat Blake was now so sick she didn't notice that a rat had gnawed off the end of one of her toes.

Some of the Dutch and Eurasian women who, according to Jessie Simons, were 'over friendly with the Japanese' now began whispering to others that the war was over.[30]

Some of the children were allowed to visit their fathers in a nearby men's camp. The women and children only discovered which men were still alive when the Japanese read out a list of the children who could *not* go.[31]

Rumours persisted about an Allied victory, but no one in the camp knew what to believe, even though the guards held a raucous party in their quarters on 21 August. The next morning, Viv was in the creek bathing with a number of women who convinced her that the war was finished. Excitedly, Viv picked up her faded top and shorts and rushed up the hill to see if the other nurses could confirm the news. No one was sure of anything.

Two days went by before Captain Seki ordered that all the prisoners assemble before him at 3 p.m. on 24 August. To make sure everyone attended he sent the guards around the camp with long sticks, though many prisoners were too sick to move.

On the parade ground, Viv and a small gathering of others looked like the living dead, dressed in tattered clothes, some barely able to stand, most unsteady on their legs. They watched the small commandant climb onto a table so a hundred or so prisoners, many barely alive and some about to die, could see him.

Seki was dressed in a pair of badly patched baggy trousers and a crumpled tunic that was tight around his middle. Behind him was a sea of banana and rubber trees. He looked exhausted as though he had been up all night, but he puffed out his chest and spoke quickly in Japanese. He waited while an interpreter relayed his speech in Malay. The interpreter was soon literally lost for words, and a Dutch woman pushed him aside to continue the translation in both Malay and English.

'Now there is peace,' Seki said in Japanese, 'and we will all soon be leaving Sumatra.'

Viv stood in stunned silence. No one cheered or clapped. They were just glad the nightmare was ending, and they hoped they and their friends in the hospital would live long enough to be liberated.

'If we have made any mistakes in the past,' Seki continued, 'we hope you will forgive us. Americano and English will be here in a few days. Now we will be friends.'[32]

Viv had news for him.

Chapter 25

THERE WAS LITTLE EMOTION from Viv and the rest of the nurses after Captain Seki's announcement. Jessie Simons sat under a rubber tree and cried for half an hour. She had heard a rumour that the Japanese were planning to shoot all the prisoners until the atomic bombs changed everything.[1]

Most of the prisoners, though, too weak to make a fuss, greeted the end of the war with stunned relief.[2] But until help and food arrived, all twenty-four of the nurses still feared joining their friends in the cemetery.

The Japanese released the pathetically thin men and boys from the male camp, and the women whose loved ones were still alive welcomed these frail, skeletal survivors with open arms. Some of the men and boys stumbled around on weary legs looking forlornly for their mothers or wives, only to be told the heartbreaking news.

The men took over the running and repairs of the camp, and a Dutchman appointed himself to organise the camp kitchen.[3]

After three years of cruelty, the women now experienced old-fashioned manners, the male former prisoners rising whenever one of the nurses shuffled into a room.

At home in Adelaide, Eva Bullwinkel cried tears of joy that the war was over. She had just written to Viv, hoping that the letter would eventually reach her. She wrote that Viv's friend Zelda Treloar had married an engineer named Alex West, and that Viv had been named godmother of their new daughter Helen.

Eva still knew nothing of the massacre on Radji Beach or the other horrors Viv had seen.

25 Blyth Street
Fullarton
Adelaide. South Australia
21st August 1945
My Darling Darling Viv,
I do not know where or how or when you will receive this but I hope it will be soon.

Oh my dear, my dear how lovely it is to know you and the other girls will all soon be free and able to come home. I am hoping and praying that you have come through the long ordeal safe and in good health … It is needless for me to say how John and I are longing for the day we will be able to welcome you home …

Mrs Drummond, although she knows Irene is not with you, is anxious about you girls as anyone. John is well and back in the bank but he is a very lucky boy to be alive …

His fighter plane was shot down in the Middle East about 8 a.m. on the 26th of October 1942. It was in flames and he had to make a parachute descent. He was severely injured as he left the plane, one leg between the knee and ankle was badly broken, a compound fracture. The other leg was badly gashed and he also had a burnt wrist, three broken ribs and one hip and ankle badly sprained. I guess that happened when he hit the ground. He was numb to the hips whilst he was coming down so he didn't feel the landing. Luckily he came down just inside our own lines manned by South Africans. Seeing he was badly injured some men raced across to him. A doctor was in attendance almost immediately.

John was in hospital in Alexandria for a month and then sent to Palestine for two months. He came home on the hospital ship [*Oranje*] a cot case and arrived in Australia at the end of February 1943. He was twenty months in

hospital and he has made a remarkable recovery and has
been back at the bank for thirteen months …

With all my love as usual, I cannot wait to see you again.
Your loving mother.[4]

A SEARCH OF THE JAPANESE quarters revealed that all the
supplies that the dead nurses had needed had been available the
whole time, along with the Red Cross parcels the guards had kept
for themselves.

The nurses were still ravenously hungry, even though their
food supplies had increased. A pair of old shorts would now buy
half a dozen eggs from the local people, and a metre of material
was worth four or five fowls.[5] Jessie Simons swapped a pair of
boots for a chicken. She was so hungry that she cut its throat
carefully to catch the blood for frying later.[6]

Viv and Betty Jeffrey joked about having a holiday in London
some time when snow was falling. Viv had always wanted to
see the places where her father had lived and meet her English
relatives. They called their dream 'Viv and Bet in Wonderland'.[7]

On 7 September, two weeks after Captain Seki's announcement, the first of the Allied soldiers reached Belalau. They were
sickened by what they saw.

Just before Japan's surrender, South African–born Major
Gideon 'Jake' Jacobs of the Royal Marines, along with two
Australian radio experts, a Dutchman and a Chinese-Javanese
soldier, had parachuted from a Catalina flying boat over Sumatra
into what was still Japanese occupied territory. The Dutchman
was Albert Happy Plesman,[8] the son of the man who in 1919
founded KLM Royal Dutch Airlines.

Their mission was to send intelligence back to Lord
Mountbatten's South-East Asian Command. After Japan
surrendered, they were ordered to make contact with Japanese
military authorities regarding the surrender of their troops,
a dangerous assignment since they were unsure whether the
thousands of Japanese troops on the island were really willing
to throw down their guns. Soon some former internees shocked

Jacobs with information about the death and misery in the prisoner-of-war camps throughout Sumatra.

Jacobs and his men began touring the island, collecting evidence of Japanese atrocities. When they reached Palembang, the Japanese told them that they had visited all the camps, and there was nothing more to see. But Jacobs began investigating reports about a remote camp at Lubuklinggau and accounts from Stoker Ernest Lloyd and others about the murder of Australian nurses on Radji Beach.

Jacobs immediately flew to Lahat with his men, then drove about 150 kilometres to Lubuklinggau, where his two Australian offsiders, sergeants Gillam and Bates, established a radio base to transmit news to their headquarters in Colombo.

At mid-afternoon on 7 September, Jacobs, the Dutch paratrooper Happy Plesman and the Chinese soldier known as Tjoeng drove into Belalau. Jacobs said it was the most appalling camp he had visited, which was really saying something. When he had earlier confronted Colonel Sada, commandant at Si Rengo Rengo in North Sumatra over his cruelty to prisoners, Sada had drawn his sword and fallen on it in a ritual suicide.[9]

On 9 September, Jacobs' two Australian radio operators sent this message to their headquarters in Colombo.

*HAVE ENCOUNTERED AMONG 250 REPEAT
250 BRITISH FEMALE INTERNEES IN
LOEBUKLINGGAU CAMP SISTER NESTA JAMES
AND 23 OTHER SURVIVING MEMBERS OF
THE AUSTRALIAN ARMY NURSING SERVICES
REMNANTS OF CONTINGENT AANS EVACUATED
FROM MALAYA IN VYNER BROOKE STOP IN
VIEW OF THEIR PRECARIOUS HEALTH SUGGEST
YOU ENDEAVOUR ARRANGE AIR TRANSPORT
DIRECT TO AUSTRALIA FROM HERE SOONEST
STOP AM COLLECTING PARTICULARS
MASSACRE OF MEMBERS AANS ON BANGKA
ISLAND FOR LATER TRANSMISSION.[10]*

Two days later, Jacobs returned to Belalau with Bates and Gillam. Viv was the first to see them, along with the Australian military badges on their berets. Breathlessly she rushed to tell the others: 'The Australians … The Australians are here!'[11]

The horrendous appearance of the women so enraged Gillam that he lined Japanese guards along the barbed-wire fence of the camp and threatened to shoot them all. Jacobs ran up to him and promised that the Japanese would pay for their cruelty through war-crimes trials.

Three days later, after Jacobs organised a food drop by a Liberator aircraft from the RAF air base on the Cocos Islands, Viv and the other nurses ate bread and Vegemite. Liberators began flying over regularly, dropping bandages, quinine, vitamin tablets, serums, powdered milk, fresh vegetables, towels, washbasins and mosquito nets.

A Japanese doctor came to the camp saying he wanted to undo at least some of the damage caused by his military masters. Butter

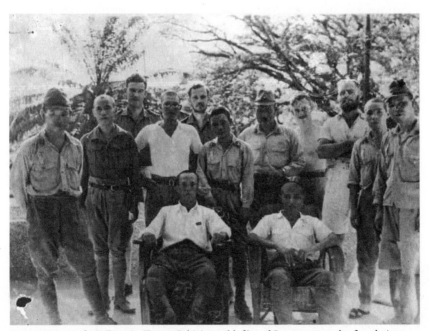

Camp commandant Captain Kazuo Seki (seated left) and Japanese guards after their surrender to Allied forces in August 1945. Seki received a fifteen-year jail sentence for his cruelty. *Muntok Peace Museum*

and sugar arrived in abundance and the nurses creamed the two ingredients and ate the concoction until they could stomach no more. Japanese guards gave many of their former prisoners their uniforms to wear and Chris Oxley was able to buy back her four back teeth on the gold bridge.

The Japanese were doing all they could to make the women look as healthy as possible before more avenging Allies arrived.

Then, on 15 September, while the nurses were plucking ducks and other fowl in preparation for a birthday party for one of the civilian internees, they received a message relayed by telephone to prepare for immediate evacuation. Feathers flew everywhere.

Viv and the other nurses made their difficult, sobbing farewells to so many with whom they had survived so much for so long. They had an emotional goodbye party and the Charitas nuns sang a Dutch farewell.

The evacuation of the nurses had been organised in part by the dogged Haydon Lennard,[12] the chief war correspondent for the Australian Broadcasting Commission and British Broadcasting Commission in the Pacific and Asia. He had been intrigued by the fate of the *Vyner Brooke* and had intensified his search for the lost nurses ever since reports filtered through that Jake Jacobs was on their trail. Lennard had heard from two officers, including Sydney solicitor Bill Tebbutt, who had been in Singapore's Changi jail, that there had been a massacre of nurses on Bangka Island and that there had been just one survivor.[13] Another inmate knew the nurses had been in Palembang because some were wearing their uniforms during a change of prison.

Lord Mountbatten approved the RAAF sending Lennard into remote Sumatra. Lennard organised a blanket censorship on the operation in case the Japanese decided to bury all the evidence of their atrocities.

There was no trace of the nurses at Palembang but at Lahat, about 220 kilometres south-west Lennard and his Adelaide pilot, Flying Officer Ken Brown, learned the women had been moved by train a further 140 kilometres north-west of Lahat, to Lubuklinggau. Brown declared the airfield at Lahat capable of accommodating a Douglas Dakota military transport plane. The news was relayed by telephone to Palembang and a call made to the women's prison to have the Australians and the most ailing of the women to be immediately airlifted to Singapore on two Dakotas.

Lennard demanded that the Japanese place a special train and a fleet of cars at their disposal. Just before daylight on 16 September, he and Brown arrived at Lubuklinggau, where they commandeered a Japanese truck at the rail terminal. They sloshed along a muddy track through the jungle to Belalau. They were horror-struck by what was waiting for them.

Brown recalled that even three weeks after the nurses had started receiving nourishment and better care, they were still 'in a terrible condition', and that the smell was 'unbelievable'.[14] For the rest of her life, when Betty Jeffrey wrote to Brown she signed her name 'Stinky'.[15]

Brown said Seki looked like the most ruthless man he had ever seen and that he and Lennard were 'the most welcome guests these poor souls had seen for many a day and they did not fail to show it'.[16]

A group of sixty-two women and children[17] were ready to leave when the first vehicles bumped through the jungle to the camp before dawn. Viv and the twenty-three other Australian nurses were proudly dressed in what remained of their uniforms, hers with the bullet hole just above the waistline. The nurses had insisted that the desperately sick should be evacuated first, so before they began their journey, thirty-eight British women and children were first helped aboard trucks and cars for the drive through pouring rain back to the train terminal.

Then the nurses, literally on their last legs, began boarding their vehicles.

Lennard noted that some were suffering badly from beri-beri, with their knees and legs hopelessly swollen and skin yellow. All they could do was shuffle towards the carriages. Joyce Tweddell had lost almost 40 kilograms since her capture and now weighed little more than 30 kilos.[18] Before the food stores had been liberated, she was probably just hours from dying. Betty Jeffrey weighed just 30 kilograms and was suffering from tuberculosis.

Viv, though, despite the same privations and an old bullet wound, was positively Amazonian by comparison, at just over 50 kilograms.[19] Her youth, athleticism and strong constitution had seen her fare much better than most of the other nurses.

Her heart was torn as she said goodbye to Little Bet Kenneison, who was now seventeen but so tiny and thin she looked like a small child. Viv choked up as she told Little Bet how grateful she was for saving her life with those limes and that she would never forget the friendship they had forged through their struggles.

Betty began to cry, the tears streaming down her thin face. Viv wiped them away and said they would meet again. They embraced for what seemed an eternity before it was time to go. Betty raised her scrawny arm to wave farewell for what she feared would be the last time.[20]

Though hobbling, Viv was among the healthiest of the prisoners. She insisted she could walk unaided to the vehicles but Lennard still helped her. As the nurses left that place of torment, one of the guards sneered in passable English, 'You might've won the war but we'll get Australia yet.'[21]

Viv saw Seki standing by the gate, scowling. The nurses flung a few rude words at the deposed commandant but as the cars and trucks trundled through the gates of Hell, most just smiled with relief at their release.

At Lubuklinggau, the women were helped onto the train by Lennard and his team. Happy Plesman had raided the station's café and gave all the women and children cakes for the journey to Lahat.

The train pulled out of Lubuklinggau at 8 a.m. to the cheers of Allied men and what Betty Jeffrey called 'the most horrible expressions of hatred' by the vanquished Japanese.

The four-hour train journey to Lahat was made through rough and muddy jungle in a tropical downpour, but Lennard said, 'even the stretcher cases would have walked; they were so overjoyed at their liberation'.[22]

'We outfitted one carriage of the train with mattresses, pillows, and sheets, which we had commandeered from the Japanese,' Lennard wrote. 'Five of the evacuees were critically ill.'[23]

Acting as both a nurse and reporter, Lennard fielded questions from all the women about the end of the war, the atomic bombs, what was happening at home, and whether or not Curtin was still prime minister. He listened intently as Viv told him about Radji Beach and thought Viv spoke levelly and unemotionally about a story of survival that was 'epic'.[24]

The nurses arrived in Lahat at midday. There had been a last-minute hitch and only one Dakota was coming. It had been delayed by a blown tyre when landing at Palembang, and it could only accommodate thirty or so passengers, so half the freed prisoners were provided beds as they waited a day for the next flight.

Viv and the other nurses, along with seven stretcher cases, were taken to Lahat airstrip where they lay on the grass under some large, shady trees, waiting for the aircraft.

Late in the afternoon, Viv heard a drone and all the nurses hushed. They scanned the sky for the approaching plane, and before long the bright afternoon sun caught the aircraft's huge wings, which glistened as the Dakota swung in to land.

There were cheers all around as Squadron Leader Fred Madsen brought the plane down between groves of palm trees and onto the Lahat runway. As the Dakota rolled towards the weary, waiting passengers, Madsen cut the motors.

A door swung open and a tall, slim Australian army medical officer, Major Harry Windsor, jumped down ahead of three nurses in tropical blouses and grey slacks. At the sight of the handsome doctor some of the nurses swooned despite their weakened condition.

Windsor had photographs of the prisoners for identification but none of this pathetic group looked anything like their studio portraits. 'Where are the Australian nurses?' he asked the ragged mob.

The women accompanying Windsor were the Australian military's Matron-in-Chief, Colonel Annie Sage,[25] her assistant,

Sister Jean Floyd, and Flight Sister Beryl Chandler of the RAAF's No. 2 Medical Air Evacuation Transport Unit. Sister Floyd had escaped Singapore on the *Empire Star*. Sister Chandler had trained with many of the Brisbane nurses, including Flo Trotter. Even in her enervated state, the skeletal and devoutly Christian Flo tut-tutted about her saviours wearing slacks instead of the regulation skirts she was used to and wondered what the army was now coming to.[26]

Sister Chandler was appalled by the condition of most of the women but pleasantly surprised by the appearance of 'a tall fair-haired nurse with her hair cut in a kind of "Eton crop"'. She said Viv had the brightest of smiles and that, despite having been shot on Bangka Island and enduring years of abuse, had retained 'such a bright personality'.[27]

Dr Windsor believed that at least five of the nurses would not have survived another week in internment and was so outraged by their appearance that he officially recommended that all of the Japanese involved in their treatment be forthwith 'slowly and painfully butchered'.[28]

Matron Sage told the Australians that she had been determined to find them ever since the sinking of the *Vyner Brooke*. Trying to hold her emotions in check as she surveyed this group of barely alive women, she spluttered, 'I am the mother of you all.'

Then she did a head count of the twenty-four nurses. 'Where are the rest of you?' she asked.[29]

Chapter 26

THE LAST TIME VIV was in Singapore there had been explosions, fires, machine-gunning, screams and misery, but this time, as the Dakota banked over the city, Viv felt only a sense of calm reassurance.

Madsen brought the plane down on the city's airfield at dusk on 16 September. On landing, the nurses were assisted into a private room at the airport, where they were met with tea and biscuits by the Australian Red Cross, as well as journalists pressing them for their stories and photographers blinding them with their flash-bulbs. Some of the Australian soldiers watching on wept openly at the sight of the emaciated women with bulging eyes and arms like sticks.

Some of the nurses found this press briefing confronting, and most were more interested in a decent meal and a hot bath than reliving their horror experiences.

Viv had already told war correspondent Haydon Lennard her story of what happened on Radji Beach and she repeated it here to other reporters. It was at odds with some of the details provided by witnesses such as Stoker Lloyd and Eric Germann, who had seen the mutilated bodies of the nurses.

She backed up Pat Blake's story to one reporter about the 'officers' club' at Irenelaan and how the nurses had escaped working there. Pat, who was keen to marry her long-time fiancé when she returned home, insisted that while none of the nurses were molested, the Japanese were 'fiendishly ingenious in discovering ways to humiliate us'.[1] Many of the nurses were planning to marry and have families, and given social mores of the times none would have wanted such things as sexual assault made public.

Years later, Mavis Hannah revealed that, in the prison camps, 'we never menstruated because we'd lost so much weight. I suppose it was nature's way of preserving us … Dr McDowell had said to me … "If anything happens to you and [you] become pregnant, I'll see what I can do." I don't suppose we would have become pregnant anyway. We weren't menstruating.'[2]

For his first report to Australia on the massacre of the nurses, Haydon Lennard quoted Viv's recollection of the murders on Radji Beach as follows:

The Japanese took out tommy-guns, set up a machine-gun, and ordered us into the sea. There was no mistaking their vicious intentions, so we ran madly into the waves. When we were thigh deep in the surf they opened up a murderous fire, mowing us down like a scene I saw in a film as a child. The women around me shrieked, stiffened, and sank. I was hit here, in the left side, under the ribs, falling unconscious in the water. I can't swim a stroke, I can't even float, but somehow I felt my body being washed about in the waves. I lost consciousness, recovered it, and lost it again. I was never clear what was happening, but a number of times I felt that I was being washed towards the beach, then snatched away again. Then I found I was on the beach. The bodies of men and women were lying around me. The Japanese bayoneted the men's bodies, but left the women's alone. That is the only reason I am alive today. I lay still, partly because something told me I would be killed if I moved, and partly because I did not care anyway.[3]

The news made headlines around the world. Newspapers published lists of the twelve nurses from the *Vyner Brooke*, now presumed to have been drowned, the twenty-one who were killed beside Viv on Radji Beach, and the eight who had died in captivity.

The eight who died in the camps were:

Pearl Beatrice Mittelheuser, 41, Bundaberg, Queensland
Winnie May Davis, 30, Ulmarra, New South Wales
Blanche Hempsted, 36, Graceville, Queensland
Gladys Laura Hughes, 36, Waikino, New Zealand
Wilhelmina Rosalie Raymont, 33, Largs Bay, South Australia
Irene Ada Singleton, 36, Maffra, Victoria
Dora Shirley Gardam, 34, Youngtown, Tasmania
Rubina Dorothy Freeman, 32, Hawthorn, Victoria

For most of the families of the dead, the newspaper reports were the first confirmation that those nurses were not coming home.

Eva Bullwinkel was aghast when she read the first articles about what Viv had survived and what so many others hadn't. She wrote immediately from her flat in Adelaide.

Viv My Darling
Oh my darling, my darling what you have suffered ...
I cannot write about your ghastly experiences and I
certainly do not want to distress you needlessly to say, the
whole world is shocked. You are considered the bravest girl
in the world. The papers have been devoting their front
pages to your story ... Everybody in Australia is talking
about you, your name is on everyone's lips throughout the
country and I believe the whole world. Everybody thinks
you are marvellous and a very brave girl. All day yesterday
at the bank John didn't do any work, for people were
ringing him all day saying how glad and thrilled they were
that you were now in safe hands and what a marvellously
brave girl you are.
    We have had telegrams galore and letters and people
have been ringing me through the phone next door.
Everyone speaks of your heroism. Yesterday I listened in to
the radio news and the first thing the announcer said was
'Sister Bullwinkel has arrived in Singapore. She stepped off

the plane in the uniform she was wearing when she was shot three and a half years ago' and then they went on with your story.

Oh darling to hear your dear name again and to know you are safe, what a load has been taken off my heart and mind but I am sad at heart when I think of all you have gone through, may the rest of your life be sweet and happy …

Darling I am waiting for one of the greatest thrills of my life … to hear your dear voice again. I received an urgent telegram from Sydney afternoon asking me to listen in to 5DN at ten o'clock tonight that Sister Bullwinkel will be sending greetings.

…. Now for your lovely voice it's ten o'clock.

…. Well darling so many spoke before you I began to fear I wasn't going to hear you. At last you spoke and it was wonderful to listen to you although it was all too short my sweet. Anyway you will be home soon. Well my sweet I will now kiss you goodnight. John joins me with fondest love to your darling self.

Your loving mother.[4]

THE NURSES WERE TAKEN from the airport back to recover at the 2/14th Australian General Hospital, which had now taken over St Pat's school, where Viv had worked before the Japanese arrived so rudely.

Many of the nurses who had left on the *Empire Star* were back to care for those of their colleagues who had not been so lucky.

Some of the male patients in the hospital were so incensed at the state of the women, they had to be restrained from getting rifles and shooting the Japanese now under guard in the city.[5]

Viv was examined and gave doctors at the 2/14th a detailed rundown of her medical history during internment from notes she had kept in a secret diary.

Her medical report that day said Viv was suffering from:

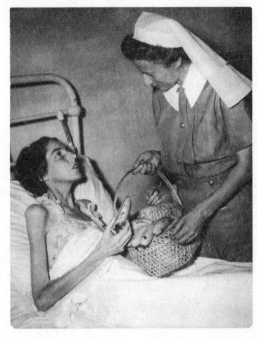

The emaciated Pat Blake was close to death by the time she arrived back in Singapore in 1945.

1. Mild debility (muscle wastage)
2. Old B.W. (bullet wound) abdominal wall
3. Scabies[6]

In her last days at the camp Viv had been vaccinated against cholera, dysentery and tuberculosis. She had mild diarrhoea and her eyesight had deteriorated.[7] She complained of tiredness and sweats at night. She noted that, consistent with the shock and starvation she had experienced, her periods had stopped for eight months after the events of February 1942. They stopped again in June 1944.[8]

Her weight had increased to 56 kilograms. Her fair hair was thin but was starting to grow back. Though Viv had lost a few fillings and was still troubled by tinea, her health was generally good with normal pulse and blood pressure of 120/70.[9] She was prescribed large doses of Vitamins B and C and a high-protein diet.

THE NURSES WERE ALL GIVEN toiletries and perfumes, baths and comfortable beds with cool white sheets. But after having spent so long sleeping on concrete, bamboo or dirt, many spent the first few nights at St Pat's sleeping on the floor until they slowly grew accustomed again to soft mattresses.

The nurses were always hungry and ate so much that some became uncomfortably distended in the belly, so rations were occasionally reduced. Perth doctor Colonel Cyril Fortune organised shampoos and manicures to take their minds off food.[10]

There was a regular procession of visitors, including men from the 8th Division, who had been patients in the hospital at the fall of Singapore and had then been captives at Changi and on the Thai–Burma 'death railway'. Like the nurses, many of them had been walking skeletons.

Within five days, some of the nurses, including Viv, had all gained weight on a diet of chicken, eggs and bananas.

Viv was examined again on 21 September and given a second vaccination against cholera. Her weight was now 60 kilograms, only a couple less than when she enlisted. 'In excellent health,' her new medical report stated. 'No ill effects from bullet wound.'[11]

The nurses learned that the bodies of Sister Gladys McDonald and two other unidentified colleagues were found on a raft in the Indian Ocean a few weeks after the sinking of the *Vyner Brooke*. Millie Dorsch's name tag was found on a Sumatran beach, leading to speculation that the raft carrying Matron Paschke made it to shore, only for the occupants to be killed by the Japanese. Viv's old commanding officer of the 2/13th AGH, Colonel Douglas Pigdon, had died at a prison camp in Manchuria just a month before the Japanese surrender.

THE NURSES' NEXT-OF-KIN were sent a message from the Commander of 2 Australian Reception Group in Singapore: 'For peace of mind of relatives of 24 sisters recovered and now in 2/14th AGH all well cared for and happy and making very good progress. None were molested by the Japanese. This information supplied by Matron-in-Charge who returned with them from Sumatra and assured me of this fact.'[12]

The government went to great pains to tell the public that

none of the Australian women had been violated. The nurses' health had improved so dramatically after two weeks of hospital treatment that on 1 October it was announced they would return to Australia that week on the hospital ship *Manunda*, which had undergone extensive repairs since the Japanese had bombed it at Darwin in February 1942.

Only five of the nurses, including Betty Jeffrey, were still in a weakened state but Eva read in her local Adelaide newspaper on 2 October that even they were 'quite well enough to travel', and would probably be 'quite fit at the end of the voyage'.[13]

The other nurses were described as being in 'fine fettle, healthy, and happy, and tripping round Singapore sightseeing and shopping, although they are not allowed night leave'. All except the five nurses who were still ailing visited the Changi camp and heard the English singer Gracie Fields, who performed exclusively for the Australians and was given 'a tumultuous reception'.[14] The nurses also watched a new Disney movie featuring Donald Duck.

Just before Viv sailed for home she heard that little Betty Kenneison had also been evacuated to Singapore and was staying at Raffles Hotel. The two met again at St Pat's and talked for several hours. Betty told Viv that a lady from the Red Cross had given her a nice floral print dress and a pair of blue shoes. The woman had told her that Betty would eventually get used to wearing wedge heels.

'It's not the heels that bother me,' Betty had told her, 'it's wearing shoes again.'[15]

The *Manunda* was readied for departure on 5 October, and even though the nurses had to wear second-hand uniforms because the shipment of new clothing had not arrived in time, the prospect of seeing Australia again far outweighed any fashion concerns. Flo Trotter even moved with the times and donned a pair of grey army trousers.

The twenty-four nurses who boarded the *Manunda*, out of sixty-five who had boarded the *Vyner Brooke* in 1942 and lived to tell the tale, were:

Vivian Bullwinkel, 29

Jean Ashton, 40

Pat Blake, 33

Jessie Blanch, 35

Veronica Clancy, 33

Cecilia Delforce, 33

Jess Doyle, 33

Jenny Greer, 32

Pat Gunther, 32

Mavis Hannah, 34

Iole Harper, 34

Nesta James, 41

Betty Jeffrey, 37

Vi McElnea, 41

Sylvia Muir, 30

Wilma Oram, 29

Chris Oxley, 33

Eileen Short, 41

Jessie Simons, 34

Val Smith, 33

Mickey Syer, 34

Flo Trotter, 30

Joyce Tweddell, 29

Beryl Woodbridge, 40

Mavis Hannah was the only one of nine nurses from the 2/4th Casualty Clearing Station on the *Vyner Brooke* to have survived. This time, as the *Manunda* motored out of Singapore with its pristine white hull and shining red cross and with more than 400 freed prisoners of war on board,[16] Viv rested her weary body. There was not a Japanese bomber in sight.

VIV'S FIRST REAL GLIMPSE of home came as the *Manunda* ploughed through the waves off Rottnest Island on 18 October. She was shifting about on the deck, her tinea still giving her grief, but buoyed by the sight of the Australian coastline.[17]

As a huge crowd of onlookers cheered and waved, the *Manunda* slowly drew into the wharf at Fremantle shortly after 6 p.m. on a glorious spring evening as the Western Command Band struck up the popular tune 'Nursie Nursie'. Men, women and children broke through barriers and ran alongside the huge vessel shouting 'coo-ees and cries of recognition'.[18] Thousands of people wept openly.[19]

The honour of being first aboard the *Manunda* went to a small red-haired son of one of the returning men, who was passed up to his father by a sailor.

After the ship berthed, Viv and the others trotted down the gangplank to meet loved ones, well-wishers and a sea of reporters, who noted that the nurses were 'gaining weight rapidly' and looking 'surprisingly fit'. Viv's progress along the wharf was likened to a 'royal procession',[20] and she was embraced by Zelda's cousin Wyn James. Sixteen Australian nurses who had been captured by the Japanese in Rabaul in January 1942 had returned to Australia a few weeks before Vivian and her comrades, but the survivor of the massacre on Radji Beach was dominating the headlines.

The nurses were escorted to a private room where Viv was the centre of attention, a role she hated. She was anxious to continue on to the *Manunda*'s next stop in Melbourne, where Eva had travelled to wait for her, but she told reporters about the massacre again, making sure all the relatives of the dead women would know that her colleagues died courageously as heroes.

She was quoted as saying: 'Not one of the girls screamed as they were shot to pieces. Australia can be mighty proud of them!'[21]

Described by the press as 'tall and slim, with her hair cut in boyish style', Viv was also quoted as saying that after the years of torture and deprivation in the Japanese camps she was now just longing to get some 'really beautiful clothes'.[22]

Flo Trotter told the pressmen, 'It is like a dream, being in Australia at last. Even on the trip home we expected to wake up and find ourselves back in Sumatra.'[23]

Cheering crowds lined the 13-kilometre route as the nurses were moved to the Hollywood Hospital in suburban Nedlands.

Staff there had decorated the ward with freshly cut wildflowers. Peggy Farmaner had been shot beside Viv on Radji Beach, and her 64-year-old mother, Flora, who had only learned of the tragedy three weeks earlier, arrived at the hospital to present each of Peggy's former colleagues with a bunch of flowers picked from the garden that Peggy had once tended. The next day, Viv was photographed at the hospital beaming as she clutched a bunch of kangaroo paws.

Iole Harper returned to her family in Perth and Mickey Syer decided to stay for a few days, but the *Manunda* continued on, bypassing Adelaide and finally docking in Port Melbourne on a wet and windy 24 October.

Viv and the other nurses passed through a guard of honour before being rushed by some of the nurses who had served alongside them in Malaya. Twenty-six of the men were taken off on stretchers, but most of the nurses looked remarkably well and some of them had put on as much as 25 kilograms in the two months since Captain Seki told them they were free.

Again, thousands of cheering people lined the pier as the nurses climbed onto a bus that led a procession of vehicles filled with returning prisoners of war through the streets of Melbourne. They stopped at Melbourne Town Hall for a brief welcome by the Lord Mayor before arriving at Heidelberg Hospital.

As Viv's bus came to a halt at the hospital, she scanned the crowd of anxious relatives and excited journalists calling out for interviews. When she walked down the stairs of the bus, cameras flashed and microphones were pushed her way, but Viv was paying no attention.

Finally, she saw Eva beaming. She forced her way through the throng and threw her arms around her mother.

'It's nice to have you home, Viv,' Eva said with lashings of understatement.[24]

Once again, Viv repeated the story of Radji Beach to reporters and again emphasised the courage of the women who had died beside her. She hoped that their loved ones would take comfort from her story.

'There was no crying from anyone,' she told the press. 'It was simply marvellous the way those girls went in with their chins up.'[25]

The *Manunda* continued on to Sydney, where just five weeks later Pat Blake married Lieutenant Keith Dixon of the AIF at the Shore Chapel in North Sydney.

The night after Viv arrived in Melbourne, she and her mother travelled to the home of her uncle Harold Harvey in Surrey Hills, where they stayed for two weeks. Viv told Eva as much as she thought she could stomach about the last three and a half years. It was not long before Eva was in tears, though Viv had not been able to cry since 1942.[26]

FIVE DAYS AFTER SHE ARRIVED in Melbourne, Viv gave evidence before Sir William Webb, Chief Justice of Queensland, who had been appointed to investigate atrocities by the Japanese armed forces. Viv was just one of hundreds of witnesses to provide evidence of Japanese war crimes.

In thirteen pages of evidence, Viv told Webb of the murders on Radji Beach, of malnutrition in the camps, of face-slapping and beatings by Japanese guards, of sick prisoners, including herself, being made to stand hatless in the sun for hours. She spoke of disease that went untreated, of sadism, cruelty and a criminal disregard for life.[27]

On the same day, an American military tribunal in Manila began hearing evidence in the trial of General Tomoyuki Yamashita, the Tiger of Malaya, whose forces had swept through Malaya and Singapore and forced General Arthur Percival into a humiliating surrender. Percival had spent the remainder of the war as a prisoner of the Japanese in Changi, Formosa and Manchuria, but after being liberated was on hand to see Yamashita taken into custody.

Chapter 27

AFTER TWO WEEKS IN MELBOURNE, Viv returned with her mother on the train to the flat in Fullarton that Eva shared with John. Despite her ordeal, the press said Viv now looked 'bright and cheerful', with a huge smile of relief. Wilma soon joined Viv for a holiday in Adelaide, and while Wilma was back at the Royal Melbourne Hospital under the army rehabilitation scheme, Viv was assigned to the Heidelberg Hospital, despite saying she felt like a break of 'four or five months'.[1]

She was given leave to visit as many families of those lost on Radji Beach as possible, and she wrote to others she couldn't see in person. She reassured all the families of the courage of the lost sisters, telling them that they had died noble deaths unmolested by the enemy. Every conversation she had with the women's loved ones was difficult.

She and her mother also went to Mount Gambier to stay for a few days with the family of Eva's younger sister, Nell Crowhurst,[2] whose husband was a mounted policeman like Viv's grandfather. The Crowhursts also had a fourteen-year-old daughter named after Viv,[3] who was following her cousin into nursing. Nell had spent much of the war years raising money for patriotic funds.

On 14 January 1946 there was a grand civic reception for Viv at the Broken Hill Town Hall, and once again she had to relive the horrors of Radji Beach and the camps for an overflowing audience.[4] She paid tribute to all the nurses who didn't come back, especially her old matron in Broken Hill, Irene Drummond.

There were meetings with old friends, relatives and the nurses at the local hospital. Zelda Treloar, now Mrs West, caught the train up from Melbourne to join her.[5] Wilma Oram was given leave as well, and she and Viv attended gatherings of the returned nurses in many towns around Australia, offering support and advice to the committees erecting monuments to their beloved local nurses who had died.

There were public calls for Viv to receive the Victoria Cross for gallantry,[6] but each time Viv would point out that she was no heroine and would instead shift her focus to the bravery of her fallen colleagues.

On 10 April, Sir William Webb's report into Japanese war crimes was tabled in parliament, with more than a thousand pages of testimony about 'sadism, torture, and sustained brutality'.[7] Massacres, beheadings, beatings, hangings, torture, starvation and other cruelties were all exposed.

'It would appear to have been the purpose of many Japanese in control of prisoners of war to ensure their slow deaths by a maximum of work, on a minimum of food and, otherwise, under heartbreaking conditions,' the report said.[8]

The trials and sometimes executions of Japanese war criminals convicted of murders were already taking place in different locations north of Australia. Some of the Australian army officers in Rabaul criticised the practice of giving sedatives, including morphine, to the condemned war criminals before they were hanged, mercies which they said had never been extended to Allied captives.[9] General Yamashita died at the end of a rope at a prison in the Philippines just four years after he had made Percival surrender Singapore.

VIV HAD MADE A RAPID RECOVERY from her mistreatment, at least physically, though she still had some pain around the area of her gunshot wound. The years of starvation had played havoc with her metabolism and by May 1946, now promoted to the rank of captain, she was 12 kilograms heavier than the 62 kilograms she had been when she enlisted.[10]

She told a doctor examining her at Heidelberg Hospital that while she was now thirty and many of her colleagues were finding husbands, she wanted to devote herself to her work as an army nurse, in memory of the friends she had left behind. She also wanted to do her best to see justice done for the atrocities committed against all the prisoners.

The medical examiner said that while Viv was 'generally fit ... her past history and privations' meant that further tropical service was 'not advisable'.[11]

Viv was made sister in charge at Heidelberg, where a rose garden had been planted in memory of the lost nurses. Servicemen were still recovering from the war there and Viv remained a casualty too, carrying emotional scars along with her bullet wound. The sight of the staff scraping leftovers into garbage bins or seeing vegetables and meat thrown out caused vicious flashbacks, and on occasion she became highly agitated, screaming that the staff were not to waste food.

Part of her rapid weight gain occurred because she insisted on cleaning her plate every time she ate. For a long time, Viv found it hard to sleep in a bed and she faced the trauma of being separated from her friends with whom she had lived through life-and-death battles for so long.

In July 1946, John Bullwinkel, now working at the Commonwealth Bank in Adelaide, announced his engagement to Laura Farrell, who had also served in the air force during the war. Many of Viv's comrades were marrying too. Cecilia Delforce and Jess Doyle married former prisoners of war, while Jenny Greer married her Singapore oilman Duncan Pemberton. Sylvia Muir, Iole Harper and Flo Trotter were making wedding plans as well, and Mavis Hannah was returning to Singapore to marry Joseph William Allgrove, a widower with a vast rubber plantation. Allgrove always called Mavis 'Nell'. While in the prison camp, starved and knocked about, Mavis had doubted she would ever be able to bear children but, as she explained years later, 'After I got back to the hospital in Singapore and was given better food ... I suddenly got funny hot flushes. Then all of a sudden I started to menstruate and it was as regular as clockwork.' Mavis's first child was born when she was thirty-eight, a second when she was forty and a third when she was forty-two.[12]

Viv's handsome friend Jim Austin had been taken prisoner in Singapore and sent to Changi prison. Back in Melbourne he started a new career in teaching and married a young librarian named Dorothy Shierson.

For now, Viv was married to her work and preserving the memory of her comrades.

BY THE MIDDLE OF 1946, Australian troops had rounded up more than 2000 suspected war criminals, and 400 had already been executed or imprisoned. Another 1600 were still being hunted, though it was suspected that most of them had already died in battle.[13]

Lieutenant Masayuki Takeuchi, commander of one of the companies on Bangka Island, had been recently identified in a prisoner-of-war camp and was now in Taiping prison in northern Malaya. Another suspect, Sergeant-Major Taro Kato, had been captured in New Guinea.

Viv read in a Melbourne newspaper that many of the Japanese division that had landed on Bangka Island at the same time as the *Vyner Brooke* survivors had been killed at Guadalcanal and in New Guinea. Captain (later Major) Masaru, who commanded the two companies at the time of the massacre on Radji Beach, had survived and fought on the Manchurian front against the Russians in 1945, but his whereabouts were unknown.[14]

While many nations were conducting their own war-crimes trials, eleven had formed an International Military Tribunal for the Far East to try the leaders of Japan for joint conspiracy to start and wage war. In October 1946, Viv sailed on the ship *Kanimbla* from Sydney with thirteen other former prisoners of war, including Nesta James, to give evidence. Bruce Hunt would give evidence about atrocities committed on the Thai–Burma Railway line. Viv was reluctant to go at first as she was 'very uncertain' as to how she would react when surrounded by

Japanese people again. But she felt she owed it to all her lost friends to see justice done.[15]

Facing court in the first round of trials in Tokyo would be twenty-eight of Japan's most senior military and government leaders, including their former prime minister, General Hideki Tojo, who had survived a self-inflicted gunshot wound at the war's end. Douglas Macarthur, the Supreme Commander for the Allied Powers, angered many senior military officials with his insistence that Emperor Hirohito should not stand trial in case it sparked another uprising.

Viv and the other prosecution witnesses arrived in the Japanese city of Kure late in October. A party of Australians hurried them through the bomb-devastated city to a ferry for the twenty-minute crossing to the island of Etajima and the former Japanese Naval Academy, which had been converted into an Allied hospital.

Viv's evidence would not be needed for several weeks and while it meant she would miss out on Christmas with her mother and John, she now had the opportunity to tour Japan. For the first couple of weeks her stomach churned if she passed groups of Japanese men, particularly if voices were raised.[16] But on her way to Tokyo by train she stopped in Hiroshima and saw the effect that the atomic bomb had on its people – children and women who probably wanted war no more than she did – and she was moved by the suffering of the Japanese civilians.[17] Amid the atomic wasteland of shattered buildings and mass destruction, Viv tried to imagine what it was like on the August day a year earlier when 100,000 people had died and others were left with lingering shock and sickness.[18] The warlords of Japan had not only caused misery for their enemies but had brought untold horrors on their people at home as well.

THE TOKYO WAR-CRIMES TRIALS were held in the former building of the Japanese Ministry of War in Tokyo. Sir William Webb, the tribunal president, took General Tojo's office as his own. The court proceedings took place on the first floor of the building in a high-ceilinged hall containing long rows of

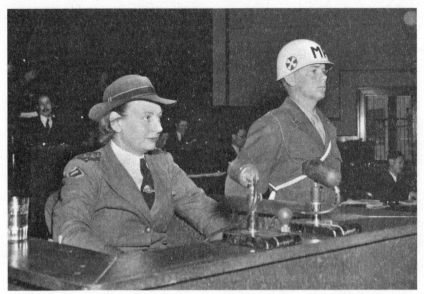

Viv giving evidence at the Tokyo war crimes trials in 1946.

tables and seating that rose in tiers from the front of the court to the back wall, above which was a public gallery.

American military police in crisp uniforms, white steel helmets, pistol belts and side arms stood at attention around the court. In two rows behind tables, Tojo and the other defendants, whose faces rarely betrayed emotion, sat staring into space, their uniforms having been stripped of military rank and decorations.

At 9.30 a.m. on 20 December, the Tokyo court rose as Sir William Webb entered the room and took his place on the judges' bench. Warrant Officer Bill Sticpewich spent much of the day relating the horrors of the Sandakan death march but, late in the afternoon, the Australian assistant prosecutor, Lieutenant Colonel Thomas Mornane, asked Webb: 'If the tribunal pleases, I now propose to call Sister Bullwinkel.' Webb nodded, and Viv, dressed in her grey Australian Army Nursing Service uniform, stepped forward and was sworn in.

Viv was afraid she might collapse on being forced to recall her sickening memories or that she might be struck dumb with stress under cross-examination.[19] But over the next ninety minutes she recounted all the horrors of Radji Beach and the prison camps where she said she and the other nurses spent much of their time digging graves.[20] When she finally finished her evidence she was shaking.[21] Webb described Viv as a model witness.

Viv's testimony and that of Nesta James would eventually see Captain Seki receive a fifteen-year prison sentence, handed down at his trial in Medan, Sumatra.[22] Guards Takeshi Shigemura and Yamada Kimihiko received sentences of six and five years.[23] Many of the Japanese war criminals insisted they were only following orders and would have been severely punished if they did not.

BACK IN AUSTRALIA IN MARCH 1947, Viv was honoured to be made an Associate of the Royal Red Cross, an award endorsed by King George VI. Jessie Blanch was given the same honour for her courage in helping others to rafts after the *Vyner Brooke* went down. The citation to Viv's award read in part: 'Lieut. Bullwinkel was a magnificent example in this period, nursing sick personnel and doing manual labour under the threat of molestation and personal violence from brutal Japanese.'[24]

Nothing came from the investigation of Lieutenant Takeuchi and Sergeant-Major Kato in connection with the massacre of the nurses, but paymaster Sukero Shibayama, one of the few survivors from the unit responsible, was transported from Tokyo on 30 May 1947 to face an interrogation by an Australian war-crimes unit in Singapore. If Shibayama was not directly implicated in the crime it was hoped that he would be able to indicate who was responsible and give information about the few remaining survivors from his unit, and especially Orita Masaru, the commanding officer, who was now believed to be a prisoner of war in Russian hands.[25]

While investigations continued, Viv was presented with the Florence Nightingale Medal in a ceremony at the Melbourne headquarters of the Australian Red Cross in July 1947. The ceremony was broadcast on ABC Radio. Viv nervously approached the microphone before taking a deep, slow breath. She said the medal was a tribute to her friends such as Matron Paschke and Matron Drummond, who 'by their ability and level-headedness in a time of crisis' were responsible for the calm behaviour of the nurses during the sinking of the *Vyner Brooke*.

That calmness and courage and the bravery of all the nurses in their final hour, Viv said, 'was forever an inspiration' to the others in their years of struggle for survival.[26]

VIV WORRIED THAT IF SHE stayed with the army she would be sent to Japan as part of the occupation force. So, in 1947, when the army handed over Heidelberg Hospital to the Repatriation Commission, Viv decided to keep working there as a civilian. She was in no hurry for a romantic relationship, later remarking that if the right man came along well and good. If not, why worry about it?[27]

Betty Jeffrey had spent two years in hospital with tuberculosis, and she and Viv now decided that they would do their utmost to create what they called a 'living memorial' to all the Australian nurses who had died in all wars. The memorial would not only honour the nurses whose lives had been sacrificed to war but continue the ongoing professional development of nurses as a centre for further education.[28] There would also be accommodation for nurses from the country or interstate awaiting their assignments.

After launching a fundraising appeal at Melbourne Town Hall on 1 December 1947, Viv and Betty spent more than a year touring Victoria in Betty's little Austin car to raise money to build the centre.[29]

Years later Viv said: 'I am not exaggerating when I say we spoke at every RSL branch, every Country Women's Association branch, every hospital, every school and at public meetings in every town in Victoria and the Riverina. The public and particularly the RSL responded magnificently and a record amount at that time of £120,000 was donated and the Nurses Memorial Centre in St Kilda Rd was established and has since served the profession well.'[30] Viv and Betty's effort became the most successful public appeal ever held in Victoria at the time,[31] and eventually the Australian Nurses Memorial Centre became one of the largest nursing scholarship contributors in Australia.[32]

The pair were backed by other founders of the memorial – Wilma Oram, Colonel Annie Sage and Edith Hughes-Jones, who owned a private hospital in Melbourne and had established the Centaur War Nurses' Memorial Trust.

Wilma was an active supporter of the fundraising but she had other pressing matters on her mind. On 5 December 1947 at East Brighton in Melbourne she married dairy farmer Alan Young, who had spent four years as a prisoner of war after seeing action in Crete in 1941.[33] Viv was Wilma's bridesmaid. The best man, John Nicholson, had also been a prisoner of war, and many of the nurses from the *Vyner Brooke* were guests.

Viv became godmother to Wilma's son, David, who has a dairy farm at Pakenham on Melbourne's southern outskirts. 'Mum and Aunty Viv were the greatest of friends,' David recalled. 'Their bond was forged by three and a half years sleeping beside each other on a slab of concrete and battling to stay alive. They had experienced part of life that hopefully not many of us will ever experience. That relationship that the nurses had, my mother and Aunty Viv particularly, was something that stood them in good stead to survive and then administer support to other veterans. They never gave up their commitment to nurse others even after they came home. That commitment to their fellow POWs, men and women, was an enduring legacy.'[34]

The wedding of Viv's brother, John, to Laura Farrell at St Peter's Church in seaside Glenelg in Adelaide on 31 January 1948 was a joyous occasion for all concerned, not least Eva, who had despaired over the fate of her two missing children during the war and now had them safe at home again.

APART FROM THE TOKYO WAR TRIALS, Australia, China, France, the Dutch East Indies, the Philippines, the United Kingdom and the United States all held separate trials that convicted more than 5500 war criminals. There were 944 executions.[35]

Australian military officials spent three and a half years searching various Allied prison camps for Orita Masaru, following his trail from Malaya through to Sumatra, Guadalcanal, Japan and China. Finally, late in 1947, Masaru was located. He was a prisoner of the Soviet Red Banner army in Siberia. It took another year to obtain his release.

Masaru was brought to Tokyo's Sugamo Prison, where General Tojo and many other major war criminals were being held under sentence of death. On the day Masaru arrived, he apparently considered his options and saw little hope. He committed suicide in his cell.[36] The date was 11 September 1948.[37]

Two days before Christmas that year, General Tojo and six other high-ranking convicted war criminals were hanged on the prison gallows.

In his final statement, Tojo apologised for the atrocities committed under his watch and urged the Americans, now occupying Japan, to show compassion towards the local people, who had also suffered much from constant aerial bombardment that culminated in two atomic bombings.

The executions did not bring closure for many of the former prisoners of war, though Viv's friend Flo Trotter, now Flo Syer, said that while she would never forget the forty-one souls from the *Vyner Brooke* who perished, she forgave everything that happened to her. 'What's the use in hating?' Flo said. 'I've seen what hate does to people and I didn't like what I saw. Far better to forgive, far better to love.'[38]

Viv was less forgiving. While she felt sorry for all the Japanese women and children damaged by war, she found the idea of Japan being invited to the 1956 Melbourne Olympics 'repugnant'.[39]

Chapter 28

IN 1950, VIV AND BETTY JEFFREY finally had the chance to make their trip to England a reality, once pressing matters at home had been finalised.

At the same Melbourne function at which cricketer Don Bradman was knighted,[1] Viv and Nesta James were presented with awards as Associates of the Order of the Royal Red Cross, and together with Ellen Savage, the only nurse to survive the sinking of the *Centaur*, Viv helped a Legacy fundraising drive for war widows and orphans.[2]

There were monuments around Australia to unveil, including one dedicated to Olive Paschke at the Memorial High School in Dimboola,[3] and the Sister Drummond Memorial Park in Broken Hill.[4]

Betty and Viv sailed for England in September 1950 on the white ocean liner SS *Arawa*. They both planned to do post-graduate courses in modern blood bank methods,[5] but they also wanted to fulfil the dream of a white Christmas in London that had been nurtured long before in the steamy jungle of Sumatra.

They stayed at the Strand Hotel while looking for cheaper lodgings and went to meet Air Commodore Modin for the first time since meeting him as prisoners at the old 'Big Hill' camp at Bukit Besar just out of Palembang not long after the killings at Radji Beach. They were honoured guests of the Marquess of Queensberry, the Duchess of Gloucester and General Arthur

Percival, who, like them, knew what it was like to be a starving prisoner of war.

They revelled in their snowy Christmas and in the New Year enjoyed a five-course lunch at the Savoy, courtesy of a women's magazine. They even went searching in vain for a glimpse of the infant Prince Charles, walking in the grounds of Buckingham Palace with his nurse.[6] At Westminster Abbey they stared solemnly at the stained-glass window installed in memory of all the nurses who lost their lives during the war, and checked for the names of the Australians on the roll of honour.

Viv and Betty then took a short holiday in Switzerland. When they returned in February 1951, they were invited to Marlborough House[7] for a meeting with 84-year-old Queen Mary.

Betty reckoned Queen Mary's eyes were so blue and so clear and her hair 'so pretty' that she really was 'the loveliest old lady I have ever seen'.[8] Queen Mary was slightly stooped but still had a firm handshake and a delightfully natural manner. She directed her two visitors to armchairs overlooking the Mall and sat between them, 'very upright'.

Queen Mary showed an amazing interest in the details of their years as prisoners. She knew about the Australian Nurses Memorial Centre in Melbourne and chuckled when Viv and Betty told her about roaring around the countryside in their little Austin car soliciting donations.[9]

They spoke for forty-five minutes. Just before they left, Queen Mary gave them both a photograph of herself, signed, 'Mary R., 1951.'[10]

Three months later, Viv and Betty were presented at court and met King George VI and Queen Elizabeth, who would soon become known as the Queen Mother when her eldest daughter ascended the throne.

Betty returned to Melbourne after a year in London but Viv stayed on, and in 1953 she took a job as a nurse-receptionist in the medical section of the Department of Immigration at Australia House.[11]

In July that year, in a giant Coronation parade of 72,000 ex-servicemen and women,[12] Viv led 200 Australian nurses marching twenty abreast past the newly crowned Queen Elizabeth II, inciting a roar of appreciation from a crowd packed in stands lining Hyde Park's East Carriage Drive.

Viv adored the theatre and the social whirl of London. She even swapped war stories with the spy Odette Churchill, who had been tortured by the Gestapo. But the call of Australia was irresistible, and in September 1953 she finally sailed for home on the *Oronsay*. When the captain heard Viv was on board he upgraded her from a tourist-class cabin to a first-class suite.[13]

EVERY YEAR ON 16 FEBRUARY, Viv would place an 'In Memoriam' notice in the *Adelaide Advertiser* newspaper honouring her friends who lost their lives.[14] While many of her fellow survivors were now raising young families, Viv remained devoted to her work back at Heidelberg Hospital. She became great friends with Ernest 'Weary' Dunlop, the surgeon who saved so many lives as a prisoner during the war. Occasionally she and Betty, who also remained single, would holiday together on Queensland's Gold Coast, but work was Viv's main priority. In 1955 she was appointed assistant matron at Heidelberg and accepted the rank of Acting Major in the Citizen Military Forces.[15] Eventually she was made a Lieutenant Colonel[16] and Commanding Officer of the Royal Australian Army Nursing Corps's Southern Command. In that capacity she was at the unveiling of the Singapore War Memorial at Kranji in 1957.[17]

Two years later, aged forty-three, Viv was awarded a diploma in nursing administration, which, in 1961, led to her becoming matron at Melbourne's Fairfield Infectious Diseases Hospital on the banks of the Yarra River.

Newspaper reports of the time focused not so much on her work but on her appearance. One pointed out that, while Viv was the first to admit she was approaching middle age, she was 'attractive, very feminine, has an engaging personality, and a very definite love for both patients and nurses'.[18]

The Fairfield hospital specialised in the treatment and control of epidemics. Despite staff shortages, Viv had taken over the hospital with a team of 217 nurses, domestics and administrative staff caring for 250 patients.

Under her guidance, Fairfield became a specialised teaching hospital for both Monash and Melbourne universities, and she encouraged registered nurses to develop their qualifications further by pursuing tertiary studies. She told all of her team that, in the modern world, nurses needed to be regarded not as submissive assistants to doctors but professionals in their own right with the highest possible qualifications. It was the only way for them to advance to senior positions within the medical profession.[19]

She had her detractors, but as Wilma Oram's son, David, pointed out: 'Throughout her life Aunty Viv was an extremely determined person who knew what she needed to do to achieve results. As well as being extremely compassionate to anyone who was in need, she was also very single-minded.'[20]

Fairfield had a severe shortage of nurses trained in the treatment of infectious diseases, but with the support of the hospital's board of management, Viv established an independent nurses' aide school, which was officially recognised and accredited by the Victorian Nursing Federation in 1964. Graduates could go on to study a specialised post-basic course followed by one specifically for fevers. This quickly gave the hospital a constant flow of highly trained staff.

Viv's nephew, John Bullwinkel, recalled that Viv was responsible for improving the lot of nurses, raising their educational standards, creating the nurses' aide position, and generally raising the profile of the nursing profession. She also broke down some of the traditional formalities that had existed in nursing. She became known as the 'Matron in Mufti', having done away with the formal matron's uniform.[21]

One of Viv's nurses at Fairfield, Joan Holland, recalled that Viv 'was just so approachable' and that she was across every problem at the hospital. She made a point of knowing every patient and every nurse and would chat with all of them.[22]

Another of Viv's team, Margaret Wiseman, said that, under Viv, Fairfield was on the front line against several epidemics such as polio and Murray Valley encephalitis, and that Viv was always coming down to the wards to ease the burden on her staff.

Viv accepted for training a lot of young women who had encountered difficult lives, and she would help them build their careers.[23] One of the young nurses Viv helped on her career path was Greek-born Olga Kanitsaki, who arrived in Melbourne in 1961 as a non-English-speaking migrant. Olga went to Fairfield looking for work as a cleaner, after a futile six-month search for employment. On arrival, Olga mistook Viv for the cleaning supervisor, and told her that she desperately wanted to become a nurse but that no hospital would take her.

Liking the youngster's enthusiasm, Viv told Olga she was actually 'Matron Bullwinkel' and gave her a start as a trainee.

'Her face was so smiling it was almost like a sun,' said the nurse who, as Dr Kanitsaki, was made a Member of the Order of Australia (AM) for her service to nursing and became Australia's first Professor of Transcultural Nursing and Head of the Department of Nursing and Midwifery at RMIT University. 'I can never stop feeling grateful,' Dr Kanitsaki said, 'because Matron Bullwinkel gave me an extraordinary chance that nobody else was prepared to do. She was a remarkable woman of extraordinary compassion and understanding who spent her life helping people.'[24]

Viv always saw her dedication to nursing as a tribute to the friends she had lost, and once, in an address to student nurses at Fairfield, she summed up her love for her calling. 'We belong to a profession,' Viv said, 'where the common language of friendliness, understanding and professional integrity bind us into a great family …

We find we belong to a profession as wide as the world and as needful as the needs of the human race. Because of the nature of our work, the confidences, respect and trust that we are privileged to have given us by all peoples, I believe that the nursing profession is one of the greatest mediums for international understanding and that it is a responsibility we should accept ... Tenacity of purpose is the only way to reach your desired goal ... As you look into the mirror and see your place in the world as a member of the Nursing Profession, remember the high ideals which motivated you to enter the Profession – whose highest ideal is 'Service'. Knowledge and technical ability [are] not enough to give the world – there must be understanding, compassion, there must be hope and faith in the future.[25]

VIV WAS ALMOST FIFTY when she was introduced to Frank Statham[26] at the Naval and Military Club in Little Collins Street. Viv loved live theatre and after seeing a show in Melbourne she would often forgo catching the late train to Fairfield and stay at the club instead.

Frank was a handsome and distinguished engineer and former army lieutenant colonel with a commanding presence and smiling eyes. Viv was immediately drawn to him.

At the time, he was an officer with the Citizen Military Force, and he told Viv of his fascinating background. Born in Toowoomba, Queensland a few months after Viv, he had been raised in the Solomon Islands, where his father was a copra planter until his death from black-water fever when Frank was eight.

Later, Frank attended North Sydney Boys' High School for a year or two, but at fourteen he became an apprentice fitter and turner while taking night classes in mechanical engineering.

During the war, Frank served at Benghazi and in the siege of Tobruk. Later, he was involved in fortifying the north-west of Australia, building airfields and gun emplacements in case of a Japanese invasion. He was awarded an OBE for his 'consistent outstanding display of ability and leadership'.[27]

In 1953 he had been appointed chief plant engineer in the Commonwealth Department of Works, and from Melbourne he supervised the construction of airports, roads, bridges and jetties throughout Australia, Papua New Guinea and the Cocos Islands.

At their first meeting, Viv and Frank chatted like old friends about their journeys through life, but eventually Viv looked at her watch and had to excuse herself. Time had gotten away and she risked being late for her show.

She asked herself if she would ever see Frank again. As it turned out, soon after, Viv was at the Puckapunyal military camp completing her fourteen days training commitment with the Citizen Military Force, and there was Frank, doing the same thing. Beside the log fire in the officers' mess, Viv and Frank drank whiskey and soda and got to know each other better.[28] It was as though they'd known each other all their lives. Viv admired everything about Frank, and it seemed his eyes were always smiling when he looked at her.

Then Frank told Viv he had a wife and two children, and that he was moving 3500 kilometres west to Perth.

Frank thought it wonderful that he and Viv could always be good friends. For Viv, the whiskey and soda suddenly didn't taste as good.

VIV'S BELOVED BROTHER, John, was just forty-six when he died suddenly after a heart attack in Adelaide on 2 November 1966. How cruel life could be. To survive a burning aircraft in the thick of war and then to die at such a young age at his desk with a young family and aged mother left to mourn him. His passing made Viv think of her dear friends in the camp who perished just before the Allies arrived with food and medicine.

Viv escorted Eva to John's funeral at the Centennial Park Cemetery in the southern Adelaide suburb of Pasadena, and then went back to Melbourne to save some more lives.

SHE WISHED FRANK STATHAM was there for her. But he was now in charge of the Western Australian region of the Commonwealth Department of Works, overseeing the planning and construction of HMAS *Stirling*, the naval base on Garden Island outside Perth. Occasionally he would visit Melbourne and

Viv would meet him at the Naval and Military Club. But it was only occasionally, and Viv was growing older and greyer.

In 1970, she retired from her role of lieutenant colonel in the army due to work commitments. Three years later, when she was President of the College of Nursing Australia, 'Miss Vivian Bullwinkel of Fairfield' was made a Member of the British Empire in the Queen's New Year's Day Honours List. Viv was surprised by the accolade and told anyone who asked that there was no award necessary because she was just doing her job.[29]

At the end of 1974, Frank was called on to coordinate the relief efforts after Cyclone Tracy had torn through Darwin. The massive clean-up would stretch well into 1975 and his visits to Melbourne became less frequent.

ON A COLD SUNDAY NIGHT in early April 1975, Viv was settled into an easy chair in front of the large log fire in her matron's apartment at Fairfield, her chihuahua, Tao, curled up at her feet. On the television was yet another news bulletin about the chaos of the war in Vietnam. Viv found the images of screaming women and children and homes on fire very unsettling. She had seen enough of all that in Singapore.

It was 10 p.m. when the telephone rang. Something about the late hour and the disturbance to her quiet time unnerved her. Viv answered the call but she could hardly believe her ears. Thirty years after Viv had come home from a war, she was now being asked to go back to another.

Chapter 29

LOOKING DOWN AT THE war-torn countryside of the Mekong Delta below, Viv's heart raced.[1] The inside of the RAAF C-130 Hercules, a military transport aircraft, was spartan and as hot as a sauna. Seated against the walls of the aircraft in drop-down aluminium seats with webbing back supports were a dozen nurses. The Hercules' four engines were so loud no one could hear each other speak. Apart from a cleared walkway through the middle of the massive aircraft, most of the interior space was stacked floor to ceiling with packing cases containing food and medical supplies for orphans.

It was 17 April 1975, and Viv, now almost sixty, was one of twelve volunteers flying through hostile air space as part of a life-saving mission to rescue Vietnamese orphans, as communist forces approached Saigon (now Ho Chi Minh City). A fighter jet was their escort.

Vulnerable to enemy anti-aircraft fire in the area, the Hercules made a steep descent into Saigon's Tan Son Nhut airfield as Viv and her colleagues prepared to race into action. Awaiting them would be harrowing scenes of distressed babies and small children, many ravaged by hunger and disease and close to death.

Viv was taking part in the second Australian mission of Operation Babylift, the name given to the mass evacuation of babies and children from South Vietnam. The rescue had started two weeks earlier, on 3 April, with the Allied forces planning to evacuate more than 3000 children to Australia, the United States, France, West Germany and Canada.

The dangers were not just from the communist forces. In the first mission of Operation Babylift, a mammoth C-5A Galaxy had experienced an explosion just twelve minutes after take-off that tore apart the lower rear fuselage. The Galaxy had landed in a rice paddy, skidded for 400 metres and became airborne again before crashing into a dam wall and bursting into flames. There were 176 survivors but 138 people, including seventy-eight children, died.

The following day, 5 April, 215 children and babies, some in cardboard boxes serving as makeshift cots, had arrived at Sydney Airport after a nine-hour flight on a chartered Qantas jumbo jet from Bangkok. The children ranged in age from three days to fourteen years. The most seriously ill travelled in a makeshift infirmary ward in the first-class cabin. When the aircraft touched down, ninety babies were rushed to the Royal Alexandra Hospital for Children (now the Westmead Children's Hospital) in a fleet of ambulances.[2] Other children, many suffering from tropical diseases, were ferried to the North Head Quarantine Station.

It was late that same evening as Viv was relaxing by the fire that she'd received a telephone call from the Fairfield hospital's medical superintendent, Dr John Forbes. He'd asked her to put together a team of volunteer nurses to travel to Saigon as soon as possible to collect 200 more war orphans. The volunteers were required to have some flying experience, some experience in South-East Asia, current cholera and smallpox inoculations and a current passport, which narrowed the field considerably.[3]

With Sydney's North Head Quarantine Station now at capacity, a new destination for the orphans was needed, and with so many again likely to be seriously ill, the Fairfield hospital was the ideal destination. Dr Forbes would lead the mission, and Viv volunteered to fly there too.

'I had no intention of staying out of this one,' Viv recalled, 'because I felt that I had experience in the tropical areas of wartime conditions and all the medical superintendent wanted of me was to be able to feed a baby and change a napkin and I said,

"Yes, I think I can do that". So I went.[4] Viv was an old hand at war conditions and evacuations under gunfire.

She did not have enough nurses at Fairfield to spare, so more were recruited from the Heidelberg Repatriation Hospital, including Phyllis Schumann, a senior operating-theatre registered nurse. Phyllis had participated in medivacs of many severely injured Australian servicemen from Vietnam to the RAAF base at Butterworth in Malaysia. With her close friend Val Seeger, a senior Fairfield nurse, Viv oversaw the packing of the necessary medical kits and nursing supplies and prepared to brief the nurses the next morning. Those who needed them were given cholera vaccinations. Then the doctors and nurses from Fairfield boarded a bus, picked up the other nurses from Heidelberg and journeyed up the Hume Highway to arrive in Sydney late that evening.

The plan was to board a flight to Bangkok the next day to meet an RAAF Hercules there for the flight to Saigon. But there was a breakdown in negotiations with the South Vietnamese government and the trip was cancelled.

Another flight was eventually rescheduled, this time with only seventy-five orphans, instead of the original 200. They were all under the age of ten years, of which 60 per cent were babies and toddlers.[5] Viv took a huge quantity of supplies and medicine with her, including anti-diarrhoeal medicines, saline solution – and a way of introducing it to babies suffering from dehydration – plus glucose and oral electrolyte fluids. There were disposable nappies, a variety of milk products, especially low-fat milk products, and plenty of feeding bottles. There were also large quantities of baby and toddler food plus meals for the older children.

The anticipated medical problems included tuberculosis, malaria, gastroenteritis, dehydration and intestinal infestation. As it turned out, the medical problems of the orphans proved to be more varied and serious.

A very early start was made on 16 April, with Viv and the others travelling to Tullamarine Airport to board another chartered Qantas jet for the 11-hour flight to Bangkok.

Passing over Derby in Western Australia and Denpasar in Indonesia, they arrived in Bangkok late that evening. Viv was immediately bowled over by the 32-degree heat and humidity of the kind she remembered on Sumatra.

An overnight stop had been arranged by the Australian Embassy, though an official seemed more concerned about the team incurring expenses rather than with their mission.[6] In any case, everyone wanted an early night, because the next day – Viv's first foray into a war zone for thirty years – would be a long one.

Viv had divided her staff into two teams. She would lead Team One, which would travel to Saigon on the Hercules the next morning to sort the orphans into broad categories based on their age and the amount of medical care they needed. Team Two would stay in Bangkok and convert the Qantas jet into a mobile hospital and nursery.

Early the next morning, Viv and eleven others in Team One departed for Saigon on the Hercules with Wing Commander John Mitchell at the controls. For two hours Viv and the other nurses endured the heat, humidity and noise inside the Hercules, as well as the clear and present danger that they could be shot out of the sky. As Wing Commander Mitchell made his final approach to Tan Son Nhut he came in low and fast to avoid possible ground fire.

As the machine rolled to a stop, the sound of gunfire echoed in the distance.[7] Reminded of Radji Beach, Viv shuddered. As soon as the doors of the aircraft were opened and the cargo ramp lowered, Wing Commander Mitchell told everyone to make a getaway as quickly as they could.

With the North Vietnamese army closing in, there were already two Hercules waiting on the tarmac. Remnants of the Australian Embassy in Saigon had already loaded the babies on one aircraft and the toddlers and children on the other. Both aircraft had their engines running and their cargo ramps down, and people were dashing everywhere. Parts of the airfield were already under attack.[8] The great propellers of the Hercules whirred to the sound of gunfire and mortars, and within minutes of the Australians arriving in Saigon both aircraft were in the air.

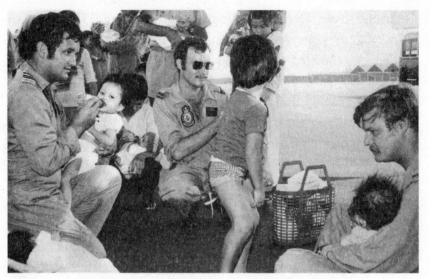

RAAF personnel with some of the orphaned children about to fly with Viv to Melbourne in 1975 during Operation Babylift. *Australian War Memorial P01973.002*

Viv would never forget the rows of cardboard cartons, in each one a small babe, in some two or even three fragile specks of humanity with pleading eyes and pot bellies of starvation and sickness. It gave her the strangest feeling to see human beings packed in cardboard.[9] Most of the babies showed glaring signs of malnourishment, a condition with which she had once been all too familiar. One baby listed as eighteen months old was in fact an undernourished three-year-old.

Viv suspected that they had all kinds of diseases – tuberculosis, worms, shigella and other parasitic conditions, scabies, boils, abscesses and infections caused by lice and by poor nutrition and hygiene. Some were beset by chickenpox and whooping cough. Some had respiratory infections. All were suffering from fear and trauma. One of the orphans, an eight-month-old boy, died on the way to Bangkok. Later, tests would show that fifteen of the orphans were carrying hepatitis B, four were carrying salmonella and one had been born with congenital syphilis. Several had pneumonia.[10]

Once in Bangkok the children were loaded onto the Qantas jet, after which the plane took off into the dark night sky, bound for Melbourne. The jet was much more comfortable than the big, loud Hercules and many of the children and babies relaxed and fell asleep. Some, though, were ravenous, gulping down the food they were offered and looking for more. All night, Viv and her team tended to the little ones, feeding, changing nappies, and making them all as comfortable and relaxed as they could.

The children were all victims of hunger, trauma and starvation. Even the toddlers had learned to fight for survival. The children gobbled down their food and some hid handfuls of rice under their seats for later use. When one of the nurses bent down to pick some up she received a karate chop to the back of the neck from an infant warning her to stay away.

After nine hours, the Qantas flight touched down at Melbourne's Tullamarine Airport in the foggy dawn of 18 April. The plane taxied to a long line of waiting ambulances. One reporter said the orphans of Saigon had arrived like ghosts in the mist.[11]

The orphans reached the Fairfield hospital at 6.30 a.m. While there was now no shortage of food, many remained severely traumatised by the war. Most wouldn't sleep near windows nor in cots. 'But as the days went by,' Viv explained later, 'they gained in confidence, and they were different kiddies. They relaxed and were gorgeous and outgoing.'[12]

The evacuation from Singapore on the *Vyner Brooke* had been a disaster but, thirty-three years later, the evacuation of the orphans was a great success. Some of the babies were already too sick to recover, however, with four of the sickest children, all in intensive care, passing away within two months of their arrival. By then, most of the seventy children who had survived were living with adoptive families. Viv stayed in touch with many of them and, as the years passed, she would delight in all their achievements.

On 24 April 1977, the day before Anzac Day, television host Roger Climpson stunned Viv by handing her an oversized folder and announcing 'Vivian Bullwinkel – This Is Your Life'. Over the next half-hour, Viv's life flashed before her as her friends including Zelda, Betty, Wilma, Mickey, Sylvia and Nesta all came through the sliding doors of the television studio to reminisce with her about what had been an extraordinary life. Viv's beloved nephew, John Bullwinkel, also appeared on the program. Eva, now eighty-nine, sent a video message from her home in Adelaide, while other guests included Ken Brown, the pilot who flew to the nurses' rescue on Sumatra, and Dr Harry Windsor, who flew with them to Singapore.

When asked to speak of her experiences in the war, though, Viv was reluctant to discuss details of the murders on Radji Beach and the atrocities in the camps. She felt that a light-entertainment television program was not the medium for those memories.

She preferred to speak about her experiences in speeches of inspiration at military and nursing functions. At one, at the Hollywood Hospital in Perth, where the nurses first landed in Australia after being freed from Sumatra, she said:

> I saw twenty-one of my colleagues murdered on a beach on Bangka Island. That incident has altered and overshadowed my life – more so than the following three and a half long years of humiliation, degradation, lack of privacy, filth, bugs, rats, slave labour, starvation, sickness and death. Yet out of that horror came courage, determination, initiative, friendship and above all a sense of humour … Throughout my professional career, I endeavoured to practise tolerance – a lesson which we learnt very quickly in prison camp. When you are in a situation of trying to survive, one's values change and we soon learnt to differentiate between what was really important and what was not. This too helped me during my career, to recognise what was really important and not to get into a hassle over things that really were petty.[13]

Viv told her audience that, despite experiencing the mass murder of her colleagues and enduring years of torture, 'I have never regretted enlisting … I loved caring for the troops … and nothing but nothing is too good for them. In the words of the National POW Association: "We remember our dead by caring for our living."'[14]

FRANK STATHAM WAS HAVING dinner with Viv at the Naval and Military Club in Melbourne about the time of her appearance on *This Is Your Life*. He was in the city for his role with the Department of Works. Viv told Frank that at the age of sixty-one she was considering retirement. The demands for her to speak at functions was increasing and she was struggling with a much-increased workload at Fairfield due to rapidly rising rates of hepatitis from illicit drug use in the community. She had already retired from the Citizen Military Forces and felt that, after making what she believed to be a considerable contribution to nursing over four decades,[15] she could do with a rest. Hazel, Frank's wife of thirty-seven years had died after a long fight with cancer in February 1977. Frank suggested that retiring might be a good idea and perhaps a change of scene might do Viv good. Perhaps she could retire to Western Australia and that they could live at his house in Nedlands as husband and wife?

At the age of sixty-one Viv had received her first marriage proposal. She caught her breath and the pair ordered a glass of port each to celebrate.

A few days later Viv proudly showed off her engagement ring to her colleagues at Fairfield. Viv had pinned the ring inside the pocket of her uniform for safekeeping and was giggling like a teenager as she showed it off.[16] She told the nurses she'd never done anything in a hurry and had finally found a wonderful man with whom she could share the rest of her days.[17]

Chapter 30

VIV MARRIED FRANK STATHAM, the love of her life, on 16 September 1977 at St Margaret's Church in Nedlands, with a reception for the two colonels at the Swan Barracks. Viv hadn't thought about hiring a professional photographer, and at the last minute asked her nephew, John, to take some photographs of the newlyweds. One of the wedding guests was Viv's dear friend, Little Bet Kenneison, now known by her married name, Edie Leembruggen.

Two days after Viv and the nurses had been evacuated from Sumatra on the Douglas Dakota in 1945, Edie and some of her fellow prisoners were flown to Singapore and lodged at Raffles Hotel. Edie had spent hours looking in the mirror trying to process a reflection she had not really seen for three and a half years. She did not recognise herself. She also did not recognise her own mother after the war and had trouble adjusting to post-war life. But she finished her schooling in Singapore, became a teacher, gained a scholarship and attended the New York State Teacher College. In 1960, she moved to Western Australia. Even as they both approached old age, Viv still called Edie 'Little Bet' and Edie would say that Viv 'always had this wide grin ... always had a big smile on her face irrespective of her situations'.[1]

Viv settled into a comfortable, easy retirement in Perth as the new Mrs Statham, and her mother, Eva, came to live with the couple for a time until she died in 1981 at the age of ninety-three. Frank served on the boards of the Princess Margaret Hospital for Children and Western Australia's state committee of the Commonwealth Scientific and Industrial Research Organisation. He then became the inaugural executive officer of the University of Western Australia's engineering foundation.[2]

FOUR YEARS AFTER VIV'S WEDDING, a junior historian at the Australian War Memorial in Canberra was sent downstairs to collect a package from an elderly member of the public. People were often bringing war relics or memorabilia to the War Memorial in the hope that they might be of some interest. The visitor was a woman with a silver perm who introduced herself as Vivian Statham. She explained that she had been a nurse during World War II and she thought the museum might like her uniform for its collection. Inside the package was the dress Viv had worn on Radji Beach. There had been some repairs, given it had been doused in salt water, oil and blood, but there was still a hole just above the waistline where a Japanese machine-gun bullet had cannoned through her body. The uniform soon became a major display at the memorial.

In 1985, Viv was appointed to the Council of the Australian War Memorial, making her the first woman trustee of the institution. For Viv, the following years were largely ones of peace and contentment, though the march of time took its toll and she eventually needed assistance walking. She and Frank took holidays to Singapore and Penang, and Viv was involved with many charities and returned services organisations. She was often called on to make speeches at nursing events, military functions and schools.

At the graduation dinner for the No. 144 Pilots Course at the RAAF base at Point Cook in 1988, Viv told the audience she was delighted to celebrate the occasion, especially as two young women, Robyn Williams and Deborah Hicks, were among the graduates as the first two women to have completed that type of pilot's training course.

Viv had a great bond with the RAAF, she said, as her late brother John had flown Kittyhawks with No. 3 Squadron in the Middle East during World War II.

'I was very proud of him,' she told the audience, 'in spite of the fact that he once forgot to look in his rear vision mirror, and as a result was shot down over the Western Desert – fortunately resulting in him only having to spend the next two years in hospital.'[3]

In 1992, Viv and Frank attended a mayoral reception in Perth for the Indonesian Ambassador to Australia. They were introduced to several Indonesian officials, one of whom mentioned the sunshine and beaches of Bangka Island and its development as a tourist destination. Viv told him the story of Radji Beach and the prison camps and said that if the area was being developed she would like to see a memorial erected to all the Australian nurses who had perished there.[4]

She suspected the idea would go nowhere but soon after that conversation Viv and Frank were invited to the Indonesian consulate in Perth to meet an entrepreneur and philanthropist who had been born on Bangka Island. He told the couple he would do all he could to see a memorial erected to the brave Australian women.

A few days later, Colonel Jim Molan, the Australian Army's attaché in Jakarta, phoned Viv to say that the relevant central and provincial governments as well as the Indonesian army and police had approved the memorial project and were asking Viv and Frank to fly to Bangka to select a suitable location for it.

In October 1992, Viv and Frank flew to Bangka Island. While there, Viv chose a site for the memorial near the old Muntok lighthouse, which had been a beacon for the nurses after their ship had gone down.

ON 2 MARCH 1993, FIFTY-ONE years after Viv was shot in the back and saw all those around her murdered, she and a small group of her fellow survivors tottered down an Indonesian jungle track. Some, including Viv, needed assistance, but they eventually emerged from the foliage to gaze upon a vivid blue sea and gentle waves lapping on a pebbled beach. This tropical paradise had once been a brief refuge for the nurses before they'd faced the viciousness of the Japanese invaders.

Now seventy-seven and carrying a small posy of jungle flowers she had picked, Viv was assisted to the waters' edge. She stepped into the cool blue waves. It was so beautiful here, she still wondered what could poison the human heart to want to commit atrocities even in a heavenly place like this. Viv closed her eyes and could see her friends all about her. Matron Drummond was telling the girls to keep their chins up and Jean Stewart was imploring them not to squeal. Over the years, Viv had often wondered 'Why me?' – why had she survived when all the others about her were killed? But being here with them again, and leaving a permanent memorial to those brave, self-sacrificing women, it felt to Viv as though they were coming home at last.[5] A tear rolled down Viv's cheek as she tossed the flowers into the waves and said goodbye to Radji Beach.[6]

Viv and six other survivors – Wilma, Mavis Allgrove (nee Hannah), Joyce Tweddell, Jean Ashton, Flo Syer (nee Trotter) and Pat Darling (nee Gunther) – then attended the unveiling of the nearby memorial honouring all sixty-five nurses on the *Vyner Brooke*. With them were Colonel Coralie Gerrard, the Australian Army's Matron-in-Chief and Director of Nursing Services, and six serving army nurses who acted as carers for the elderly women.[7]

It was a quiet, dignified ceremony. Colonel Molan read out the names of the nurses' lost friends, while some of the women read from the Bible and others offered prayers from the heart.[8] Viv laid a wreath at the base of the monument, in which was embedded a stone from one of the prisoner-of-war camps.[9]

Mavis Allgrove, the only survivor from her unit, said later that she wept the whole day of the ceremony. 'I could see all those lovely sisters who didn't have a chance to live their lives,' she said. 'I've been very, very lucky to have lived and to have had a family. I think of my lovely girls laughing, beautiful happy girls cut off like that. I always think of them as young and beautiful and hope that they see me from wherever they are and see the love we all had for them.'

During the trip the women also travelled to Jakarta to pay tribute to the eight nurses who died in the camps and who are now buried in the Commonwealth War Graves Commission Cemetery.

SIX MONTHS AFTER VIV'S return to Radji Beach, Yuki Tanaka, a lecturer teaching at Melbourne University, delivered a paper to an international conference on Japan claiming that the nurses on Radji Beach 'almost certainly were raped by soldiers before being killed, but the rape was covered up to protect their memory'.[10]

His paper suggested that Viv, who had been made an Officer of the Order of Australia that year, 'did not tell the truth at the investigation in order to save her dead colleagues from the disgrace [of] being known as victims of rape'.

According to Tanaka it was 'quite possible that the Australian nurses were raped before they were killed'. He said it was 'significant that the bodies of bayoneted British soldiers were left on [Radji Beach], but that the Japanese had made sure that the evidence of the women's bodies would not be left behind'.[11]

Another shipwreck survivor had claimed that a group of imprisoned Australian soldiers were rounded up by the Japanese and ordered to carry the bodies of the massacred men and nurses from Radji Beach to be burned. They had to collect wood and debris, build a large funeral pyre and then place all the bodies – men and women – one by one on the fire until only the ashes remained.[12]

Tanaka had also documented Japanese research that pointed to Australian troops being involved in the systematic rape of Japanese civilians at Kure in Japan in October 1945.

There was no conclusive proof that the nurses on Radji Beach had been raped, however, and Viv did not respond to the claims, though they would resurface again and again over the years. Viv's nephew, John Bullwinkel, said that, while she spoke openly of the atrocities and humiliations she and the others had endured, she 'never once' said anything to her family about her or the other nurses being molested before the murders.[13]

VIV'S FINAL DAYS WERE blighted by ill-health and she was often confined to a wheelchair. In September 1994 she launched the frigate HMAS *Anzac* in Melbourne but the following year, back in Perth, she suffered a stroke and was rushed to the Hollywood Hospital. She underwent months of therapy to learn to walk and talk again. Frank became her full-time carer and the couple moved into a smaller home in a retirement village at Claremont. They travelled to Canberra in 1997, where a frail Viv was photographed shedding a silent tear at the dedication of the site to house the Australian Service Nurses National Memorial on Anzac Parade.[14]

Viv was back at home in Claremont the following year when she received a letter from a man she first met on the *Vyner Brooke* as it readied to sail out of Singapore in 1942. She remembered him as a big, burly action-man with an American accent. On Bangka Island, he had helped carry wounded nurses to Radji Beach on a makeshift stretcher before being marched off to his death by the Japanese and run through with a bayonet not long before the soldiers returned to shoot Viv and the twenty-two other women.

In a letter dated 15 December 1998, the former brewer wrote to Viv from his home in Boynton Beach, Florida.[15]

> Speaking of shades of Christmases past, here is one of a February day of many years ago – and the ones which followed, come to visit you.
>
> I am Eric H. Germann, an American, 85, a widower and retiree, living in south Florida now, but at one time, a fellow passenger with you aboard the *Vyner Brooke* and a near lost soul companion afterward on that miserable Banka beach.
>
> An account of your experience, before, and after those days ... recently appeared in an issue of *The Nursing History Review*, published by the American Association for [the] History of Nursing, here in the States ...
>
> Blessed with the longevity given us – there must be few of our companions left anywhere anymore, and more it

seems are leaving us yearly – so I believe it time to finally reintroduce myself, and also congratulate you for your survivability; the estimable dedication to your profession all these years, and I wish you a few more additional 'golden years'.

We've taken rather diverse routes for our lives, since those days, often pragmatically, suppressing the worst memories of them, just to face the everyday ordeals of daily living …[16]

After surviving the bayonet attack and eventually being liberated from his prisoner-of-war camp on Sumatra, Germann had continued working as a brewer in New York, and then in Ecuador, where he married. He then worked in Costa Rica, Puerto Rico, Spain, the Netherlands and Nigeria. In 1974 he retired to Florida with his wife, Connie, and stayed fit playing badminton in Boca Raton.[17]

Germann told Viv he had long wondered about the fate of that 'vivacious fiery redhead' [Vima Bates, lost at sea] and the 'young naval stoker Ernest Lloyd, the only other man beside myself to have survived the butchery on the beach, by dashing into the sea and swimming away'.[18]

He was unaware that Lloyd had died in March 1991, aged seventy-four, after living at Gwent in Wales for most of his life.[19]

IN 1999 VIV AND FRANK were travelling to Canberra again for the unveiling of the Australian Service Nurses National Memorial, when Frank took ill and had to return to Perth. Viv was by his side when her husband of twenty-two years died on 3 December 1999.

Viv had been able to survive a machine-gun bullet and starvation but now, aged eighty-four, the loss of Frank was too much. She underwent a complicated operation on her leg in June 2000 and a few days later, on 3 July, the huge heart that had defied death so many times finally gave out.

Australia had lost a national treasure.

A week later, four of Viv's surviving comrades, Wilma, Flo Syer, Pat Darling and Jessie Hookway (nee Simons), flew in from around Australia to attend a State Service at Saint George's Cathedral in Perth. Hundreds of people braved stormy weather to farewell one of Australia's great heroes, admired not just for her extraordinary survival during the war but for her compassion and dedication to nursing in the decades that followed.

A devastated Betty Kenneison said she felt lost that she would never see this remarkable woman again, 'a wonderful person and a carer in the true sense of the word'.[20] Bishop Brian Kyme told the mourners that Viv had made a 'monumental contribution to easing the suffering of the sick and dying during and after the war'.

Viv's old friends placed poppies on the flag-draped casket, upon which rested Viv's white nurses veil, her scarlet cape and her medals and decorations.

Members of the Australian Defence Force and service organisations carried Viv's casket to the hearse. Flags flew at half-mast, police stopped the traffic along Saint George's Terrace and onlookers bowed their heads as the funeral procession made its way to the Karrakatta Crematorium for a private committal.

Years later, General Peter Cosgrove, who would become Australia's Governor-General, said that Viv and her comrades had fought not against a physical enemy but 'against anything which threatened to destroy life. Theirs was a courage not stimulated by the lust for battle but borne of women's natural instinct to tend the sick, the helpless, the suffering and the fearful.'[21]

Epilogue

IN 2023, VIVIAN BULLWINKEL became a permanent symbol of strength and compassion for all Australia. She had gained enormous respect in a life of self-sacrifice, and now her form, cast in bronze, stands in the grounds of the Australian War Memorial.

More than eighty years after the horrors of Radji Beach, a large crowd of dignitaries from government, nursing and the military, along with descendants of nurses from the *Vyner Brooke*, gathered together under leaden skies to see the unveiling of a monument that not only honoured Viv and the nurses who did not return home but all those nurses who have risked their lives to help others in warfare.

John Bullwinkel was one of three generations of Viv's family among the hundreds of invited guests who, on a cold winter's morning of 2 August 2023, witnessed the dedication of the bronze statue. John, who had donated all of Viv's medals and awards to the War Memorial, said Viv would probably have been a little embarrassed by all the fuss and fanfare, as she was never one to seek the limelight. Viv was humble, he said, compassionate, and self-effacing. She learned to use humour whenever she could in the prison camps, once recalling that a Japanese guard had tossed her half a coconut shell on a stick and told her to empty a 10-by 20-metre overflowing cesspit infested with dysentery. To stop herself from going mad she told herself that it was 'either funny ridiculous or ridiculously funny'.[1]

'She had a great sense of humour and she loved to party,' John explained. 'She was always trying to help people. She lived her life as a tribute to friends who would never return home.'

Governor General David Hurley also spoke, saying he would try to do Viv justice by his words, though he conceded that Viv 'was a giant'.

Brisbane-based artist Dr Charles Robb's sculpture depicts Viv standing in her nurse's uniform, hands gently clasped to reflect her dignified composure, determination and strength of character. More than 3 metres high so now everyone must look up to her, Viv gazes placidly across at the powerful but benign figure of Weary Dunlop, a man with a similar reputation for strength and kindness. The first statue of a woman at the War Memorial, it was designed to capture the spirit of nurses everywhere.

The War Memorial had attracted criticism for not funding the statue itself. Instead the $500,000 needed was raised from a tireless campaign spearheaded by Adjunct Professor Kylie Ward, the CEO of the Australian College of Nursing, who had been overwhelmed by emotion on her own visit to Radji Beach.

Donations came from both big corporations and cake stalls as Professor Ward mirrored the actions of Viv and Betty in their fundraising drive fifty years earlier for the nurses memorial centre. Professor Ward insisted that a statue of a woman at the War Memorial was long overdue, considering that it already had statues of a digger's dog and Simpson's donkey.

'We lost our sons but we also lost our nation's daughters, and I think the brutality of what these nurses experienced, and what Vivian fought to get them recognition for, came to the forefront today in our hearts,' Professor Ward said at the unveiling.[2]

'I think that Vivian Bullwinkel should have been a household name to me when I was growing up – to every Australian – so why don't we know the names of our women that have shaped our country and our culture?'

Professor Ward also announced that the Australian College of Nursing would introduce twenty-two scholarships to honour all the nurses who were shot by the Japanese on Radji Beach. 'Vivian

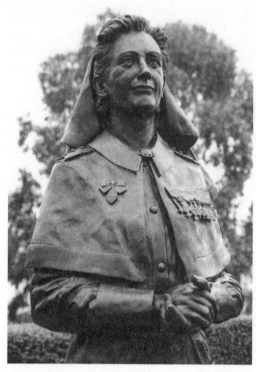

Viv was honoured in 2023 as the subject for the first statue of a woman at the Australian War Memorial. *Australian College of Nursing*

Bullwinkel devoted her life to ensuring the nurses would not be forgotten, and the ACN Foundation intends to carry on her work and legacy,' she said.

Michael Noyce, brother of Hollywood film director Phil Noyce and the nephew of Kathleen Neuss, who was killed on Radji Beach, makes a yearly pilgrimage to the pebbled sand to honour the memory of the fallen nurses.

He says their stories must never be forgotten. 'To imagine what happened there all those years ago is quite chilling,' he said. 'The more the stories of all these people can be told the better we all are.'[3]

TIME EVENTUALLY CAUGHT up with all of Viv's fellow survivors from Sumatra. Betty Jeffrey died a few months after Viv in 2000, Wilma Young a year later, Flo Syer in 2002, and Little Bet Leembruggen in 2008. Cecilia McPhee (nee Delforce) was the last of the *Vyner Brooke* nurses, passing away on the Gold Coast in 2011 at the age of ninety-eight. Cecilia had asked for no flowers at her funeral in remembrance of all her friends who had died without flowers in 1942.

TWO DECADES AFTER Viv died in Perth, speculation continued in regard to the events on Radji Beach and whether she had told the whole, awful truth about the massacre. Some writers have claimed that the Australian Government 'gagged' her, preventing Viv from revealing that the nurses on Radji Beach, including herself, were raped before being slaughtered.

In an article for the website *Independent Australia* in 2017, journalist Tess Lawrence said she had met Viv in Melbourne on several occasions, 'at least twice at the now defunct Naval and Military Club in Little Collins Street'.[4] Lawrence claimed that Viv told her that she and most of the other women had been 'violated' by the Japanese soldiers before being shot and that she was under 'great mental and emotional anguish and distress' because she had been gagged at the war-crimes tribunal.[5]

But John Bullwinkel is sceptical that his aunt would confide in a writer she'd met a few times rather any of her close family members. And he asks that, even if she had felt frustrated and gagged by army officials in 1946, as some journalists contend, why didn't she reveal the truth in a public forum at some time during the fifty-five years she was alive following the end of the war? She must have given hundreds of interviews and speeches over the years.

Noted military historian Lynette Silver said she had uncovered a key witness to whom Vivian Bullwinkel disclosed the rapes – the now retired Australian Army major Patricia Hincks. The revelation was said to have occurred in 1991 in the Officers' Mess in Fremantle's Leeuwin Barracks, where Viv apparently told Major Hincks, whom she had just met, that the nurses 'were actually tortured and raped – and then they marched [us] out to sea'.[6] Ms Hincks says she has 'no idea' why Vivian would confide such delicate, personal information to someone she had just met in passing. 'I had never met her before. I don't know why we had that brief conversation,' Ms Hincks said. 'But Vivian told me that the abuse was a secret among the nurses and that they had all been sworn to secrecy.'[7]

Lynette Silver surmised that 'Senior Australian Army officers wanted to protect grieving families from the stigma of rape'.[8] There have also been claims that, because Viv had stopped menstruating while she was in the prison camps, she may have even fallen pregnant, though many of the nurses revealed that the combination of shock and extreme hunger that they experienced in captivity had disrupted monthly cycles for all of them.

John Bullwinkel says some writers seem to be drawing 'a very long bow' to make events fit a narrative of rape and cover-up. Some have even speculated that Viv's tinea may have actually been syphilis[9] and that repairs to Viv's tattered uniform may have been necessitated because it was torn open by a rapist.[10]

The Japanese were notorious for using rape as a weapon of war. Viv never spoke publicly of the Japanese molesting the nurses on Radji Beach or in the prison camps. It seems almost certain, though, that Viv did her best to spare the relatives of the dead nurses, her dear friends, the most horrific details of the murders. The killers on Radji Beach were from the same unit that had a reputation for rape and murder. Witnesses who saw the bodies after the massacre said some of the women were naked, and that, contrary to Viv's claims that they had all marched calmly into the water, it seemed obvious that some had run for their lives and been slashed by bayonets. It appeared one had been killed by a sword.

The events on Radji Beach were some of the darkest for Australia during World War II. No one can be certain of what happened on Radji Beach before the shooting began but there is no dispute that twenty-two Australian nurses and poor old Mrs Carrie Betteridge were machine-gunned, and that only Viv survived.

JOHN BULLWINKEL CHOKED on his words at the dedication of Viv's statue when he remembered the courage of his aunt and the tragedy of what happened to forty-one of her colleagues.

Professor Ward told the audience she was inspired by the thought that generations of children to come would see a figure in bronze of a nurse and midwife at the Australian War Memorial. The sculpture would be a powerful and long-lasting symbol of the selfless service to Australia and its citizens that nurses have always provided, whether in war or in peace.

Addressing 'Dearest Vivian' in her speech, Professor Ward said, 'I imagine you are probably looking down wondering what all the fuss is about and why for goodness' sake we have fought so hard to get a larger-than-life statue of you in such a prominent position here on the grounds of the Australian War Memorial. I want you to know that this statue and you are a symbol for all [that] I hope nursing continues to be – proud, determined, tenacious, disciplined, educated, dignified, brave, selfless and formidable ... Viv, you gave great sacrifices for your profession and for your country. You were a great Australian, a great leader and an inspiration to all.'[11]

It had been an emotional ceremony, the speakers all moved by the memories of Viv's courage and the tragic loss of so many lives, so many wonderful, brave, caring women cut down as innocent victims during the insanity of war.

All morning it had threatened to rain on Viv's parade but the rain stayed away through the 'Ode of Remembrance', 'The Last Post', a minute's silence and then the military band's rendition of 'Advance Australia Fair'.

As the guests shook each other's hands at the end of the ceremony and told stories about Viv and the shining light she had been for all those she met and for the country she loved, some in the audience turned their faces to the mountains behind the city. After a morning of threatening rain there had been a break in the storm clouds.

A brilliant, shining rainbow emerged from the darkness.

Acknowledgements

VIVIAN BULLWINKEL knew the importance of teamwork and this book would not have been possible without the assistance of so many wonderful people.

Viv was a remarkably selfless woman who devoted her life to helping others, and I received priceless assistance from so many people in telling her story.

I am indebted to the unstinting generosity of Viv's nephew John Bullwinkel and his wife Melissa who shared with me, not only so many valuable memories, but so much of Viv's correspondence and private possessions, including her own family photo albums kept from the days of her childhood.

I am very grateful for the support of Associate Professor Kylie Ward, the Chief Executive Officer of the Australian College of Nursing, whose extraordinary drive resulted in the erection of the Australian War Memorial's remarkable statue of Vivian.

Thank you also to David Young, son of Viv's great friend Wilma Oram, Emily Malone, the great niece of Betty Jeffrey, and Michael Noyce, nephew of Kathleen Neuss. The meticulous research of historian Michael Pether provided so much important information about the events surrounding Radji Beach and their aftermath.

Thanks also to Dr Olga Kanitsaki for sharing with me her memories of Viv's kindness and diligence.

I am greatly indebted to the work of Norman Manners, Betty Jeffrey, Jessie Simons and Pat Gunther whose books shone so much light on the life of Viv and her colleagues.

Luke Slatter, Samantha McCrossen, and Lauren Watkins from the Australian War Memorial gave me great assistance as did the staff at the National Library of Australia, and the State Libraries of Queensland, New South Wales, Victoria and South Australia.

This book would not have been possible without the extraordinary support of the marvellous editorial team at HarperCollins/ABC Books, including Roberta Ivers, Lachlan McLaine, Brigitta Doyle, Helen Littleton, Hannah Lynch, Nicolette Houben, Jacqui Furlong and Erin Dunk, as well as my tireless editor Jude McGee.

Thank you all, very much.

Grantlee Kieza, January 2024

Bibliography

BOOKS

Barbara Angell, *A Woman's War: The Exceptional Life of Wilma Oram*, New Holland, 2011

Ralph Armstrong, *A Short Cruise on the Vyner Brooke*, George Mann, 2003

Lex Arthurson, *The Story of the 13ᵗʰ Australian General Hospital*, pows-of-japan.net

Jean Ashton, *Jean's diary: a POW diary, 1942–1945*, Jill Ashton, 2003

Colin Burgess, *Sisters in Captivity*, Simon & Schuster, 2023

Iris Chang, *The Rape of Nanking: The Forgotten Holocaust of World War II*, Basic Books, 2011

Winston S. Churchill, *The Second World War*, vol. 4, Cassell & Co., 1951

Pat Darling, *Portrait of a Nurse*, Don Wall, 2001

Susannah de Vries, *Heroic Australian Women in War*, HarperCollins, 2004

Henry Taprell Dorling, *Blue Star Line at War*, 1939–45, W. Foulsham & Co, 1973

Gideon Francois Jacobs, *Prelude to the Monsoon*, Purnell & Sons, 1966

Betty Jeffrey, *White Coolies*, Angus & Robertson, Sydney, 1954

Catherine Kenny, *Captives: Australian Army Nurses in Japanese Prison Camps*, University of Queensland Press, 1986

Beryl Maddock, (nee Chandler), *Flight Sister*, unpublished book

Norman G Manners, *Bullwinkel*, Hesperian Press, 1999

William H. McDougall, *By Eastern Windows*, Charles Scribner's Sons, 1949

Hank Nelson and Gavin McCormack (eds), *The Burma–Thailand Railway: Memory and History*, Allen & Unwin, 1993,

Willem Remmelink (ed), *The Operations of the Navy in the Dutch East Indies and the Bay of Bengal*, Leiden University Press, 2018

Jessie Simons, *While History Passed*, Heinemann, 1954

Ian W. Shaw, *On Radji Beach*, Pan Macmillan Australia, 2010 (Kindle edition)

Ian W. Shaw, *Operation Babylift*, Hachette, 2019 (Kindle edition)

Peter Thompson, *The Battle for Singapore*, Portrait Books, 2005

Otto D. Tolischus, *Through Japanese Eyes*, The Infantry Journal, 1946

Ian Townsend, *Line of Fire*, Fourth Estate, 2017.

NEWSPAPERS and MAGAZINES

Army Magazine
Australian Nursing and Midwifery Journal
Barrier Daily Truth (Broken Hill)
Barrier Miner (Broken Hill, NSW)
Brisbane Telegraph
Cairns Post
Chronicle (Adelaide)
Commonwealth of Australia Gazette
Huon and Derwent Times (Tasmania)
Inverell Times (NSW)
Journal of Contemporary History
Kapunda Herald (SA)
Launceston Examiner (Tasmania)
News (Adelaide)
Northern Star (Lismore, NSW)
Northern Territory News
Pacific Historical Review
Recorder (Port Pirie, SA)
Remembrance: Official Magazine of the Shrine of Remembrance Melbourne
Sporting Globe (Melbourne)
The Advertiser (Adelaide)
The Armidale Express and New England General Advertiser (NSW)
The Age (Melbourne)
The Argus (Melbourne)
The Australian Women's Weekly
The Bulletin
The Canberra Times
The Catholic Press (Sydney)
The Courier-Mail
The Daily Mirror (Sydney)
The Daily Telegraph (Sydney)
The Herald (Melbourne)
The Horsham Times
The Journal (Adelaide)
The Mercury (Hobart)
The Narracoorte Herald (Naracoorte, SA)
The Newcastle Sun (NSW)
The Register (Adelaide)
The Riverine Herald (Echuca, Vic)
The Sarawak Gazette
The Sun (Sydney)

The Sun-Herald (Sydney)
The Sunday Mail (Brisbane)
The Sydney Morning Herald
The Telegraph (Brisbane)
The West Australian (Perth)
Transcontinental (Port Augusta, SA)
Woman's Day and Home

INTERNET
229battalion.org.au
abc.net.au
aircrewremembered.com
ancestry.com
angellpro.com.au
anzacportal.dva.gov.au
Australian College of Nursing, acn.edu.au
Australian Dictionary of Biography
australiannursesmemorialcentre.org.au
Australian War Memorial, awm.gov.au
bbc.com
brokenhill.nsw.gov.au
Hansard
Imperial War Museums, iwm.org.uk
independentaustralia.net
jahis.law.nagoya-u.ac.jp.
malayanvolunteersgroup.org.uk
muntokpeacemuseum. org
Museums of History NSW, mhnsw.au
National Archives of Australia
National Library of Australia, nla.gov.au
National Museum of Australia, nma.gov.au
Pows-of-japan.net
Prospect Public School, prospectps.sa.edu
Sarah Fulford, 'Training, Ethos, Camaraderie and Endurance of World
    War Two Australian POW Nurses', Department of Social Sciences and
    Security Studies, Curtin University, espace.curtin.edu.au
singingtosurvive.com
Southern Grampians Shire Council, sthgrampians.vic.gov.au
southwalesargus.co.uk
themonthly.com.au
warfarehistorynetwork.com

Endnotes

Prologue

1 Sister Vivian Bullwinkel's testimony, Australian War Crimes Board of Inquiry, Melbourne, 29 October 1945, p. 4, Australian War Memorial, AWM 54, 1010/4/24, Part 2.

2 'The Sinking of SS *Vyner Brooke* and the Banka Island Massacre', awm.gov.au

3 'Brutality of Japanese at Hong Kong', *The Argus* (Melbourne), 19 December 1946, p. 5.

4 Sister Vivian Bullwinkel's testimony, Australian War Crimes Board of Inquiry, Melbourne, 29 October 1945, p. 4, AWM 54, 1010/4/24, Part 2.

5 *Ibid.*

6 Vivian Bullwinkel interview, *Vivian Bullwinkel: An Australian Heroine*, Waterbyrd Filmz, 2007.

Chapter One

1 'Family Notices', *The Advertiser* (Adelaide), 24 December 1915, p. 6.

2 Eva Kate Bullwinkel (nee Shegog), b. 13 February 1888 (Port Augusta, SA), d. 3 September 1981 (Adelaide, SA).

3 George Albert Bullwinkel, b. 19 March 1879 (Leytonstone, UK), d. 19 September 1934 (Broken Hill, NSW).

4 William Lyle Shegog, b. 13 April 1856 (Londonderry, Ireland), d. 28 March 1930 (Prospect, SA).

5 'Obituary', *Launceston Examiner* (Tasmania), 27 April 1896, p. 6.

6 'Personal', *The Advertiser* (Adelaide), 29 June 1920, p. 4.

7 Emily Shegog (nee Robinson), b. 1860, d. 21 June 1931 (Prospect, SA).

8 'North-West Police', *The Register* (Adelaide), 12 May 1924, p. 13.

9 'Personal', *The Advertiser* (Adelaide), 29 June 1920, p. 4. Some of the places were Farina, Maree, Beltana, Blinman, Melrose, Carrieton, Teetulpa, Yongala, Peterborough, Cockburn, Tanunda, Kapunda, Renmark and Kingscote.

10 'Wreck of the *Loch Sloy*: Ashore off Kangaroo Island', *The Argus* (Melbourne), 10 May 1899, p. 5.

11 William Lyle Shegog Jnr, b. 20 January 1886 (Port Augusta, SA), d. 5 September 1968 (Brighton, SA).

12 'Dispatch Bag', *Chronicle* (Adelaide), 7 September 1901, p. 47.

13 'Out Among the People', *The Advertiser* (Adelaide), 14 December 1945, p. 12.

14 'News from Broken Hill', *Recorder* (Port Pirie), 24 September 1934, p. 2.

15 'History', brokenhill.nsw.gov.au

16 Auguste Joseph François de Bavay, b. 9 June 1856, d. 16 November 1944.

17 'Norths Soccer Club Meeting', *Barrier Miner* (Broken Hill, NSW), 1 May 1913, p. 3.

18 'Family Notices', *Chronicle* (Adelaide), 9 May 1914, p. 35.

19 Nicholas Shakespeare, 'Outback Jihad: How World War One came to Broken Hill', themonthly.com.au, November 2014.

20 'War at Broken Hill', *The Narracoorte Herald* (Naracoorte, SA), 5 January 1915, p. 3.

21 'Barrier Casualties', *The Register* (Adelaide), 14 January 1915, p. 7.

22 'Battle Of Broken Hill', *The Journal* (Adelaide), 5 January 1915, p. 2.

23 'Football', *Barrier Miner* (Broken Hill), 19 March 1915, p. 1.

24 *Ibid.*

25 'British Association', *ibid.*, 11 July 1919, p. 3.

26 John Monash to his wife Victoria, 20 December 1915, War Letters of General Monash, Vol 1, 24 December 1914 – 4 March 1917, Australian War Memorial, awm.gov.au, 3DRL/2316.

27 'The Australian Exodus', *Chronicle* (Adelaide) 8 January 1916, p. 37.

Chapter Two

1 Papers of Vivian Bullwinkel, Album 3, Australian War Memorial, PR01216.

2 'War Memorial Unveiled by Sir John Monash', *Barrier Miner* (Broken Hill), 12 October 1925, p. 3.

3 'Broken Hill Stamp Club', *ibid.*, 1 July 1916, p. 6.

4 'Collapsed In Taxi', *ibid.*, 19 September 1934, p. 1.

5 'Ancient Order of Foresters: Court Stewart', *ibid.*, 8 March 1915, p. 4.

6 Norman G Manners, *Bullwinkel*, Hesperian Press, 1999, p. 3.

7 'Presentation to Sgt. Shegog', *Kapunda Herald*, 20 July 1917, p. 2.

8 'Concerning People', *The Register* (Adelaide), 30 June 1919, p. 6.

9 *Transcontinental* (Port Augusta), 2 July 1920, p. 3.

10 'Broken Hill: City of Depression', *The Inverell Times* (NSW), 12 April 1921, p. 7.

11 John William Bullwinkel, b. 19 April 1920 (Broken Hill, NSW), d. 2 November 1966 (Rosslyn Park, SA).

12 *The Bulletin*, 7 April 1921, p. 12.

13 'School History', prospectps.sa.edu

14 'North and Northwest Police', *The Register* (Adelaide), 7 June 1924, p. 14.

15 'The Motoring World', *ibid.*, 5 November 1924, p. 5

16 'De Bavay's Plant Closed', *Barrier Miner* (Broken Hill), 17 April 1925, p. 2.

17 John Monash to his wife Victoria, 16 March 1917, War Letters of General Monash, awm.gov.au, 3DRL/2316.

18 'Broken Hill', *Chronicle* (Adelaide), 17 October 1925, p. 35.

19 'War Memorial Unveiled by Sir John Monash', *Barrier Miner* (Broken Hill), 12 October 1925, p. 3.

20 *Ibid.*

21 'Skint! Making Do In the Great Depression', Museums of History NSW, mhnsw.au

22 'School Sport', *Barrier Miner* (Broken Hill), 3 May 1928, p. 3.

23 'Speech Night at High School', *ibid*, 12 Dec 1933, p. 3.

24 'Headmaster Farewelled', *Northern Star* (Lismore), 27 February 1930, p. 4.

25 Manners, *Bullwinkel*, p. 1.

26 Zelda Emily Treloar, b. 1915 (Broken Hill, NSW), d. 5 February 2009 (Windsor, Vic).

27 'Protest By Teachers', *The Newcastle Sun* (NSW), 18 August 1932, p. 1.

28 On 15 May 1932.

29 Manners, *Bullwinkel*, p. 2.

30 *Ibid.*

31 *Ibid.*

Chapter Three

1 'High School Prefects', *The Barrier Miner*, 18 February 1932, p. 3.

2 'High School Staff and Prefects', *ibid.*, 23 November 1932, p. 4.

3 High School Prefects', *ibid.*, 14 February 1933, p. 3.

4 'High School Sport', *ibid.*, 7 December 1933, p. 5.

5 'Visiting Lodge Officers', *ibid.*, 22 May 1933, p. 3.

6 'Adolf Hitler', *ibid.*, 16 June 1933, p. 2.

7 'Speech Night at High School', *ibid.*, 12 December 1933, p. 3.

8 'The Leaving Certificate', *ibid.*, 16 January 1934, p. 4.

9 Manners, *Bullwinkel*, p. 3.

10 'Examination No. 1869', *Commonwealth of Australia Gazette*, 11 January 1934, p. 43.

11 Rachel Isabella Charlton Hunter, b. 1897 (Grenfell, NSW), d. 1972 (Blacktown, NSW).

12 Irene Melville Drummond, b. 26 July 1905 (Ashfield, NSW), d. 16 February 1942 (Bangka Island, Indonesia).

13 'Firing During Shifts at South', *The Barrier Miner*, 18 September 1934, p. 1.

14 'Woman Dies from Wounds', *The Barrier Miner (Broken Hill)*, 18 September 1934, p. 1.

15 Vivian Ramsay Smith, b. 1890 (Edinburgh, UK), d. 28 September 1956 (Adelaide, SA).

16 'Temperatures', *The Barrier Miner*, 18 September 1934, p. 1.

17 'Collapsed In Taxi', Death of Mr. G. Bullwinkel, 19 September 1934, p. 1.

18 'The Late Mr. Bullwinkel', *The Barrier Miner*, 21 September 1934, p. 2.

19 'Architect Condemns Hospital Building: Complete Rebuilding Only Remedy', *ibid.*, 6 June 1935, p. 4.

20 'Shortage Of Doctors', *ibid.*, 6 October 1934, p. 13.

21 Vivian Bullwinkel Interview, 1993, *Vivian Bullwinkel: An Australian Heroine*, Waterbyrd Filmz, 2007.

22 Dr Gavin Murray Crabbe, b. 26 November 1901 (North Adelaide, SA), d. 14 November 14, 1951 (Hobart, Tas.).

23 'Hospital Medical Staff', Barrier Miner (Broken Hill), 9 August 1937, p. 3.

24 'Nurses' Examinations', *ibid.*, 17 December 1937, p. 3.

25 Constance Eva Sampson, b. 23 June 1912 (Laura, SA), d. 28 September 2004 (Crystal Brook, SA).

26 Mabel Gwendoline McMahon, b. 21 October 1914 (Ballarat, Vic.), d. 29 March 2002 (Millicent, SA).

27 'Nanking Terror: Japanese Barbarity, Slaughter, Rape and Looting', *The West Australian* (Perth), 29 January 1938, p. 19.

28 Iris Chang, *The Rape of Nanking: The Forgotten Holocaust of World War II*, Basic Books, 2011, pp. 103–104.

29 Otto d. Tolischus, *Through Japanese Eyes*, The Infantry Journal, 1946, p. 200

30 'Ex-Missionary Reports Cannibalism by Japs', *The Daily Telegraph* (Sydney), 11 December 1943, p. 3.

31 *Ibid.*

32 'Menzies has Killed "Pig Iron Bob"', *The Daily Telegraph* (Sydney), 3 April 1949, p. 12.

33 'Country', *The Sydney Morning Herald*, 16 December 1938, p. 3.

34 Barbara Helen Crowhurst (nee Shegog), b. 11 August 1890 (Port Augusta, SA), d. 29 May 1950 (Adelaide, SA).

35 Southern Grampians Shire Council, sthgrampians.vic.gov.au

36 Winifred 'Wyn' Frances James (nee Milner), b. 27 January 1902 (Buninyong, Vic), d. 18 May 1973 (Perth, WA).

37 Vivian Bullwinkel to Wyn James, 12 May 1939, Australian War Memorial, AWM2018.179.1.

38 'Far East Situation', Hansard, July 24, 1939.

39 Menzies, Robert, Papers of Sir Robert Menzies, National Library of Australia, nla.gov.au/nla.obj-233710278.

40 Second World War Official Histories, 'The Australian Army Nursing Service', p. 428, awm.gov.au, RCDIG1070406.

Chapter Four

1 Ibid.

2 Olive Dorothy Paschke, b. 19 July 1905 (Dimboola, Vic), d. 15 February 1942 (Bangka Strait, Indonesia).

3 Janice McCarthy, 'Paschke, Olive Dorothy (1905–1942)', *Australian Dictionary of Biography*, Vol. 15, Melbourne University Press, 2000.

4 Bullwinkel, John William: Service Number 407780, NAA: A9301, 407780, p. 42.

5 *Ibid.*, p. 46.

6 Manners, *Bullwinkel*, p. 7.

7 Interview, Vivian Bullwinkel, 1993 from *Vivian Bullwinkel: An Australian Heroine*, Waterbyrd Filmz, 2007.

8 Sampson, Constance Eva, Service Number 500024, National Archives of Australia, National Archives of Australia: A9300, p. 23.

9 David Day, *Menzies and Churchill at War*, Oxford University Press, 1993, pp. 9–26.

10 She joined on 23 July 1940 as a staff nurse. Paschke, Olive Dorothy, Service Number VX38812, National Archives of Australia (NAA) B883, p. 4.

11 'A Tokio Denial', *The West Australian* (Perth), 17 Apr 1941, p. 8.

12 Bullwinkel, John William: Service Number 407780, NAA: A9301, 407780, p. 33.

13 *Ibid.*, p.19–20.

14 Statham, Vivian (nee Bullwinkel), Service Number: VFX61330, NAA: A14472, VFX61330, p. 66.

15 *Ibid.*
16 Second World War Official Histories, 'The Australian Army Nursing Service', p. 428, awm.gov.au, RCDIG1070406, p. 429.
17 'Greek Campaign, 1941', awm.gov.au
18 Takeo Yoshikawa (March 7, 1912 – February 20, 1993).
19 'She's Met the Boys in Malaya', *The Australian Women's Weekly*, 5 April
20 '"They Treat Us Like Film Stars" Says A.I.F. Matron in Malaya', *The Australian Women's Weekly*, 3 May 1941, p. 7.
21 *Ibid.*
22 *Ibid.*

Chapter Five
1 Viv to Eva Bullwinkel, 20 May 1941, Papers of Vivian Bullwinkel, Australian War Memorial, PR01216, Series 2/1.
2 *Ibid.*
3 *Ibid.*
4 Clarice Isobel Halligan, b. 17 September 1904 (Ballarat, Vic), d. 16 February 1942 (Bangka Island, Indonesia).
5 Lorraine Clarice Curtis (nee Halligan), 'My Story of Aunt, Clarice Isobel Halligan', p. 2. muntokpeacemuseum. org
6 *Ibid*, p. 13.
7 *Ibid*, p. 10.
8 James Ronald Austin, b. 26 December 1919 (Melbourne, Vic.), d. 4 January 2006 (Melbourne, Vic.).
9 Austin, James Ronald, Service Number: VX25306, NAA: B883, p. 3.
10 Viv to Eva Bullwinkel, 20 May 1941, Papers of Vivian Bullwinkel, Australian War Memorial, PR01216, Series 2/1.
11 Bullwinkel, John William: Service Number 407780, NAA: A9301, 407780, p. 33.
12 'Hostel for Army Nurses: Gift to Red Cross Society', *The Age* (Melbourne), 12 December 1940, p. 3.
13 The house sold for $18 million in 2021.
14 'Matron for War Nurses Hostel', *The Argus* (Melbourne), 1 February 1941, p. 9.
15 *Ibid.*
16 '2/13th Australian General Hospital', Australian War Memorial, awm.gov.au
17 Bullwinkel, Vivian, Service Number VX61330, NAA: B2458, F31029, p. 1.

18 'Luxury Ship: Wanganella As a Hospital', *The Age* (Melbourne), 25 July 1941, p. 4.
19 *Ibid.*
20 'Conference Fails: Dock Yard Strike', *The Age,* 28 August 1941, p. 6.
21 On 25 August.
22 Mary Eleanor McGlade, b. 2 July 1902 (Armidale, NSW), d. 16 February 1942 (Bangka Island, Indonesia).
23 'The White Plague', *The Armidale Express and New England General Advertiser*, 26 September 1905, p. 5.
24 'In the Armidale Diocese', *The Catholic Press* (Sydney), 15 December 1910, p. 35.
25 'Service for Former St. Ursula Pupil', *The Armidale Express and New England General Advertiser*, 17 October 1945, p. 8.
26 Ian W. Shaw, *On Radji Beach,* Pan Macmillan Australia, 2010, ebook ed.
27 Janet 'Jenny' Kerr, b. 8 August 1910 (Monteagle, NSW), d. 16 February 1942 (Bangka Island, Indonesia).
28 Mona Margaret Anderson Tait, b. 6 February 1915 (Booval, Qld), d. 16 February 1942 (Bangka Island, Indonesia).
29 Mona Margaret Wilton, b. 8 September 1913 (Willaura, Vic), d. 14 February 1942 (lost at sea off Bangka Island, Indonesia).
30 Wilma Elizabeth Forster Young (nee Oram), AM, [Member of the Order of Australia] b. 17 August 1916 (Glenorchy, Vic), d. 28 May 2001 (Richmond, Vic.).
31 Kathleen 'Kit' Kinsella, b. 18 March 1904 (South Yarra, Vic.), d. 14 February 1942 (Bangka Island, Indonesia)
32 'A Doctor Enlists', *Huon and Derwent Times* (Tas), 4 September 1941, p. 1.
33 Irvine H. Anderson, Jnr, 'The 1941 De Facto Embargo on Oil to Japan: A Bureaucratic Reflex', *Pacific Historical Review,* Vol. 44, No. 2 (May 1975), University of California Press, p. 201.

Chapter Six
1 Major Bruce Atlee Hunt MBE, b. 23 February 1899 (Glebe, NSW), d. 29 October 1964 (West Perth, WA).
2 'Major Bruce Atlee Hunt', pows-of-japan.net.
3 Hunt, Bruce Atlee, Service Number: WX11177, NAA B883, p. 20.

4   Alma May Beard, b. 14 January 1913 (Toodyay, WA), d. 16 February 1942 (Bangka Island, Indonesia).

5   Minnie Ivy Hodgson, b.16 August 1908 (Perth, WA), d 16 February 1942 (Bangka Island, WA).

6   Iole Harper (later Burkitt), b. 15 March 1911 (East Guilford, WA), d. 4 September 1998 (Guilford, WA).

7   Wilfred Tuthill (Bill) Harper, b. 21 April 1921 (East Guildford, WA), d. 26 July 1943 (off coast of the Netherlands).

8   Later Lieutenant General Henry Gordon Bennett, b. 15 April 1887 (Balwyn, Vic) d. 1 August 1962 (Dural, NSW).

9   Douglas Clelland Pigdon, b. 6 December 1891 (Carlton North, Vic), d. 6 July 1945 (Prison camp at Hoten, Manchuria, China)

10 Pigdon, Douglas Clelland: Service Number –VX39275, NAA B883, p. 36.

11 Lieutenant-General Arthur Ernest Percival OBE, b. 26 December 1887, d. 31 January 1966.

12 'Singapore Was Not a Fortress', Imperial War Museums, iwm.org.uk

13 Peter Thompson, *The Battle for Singapore*, Portrait Books, 2005, p. 42.

14 Vivian Bullwinkel diary, AWM, PR01216, Series 1, 1/1/3.

15 Later Sir Wilfrid Selwyn 'Bill' Kent Hughes, b. 12 June 1895, d. 31 July 1970.

16 Mary Eileen (Maisie) Cooper (nee Rayner), b. 5 August 1912 (Strahan, Tas), d. 2 November 1990 (Beaconsfield, Tas).

17 Nancy Harris, b. 15 January 1913 (Guyra, NSW), d. 16 February 1942 (Bangka Island, Indonesia).

18 Later Lieutenant-Colonel Clement Polson Manson, b. 24 May 1909 (Newry, Vic), d. 14 May 1943 (killed in action aboard the *Centaur* off Brisbane).

19 Mollie Marie Gunton, b. 17 October 1913 (Mangana, Tas), d. 10 December 1994 (Hobart, Tas.).

20 Harley Rosalind Brewer, b. 6 December 1916 (Launceston, Tas) d. 5 August 2005 (Sydney, NSW).

21 Nesta Gwyneth Lewis Noy (nee James), b. 5 December 1903 (Carmarthen, UK) d. 12 February 1984 (Kew Vic.).

22 'The Building in Malaya Used as the 2/10th Australian General Hospital (AGH)', awm.gov.au/collection/ C1370991.

23 Agnes Betty Jeffrey, OAM, b. 14 May 1908 (Hobart, Tas.), d. 13 September 2000 (Melbourne, Vic.).

24 Jeffrey, Agnes Betty: Service Number: VX53059, NAA, B883, p. 6.

25 John George Glyn White, b. 9 April 1909 (Drummond North, Vic.), d. 2 November 1987 (East Melbourne, Vic.).

26 David F. Elder, 'White, John George Glyn (1909–1987)', *Australian Dictionary of Biography*, Vol. 18, Melbourne University Press, 2012.

27 Alfred Plumley Derham, b. 12 September 1891 (Camberwell, Vic), d. 26 June 1962 (Heidelberg, Vic).

28 Lieutenant Colonel Charles Harwood Osborn, b. 10 July 1897 (Boort, Vic), d. 27 December 1982 (Melbourne, Vic.).

29 Florence Elizabeth Syer (nee Trotter), b. 4 October 1915 (Eastwood, NSW), d. 31 July 2002 (Greenslopes, Qld).

30 Jean 'Jenny' Keers Pemberton (nee Greer), b. 21 October 1912 (Petersham, NSW), d. 7 December 2001 (Chichester, UK).

31 John Curtin, b 8 January 1885 (Creswick, Vic), d. 5 July 1945 (Canberra, ACT).

Chapter Seven

1   Phyllis Bronwyn Campbell (nee Pugh), b. 29 January 1916 (Brisbane, Qld), d. 19 October 1998 (Brisbane, Qld).

2   Shaw, *On Radji Beach*, ebook ed., loc. 756.

3   Sub-Lieutenant James William Miller, b. 1912 (Oamaru, NZ), d. 16 February 1942 (Bangka Island, Indonesia).

4   'S.S. Vyner Brooke', *The Sarawak Gazette*, 1 November 1927, p. 279.

5   Charles Vyner de Windt Brooke, known as Vyner, Rajah of Sarawak, b. 26 September 1874 (Greenwich, UK), d. 9 May 1963 (Bayswater, UK)).

6   Vivian Bullwinkel diary, AWM, PR01216, Series 1, 1/1/3.

7   Sultan Sir Ibrahim Al-Masyhur Ibni Almarhum Sultan Abu Bakar Al-Khalil Ibrahim Shah, b. 17 September 1873, d. 8 May 1959.

8   Eliza Margaret Bullwinkel (nee Matthews), b. c. 4 August 1852 (Sydenham, UK), d. January 1943 (Hackney, UK).

9   Dudley Walter Bullwinkle, b. 20 November 1884 (West Ham, UK), d. 20 December 1943 (Essex, UK).

10 John Bullwinkel to Vivian, 30 November 19141, AWM, PR01216, Series 2.

11 Bud Flanagan (born Chaim Weintrop, 1896–1968) and Chesney Allen (1894–1982).

12 John Bullwinkel to Vivian, 30 November 19141, AWM, PR01216, Series 2.

13 *Ibid.*

14 Hideki Tojo, b. 30 December 1884 (Kojimachi Ward, Japan), d. 23 December 1948 (executed by hanging, Sugamo Prison, Japan).

15 Tomoyuki Yamashita, b. 8 November 1885 (Otoyo, Kochi, Japan), d. 23 February 1946, (executed by hanging, Los Baños, Laguna Prison Camp, Philippines).

16 Bessie Wilmott, b. 24 May 1913 (Claremont, WA), d. 16 February 1942 (Bangka Island, Indonesia).

17 Peggy Everett Farmaner, b. 8 March 1913 (Claremont, WA), d. 16 February 1942 (Bangka Island, Indonesia).

18 Millicent Hulda Maria Dorsch, b. 25 February 1912 (Brighton, SA), d. 14 February 1942 (lost at sea off Bangka Island, Indonesia).

19 Wilhelmina (Mina) Rosalie Raymont, b. 7 December 1911 (Adelaide, SA), d. 8 February 1945 (Muntok, Indonesia).

20 'Australians Asked to Share Stories of Bangka Island World War II Nurses', Australian College of Nursing, acn.edu.au

21 Raymont, William Ernest, Service Number: 1172, NAA: B2455, p. 35.

22 Shaw, *On Radji Beach*, ebook ed., loc. 840.

23 Manners, *Bullwinkel*, p. 24.

24 Beryl Woodbridge, b. 11 February 1905 (Melbourne, Vic.), d. 29 September 1986 (Canterbury, Vic.).

25 Manners, *Bullwinkel*, p. 27.

26 David H. Lippman, 'The Fall of Malaya: Japanese Blitzkrieg on Singapore', warfarehistorynetwork.com.

Chapter Eight

1   Pauline Blanche Hempsted, b. 9 September 1908 (Brisbane, Qld), d. 19 March 1945 (Muntok, Indonesia). Her surname is often recorded as 'Hempstead' in accounts of the war.

2   Valrie Elizabeth Smith, b. 2 February 1912 (Wondecla, Qld), d. 7 June 1995 (Herberton, Qld). Sometimes recorded as 'Valerie' Smith.

3   Sarah Fulford, 'Training, Ethos, Camaraderie and Endurance of World War Two Australian POW Nurses', Department of Social Sciences and Security Studies, Curtin University, espace.curtin.edu.au

4   Manners, *Bullwinkel*, p. 31.

5   Vivian Bullwinkel diary, AWM, PR01216, Series 1, 1/1/4.

6   *Ibid.*

7   The *Awazisan Maru, Ayatosan Maru* and *Sakura Maru.*

8   Oscar Nathan Diamond b. 27 October 1916 (New Farm, Qld), d. 25 August 2003 (Brisbane, Qld).

9   'Seventy Minutes Before Pearl Harbor: The landing at Kota Bharu, Malaya, on December 7th 1941', warfare.gq/ dutcheastindies.

10 Catriona Mathewson, 'Dry-cleaner Sank First Japanese Boat of the War', *The Courier-Mail*, 4 September 2003.

11 *Ibid.*

12 Singapore Was Not a Fortress', Imperial War Museums, iwm.org.uk.

13 Manners, *Bullwinkel*, p. 32.

14 Shaw, *On Radji Beach*, ebook ed., loc. 939.

15 Singapore was not a fortress', Imperial War Museums, iwm.org.uk

16 'Prince Of Wales and Repulse Sunk', *The Age* (Melbourne), 11 December 1941, p. 5.

17 Vivian to Eva Bullwinkel, 11 December 1941, AWM, PR01216, Series 2.

18 Shaw, *On Radji Beach*, ebook ed., loc. 991.

19 Austin, James Ronald, Service Number: VX25306, NAA: B883, p. 5.

20 Manners, *Bullwinkel*, p. 36.

21 Yi Hak Nae, 'The Man Between: A Korean Guard Looks Back', in Hank Nelson and Gavin McCormack

(eds), *The Burma–Thailand Railway: Memory and History,* Allen & Unwin, 1993, p. 121.

22 'Burma–Thailand Railway and Hellfire Pass 1942 to 1943: The Enemy', anzacportal.dva.gov.au

23 *Ibid.*

24 Charles G. Roland, 'Massacre and Rape in Hong Kong: Two Case Studies Involving Medical Personnel and Patients', *Journal of Contemporary History,* Vol. 32, pp. 52–61.

25 War of 1939–45, War Crimes Papers [WO 235], [Public Record Office 6995–7004], file 1107, Testimony of S.D. Begg, p. 72, State Library of Victoria.

26 'Apprehension of Suspected War Criminals', Supreme Commander of the Allied Powers, 15 July 1946, jahis.law. nagoya-u.ac.jp.

Chapter Nine

1 *Ibid.*

2 'The Ambush at the Bridge Over the Gemencheh River, Beyond Gemas, 14th January 1942', awm.gov.au

3 Shaw, *On Radji Beach,* ebook ed., loc. 1106.

4 'Popular Matron Awarded Royal Red Cross', *The Argus* (Melbourne), 16 January 1942, p. 6.

5 Manners, *Bullwinkel,* p. 38.

6 *Ibid.*

7 Lieutenant Colonel Charles Groves Wright Anderson, VC, MC, b. 12 February 1897 (Cape Town, South Africa), d. 11 November 1988 (Red Hill, ACT).

8 Count Hisaichi Terauchi, b. 8 August 1879, d. 12 June 1946.

9 'Records of the Air Operations in the Dutch East Indies Operation', compiled by Lt Col. Miyashi Minoru, chief of operations staff of the [Army] Third Air Force based on contemporary materials, from *The Operations of the Navy in the Dutch East Indies and the Bay of Bengal* (edited and translated by Willem Remmelink), Leiden University Press, 2018, p. 266.

10 *Ibid.*

11 Elaine Lenore 'Lainie' Balfour-Ogilvy, b. 11 January 1912 (Renmark, SA),

d. 16 February 1942 (Bangka Island, Indonesia).

12 'The Battle of Muar', 229battalion.org.au

13 Two Australians managed to escape the massacre by playing dead. Lt Ben Hackney crawled through the jungle for six weeks with two broken legs before he was recaptured. He spent the rest of the war in a hellish prison camp.

14 Vivian Bullwinkel diary, AWM, PR01216, Series 1, 1/1/4.

15 Carrie Jean Ashton, b. 31 May 1905 (Woodside, SA), d. 7 December 2002 (Westbourne Park, SA). Sometimes called Jenny Ashton.

16 Manners, *Bullwinkel,* p. 40.

17 'Singapore Was Not a Fortress', Imperial War Museums, iwm.org.uk.

Chapter Ten

1 Austin, James Ronald, Service Number: VX25306, NAA: B883, p. 5.

2 Shaw, *On Radji Beach,* ebook ed., loc. 1418.

3 'Singapore Was Not a Fortress', Imperial War Museums, iwm.org.uk.

4 Kathleen Margaret Neuss, b. 16 October 1911 (Ballarat, Vic), d. 16 February 1942 (Bangka Island, Indonesia)

5 Claire Hunter, 'Guess You Will Be Thinking I've Gone Up In Smoke', awm.gov.au, 20 June 2018.

6 *Ibid.*

7 Barbara Angell, *A Woman's War: The Exceptional Life of Wilma Oram,* New Holland, 2011, p. 45.

8 Janet Patteson Darling (nee Gunther), b. 31 August 1913 (Casino, NSW), d. 2 December 2007 (Mosman, NSW).

9 I.R. Hanger, '2nd Report of Work of YMCA with the AIF in Malaya', AWM 3DRL/1836.

10 Vivian Bullwinkel diary, AWM, PR01216, Series 1, 1/1/4.

11 Peter Luby, 'Passage On the Empire Star', *Remembrance: Official Magazine of the Shrine of Remembrance Melbourne,* November 2022, pp. 50–61.

12 Churchill to Wavell, The War Office to C-in-C, S.W. Pacific, Most Secret Cipher Telegram, 10/2/42, Churchill Trust, (CAC, CHAR 20/70/9).

13 On 9 February 1942.

14 Pearl Beatrice Mittelheuser, b. 28 April 1904 (Bundaberg, Qld), d. 18 August 1945 (Sumatra, Indonesia).

15 Wilton, note to parents, AWM PR89/92.

16 Vivian Bullwinkel diary, 10 February 1942, AWM, PR01216, Series 1, 1/1/4.

17 Jessie Elizabeth Hookway (nee Simons), b. 23 August 1911 (Launceston, Tas.), d. 23 December 2004 (Launceston, Tas.).

18 Jessie Elizabeth Simons, *While History Passed: The Story of the Australian Nurses who Were Prisoners of the Japanese for Three and a Half Years,* Heinemann, 1954, p. 7.

19 Selwyn Norman Capon, b. 15 April 1890 (Acle, UK), d. 23 October 1942 (lost at sea on the MV *Empire Star*).

20 Peter Luby, 'Passage on the Empire Star', *Remembrance: Official Magazine of the Shrine of Remembrance Melbourne,* November 2022, pp. 50–61.

21 *Ibid.* The toy rabbit is on display at Melbourne's Shrine of Remembrance.

22 Taffrail (Henry Taprell Dorling), *Blue Star Line at War,* 1939–45, W. Foulsham & Co, 1973, p. 61.

23 'Blitzer' became a prize possession of Maude's granddaughter.

24 'A Bitter Fate – Australians In Malaya & Singapore', anzacportal.dva.gov.au

25 Howgate, diary entry, 12 February 1942, AWMPR91/045.

26 Margaret Irene O'Bryan (nee Anderson) (George Medal), b. 11 December 1915 (Melbourne, Vic.), d. 16 July 1995 (Melbourne, Vic.).

27 Vera Alexandra 'Vee' Berry MBE (nee Torney), b. 27 July 1916 (Saint Arnaud, Vic.), d. 19 June 2006 (Vic.).

28 'Bravery of Nurses On Bombed Ship', *The Argus* (Melbourne, Vic.), 23 September 1942, p. 1.

29 They would eventually become Prisoners of War at Changi with some of the men they had left behind in Singapore.

30 Peter Luby, 'Passage On the Empire Star', *Remembrance: Official Magazine of the Shrine of Remembrance Melbourne,* November 2022, pp. 50–61.

Chapter Eleven

1 Vivian Bullwinkel diary, 12 February 1942, Australian War Memorial (AWM), PR01216 Series 1, AWM2020.22.50.

2 Betty Jeffrey, *White Coolies,* Angus & Robertson, Sydney, 1954.

3 Brian Crisp, 'Thoughts of a Brave Lady', *Army Magazine,* 1 December 1992, p. 30.

4 *Ibid.*

5 Manners, *Bullwinkel,* p. 55.

6 'The Ships', muntokpeacemuseum.org

7 Vivian Bullwinkel diary, 12 February 1942, AWM, PR01216 Series 1, AWM2020.22.50.

8 Ellen Mavis Allgrove (nee Hannah), b. 12 October 1910 (Claremont, WA), d. 29 October 1993 (Dedham, UK). Sometimes referred to as Nell, the name she preferred in later years.

9 'HMS Vyner Brooke', malayanvolunteersgroup.org.uk

10 'HMS Vyner Brooke: Passenger List (Recreated)', muntokpeacemuseum.org

11 Isidore Warman, b. 5 February 1939 (Shanghai, China).

12 Eric Harrison August Germann, b. 7 October 1913 (Winnipeg, Canada), d. 9 November 2000 (Palm Beach, Fla, USA).

13 William H. McDougall, *By Eastern Windows: The Story of a Battle of Souls and Minds in the Prison Camps of Sumatra,* Charles Scribner's Sons, 1949, p. 140.

14 Simons, *While History Passed,* p. 8.

15 William Alston Tebbutt, b. 19 February 1898 (Sydney, NSW), d. 29 June 1960 (Sydney, NSW).

16 Tebbutt, William Alston, Service Number: NX70344, NAA: B883, NX70344.

17 'Defence Medal: Sister J.K. Greer, Australian Army Nursing Service', awm.gov.au.

18 Vivian Bullwinkel diary, 12 February 1942, AWM, PR01216 Series 1, AWM2020.22.50.

19 Richard Edward Borton, b. 4 July 1887 (Ramsgate, UK), d. 1965 (Leeds, UK).

20 William Sydney Sedgeman, b. March 1911 (Haverfordwest, UK), d. 16 February 1942 (Radji Beach on Bangka Island, Indonesia).

21 Vivian Bullwinkel diary, 12 February 1942, AWM, PR01216 Series 1, AWM2020.22.50.
22 *Ibid.*, 13 February 1942.
23 Simons, *While History Passed*, p. 9.
24 Vivian Bullwinkel diary, 12 February 1942, AWM, PR01216 Series 1, AWM2020.22.50.
25 Manners, *Bullwinkel*, p. 66.
26 Vivian Bullwinkel diary, 13 February 1942, AWM, PR01216 Series 1, AWM2020.22.50.
27 *Ibid.*, 14 February 1942.
28 Violet 'Vi' Irene McElnea, b. 14 February 1904 (Ingham, Qld), d. 17 September 1959 (Chatswood, NSW).
29 The 'Fighting' McElneas from North Queensland included Vi, Henry, Joseph, Robert, Edith, Dorothy and Keith.
30 Lorna Florence Fairweather, b. 31 January 1913 (Stirling West, SA), d. 16 February 1942 (Radji Beach on Bangka Island, Indonesia).
31 Manners, *Bullwinkel*, p. 68.
32 Ethel Mannin, *Cactus*, Jarrolds, 1935.
33 Vivian Bullwinkel diary, 14 February 1942, AWM, PR01216 Series 1, AWM2020.22.50.
34 *Ibid.*
35 'Officer's Investigation of Banka Island Massacre', *The Advertiser* (Adelaide), 18 September 1945, p. 4.
36 Kathleen Constance 'Pat' Dixon (nee Blake), b. 16 July 1912 (Chatswood, NSW), d. 7 April 1998 (Sydney, NSW).

Chapter Twelve

1 Lt Col (Retired) Peter Winstanley OAM RFD JP, Recollections of Florence Elizabeth Syer (nee Trotter), Lieutenant Australian Army Nursing Service (AANS) 2/10th Australian General Hospital (AGH), pows-of-japan.net. Others on board remembered there being nine aircraft in total.
2 Vivian Bullwinkel diary, 14 February 1942, AWM, PR01216 Series 1, AWM2020.22.50
3 Florence Elizabeth Syer (nee Trotter), b. 4 October 1915 (Eastwood, NSW), d. 31 July 2002 (Brisbane, Qld).
4 Frances Whiting, 'They Machine Gunned Us in the Water', *The Sunday Mail* (Brisbane), 20 January 2002.
5 *Ibid.*
6 'White Coolies', *Brisbane Telegraph*, 1 March 1954, p. 11.
7 Vivian Bullwinkel diary, 14 February 1942, AWM, PR01216 Series 1, AWM2020.22.50.
8 Louvima 'Vima' Mary Isabella Bates, b. 1 January 1910 (Fremantle, WA,) d. 14 February 1942 (lost at sea near Bangka Island, Indonesia). Sometimes referred to as Louvinia Bates.
9 Sylvia Jessie Mimmie McGregor (nee Muir), b. 24 August 1915 (Longreach, Qld), d. 18 February 1996 (Brisbane, Qld).
10 Mary Elizabeth Cuthbertson, b. 5 March 1910 (Stirling, SA), d. 16 February 1942 (Radji Beach on Bangka Island, Indonesia).
11 Sister Caroline Mary Ennis, b. 13 August 1913 (Swan Hill, Vic.), d. 14 February 1942 (lost at sea near Bangka Island, Indonesia).
12 Rosetta Joan Wight, b. 3 December 1908 (Fish Creek, Vic.), d. 16 February 1942 (Radji Beach on Bangka Island, Indonesia).
13 Florence Rebecca Casson, b. 6 March 1903 (Warracknabeal, Vic.), d. 16 February 1942 (Radji Beach on Bangka Island, Indonesia).
14 The Pinnaroo Soldiers Memorial Hospital.
15 Claire Hunter, 'Guess You Will Be Thinking I've Gone Up in Smoke', awm.gov.au, 20 June 2018.
16 Veronica Ann Turner (nee Clancy), b. 29 June 1912 (Eurelia, SA), d. 9 October 1997.
17 McDougall, *By Eastern Windows*, p. 142.
18 Sister Vivian Bullwinkel's testimony, Australian War Crimes Board of Inquiry, Melbourne, 29 October 1945, p. 1, AWM 54, 1010/4/24, Part 2.
19 Florence Aubin Salmon, b. 20 October 1915 (Sydney, NSW), d. 16 February 1942 (Radji Beach on Bangka Island, Indonesia).
20 McDougall, *By Eastern Windows*, p. 143.
21 Whiting, 'They Machine Gunned Us in the Water', *The Sunday Mail* (Brisbane), 20 January 2002.
22 Winnie May Davis, b. 7 July 1915 (Cowper, NSW), d. 19 July 1945 (Sumatra, Indonesia).

23 Manners, *Bullwinkel*, p. 72.
24 Wilma Elizabeth Forster Young
    (Oram), interviewed 20 January 1983
    by Margaret Evans, 'Prisoners of War:
    Australians under Nippon', AWM,
    S02947.
25 *Ibid.*
26 *Ibid.*
27 Whiting, 'They Machine Gunned Us in
    the Water', *The Sunday Mail* (Brisbane),
    20 January 2002.
28 Winstanley, Recollections of Florence
    Elizabeth Syer (nee Trotter), pows-of-
    japan.net
29 Joyce Tweddell, b. 3 July 1916,
    (Brisbane, Qld), d. 14 November 1995
    (Caloundra, Qld).
30 Jessie Jane Eaton-Lee (nee Blanch),
    b. 18 March 1910 (Bangalow, NSW),
    d. 15 May 1999 (Alstonville, NSW).
31 Winstanley, Recollections of Florence
    Elizabeth Syer (nee Trotter), pows-of-
    japan.net
32 Vivian Bullwinkel's testimony,
    Australian War Crimes Board of Inquiry,
    Melbourne, 29 October 1945, p. 1,
    AWM 54, 1010/4/24, Part 2.
33 Manners, *Bullwinkel*, p. 73.
34 Annie Merle Trenerry, b. 31 March
    1909 (Moonta Mines, SA),
    d. 14 February 1942 (Bangka Island,
    Indonesia).
35 Gladys Myrtle McDonald, b. 17 July
    1909 (Brisbane), d. 14 February 1942
    (Bangka Island, Indonesia).
36 Mary Dorothea Clarke, b. 20 July 1911
    (Rylstone, NSW), d. 14 February 1942
    (Bangka Island, Indonesia).
37 'White Coolies', *The Mail* (Adelaide), 3
    April 1954, p. 33.
38 'A Nursing Sister's Account of Life as
    a Prisoner of the Japanese', pows-of-
    japan.net
39 Vivian Bullwinkel's testimony,
    Australian War Crimes Board of Inquiry,
    Melbourne, 29 October 1945, p. 2,
    AWM 54, 1010/4/24, Part 2.
40 Gladys Laura Hughes, b. 19 September
    1908 (Waikino, NZ), d. 31 May 1945
    (Sumatra).
41 Dora Shirley Gardam, b. 24 August
    1910 (Ulverstone, Tas.), d. 4 April 1945
    (Muntok, Bangka Island, Indonesia).

42 Mrs Bull and Hazel spent the war
    in prison camps but were eventually
    reunited with the two other children in
    1946. The 'lost children' Robin and Molly
    had been rescued by a Thai woman who
    cared for them until the war's end.
43 Evelyne Frances Madden (nee Thyme),
    widow of Lewis John Butler Madden.
    Died 22 April 1945 (Belalau Prison
    Camp, Sumatra, Indonesia).
44 'HMS Vyner Brooke: Passenger List
    (Recreated)', muntokpeacemuseum.org.
45 Recollections of Veronica Ann Turner
    (nee Clancy), AWM, MSS 1086
46 Simons, *While History Passed*, p. 22.

Chapter Thirteen
1   Sister Vivian Bullwinkel's testimony,
    Australian War Crimes Board of Inquiry,
    Melbourne, 29 October 1945, p. 2,
    AWM 54, 1010/4/24, Part 2.
2   *Ibid.*
3   *Ibid.*
4   Esther Sarah Jean Stewart,
    b. 15 October 1904 (Brisbane, Qld),
    d. 16 February 1942 (Radji Beach,
    Bangka Island, Indonesia).
5   Ellen 'Nell' Louisa Keats, b. 1 July 1915
    (Adelaide, SA), d. 16 February 1942
    (Radji Beach, Bangka Island, Indonesia).
6   'Mother Perpetuates Memory of Heroic
    Army Nurse Shot by Japs', *The Courier-
    Mail* (Brisbane), 29 January 1946, p. 1.
7   McDougall, *By Eastern Windows*, p. 146.
8   *Ibid.*
9   Ellenor Calnan, b. 4 March 1912
    (Culcairn, NSW), d. 14 February 1942
    (Bangka Island, Indonesia).
10 Lavinia Jean Russell, b. 21 December
    1909 (Sydney, NSW), d. 14 February
    1942 (Bangka Island, Indonesia).
11 Marjorie Schuman, b. 28 January 1911
    (Inverell, NSW), d. 14 February 1942
    (Bangka Island, Indonesia).
12 Winstanley, Recollections of Florence
    Elizabeth Syer (nee Trotter), pows-of-
    japan.net
13 *Ibid.*
14 Wilma Elizabeth Forster Young
    (Oram), interviewed 20 January 1983
    by Margaret Evans, 'Prisoners of War:
    Australians under Nippon', AWM,
    S02947.

15 Cecilia May McPhee (nee Delforce), b. 7 September 1912 (Augathella, Qld), d. 7 March 2011 (Broadbeach Waters, Qld).

16 Manners, *Bullwinkel*, p. 76.

17 McDougall, *By Eastern Windows*, p. 177.

18 *Ibid.*

19 Sister Vivian Bullwinkel's testimony, Australian War Crimes Board of Inquiry, Melbourne, 29 October 1945, p. 2, AWM 54, 1010/4/24, Part 2.

20 Ada Joyce Bridge, b. 6 July 1907 (Scone, NSW), d. 16 February 1942 (Radji Beach, Bangka Island, Indonesia).

21 Sister Vivian Bullwinkel's testimony, Australian War Crimes Board of Inquiry, Melbourne, 29 October 1945, p. 2, AWM 54, 1010/4/24, Part 2.

22 'Churchill Announces Fall of Singapore', *The Telegraph* (Brisbane), 16 February 1942, p. 1.

23 Winston S. Churchill, *The Second World War*, vol. 4, 'The Hinge of Fate', Cassell & Co., 1951, p. 81.

24 Cecil Gordon Kinsley, b. January 1909 (Skirlaugh, UK), d. 24 March 1942 (Muntok, Bangka Island, Indonesia)

25 Vivian Bullwinkel interview, 1993, from *Vivian Bullwinkel: An Australian Heroine*, Waterbyrd Filmz, 2007.

Chapter Fourteen

1 McDougall, *By Eastern Windows*, p. 178.

2 Manners, *Bullwinkel*, p. 78.

3 Sister Vivian Bullwinkel's testimony, Australian War Crimes Board of Inquiry, Melbourne, 29 October 1945, p. 2, AWM 54, 1010/4/24, Part 2.

4 Manners, *Bullwinkel*, p. 78.

5 Carrie Rose Betteridge (nee Faraday), d. 16 February 1942 (Radji Beach, Bangka Island, Indonesia).

6 Thomas Daniel Betteridge, b. June 1880 (West Derby, Lancashire), d. 16 February 1942 (Radji Beach, Bangka Island, Indonesia).

7 'HMS Vyner Brooke', muntokpeacemuseum.org

8 John Gallagher Dominguez, 6 March 1879 (Wandiligong, Vic.) d. 11 September 1944 (Muntok POW Camp, Bangka Island, Indonesia)

9 Agnes Gertrude 'Gerte' Dominguez (nee Dunphy) b. 1881 (Buckland, Vic.),

d. 9 November 1944 (Muntok POW Camp, Bangka Island, Indonesia).

10 'Officer's Investigation of Banka Island Massacre,' *The Advertiser* (Adelaide), 18 September 1945, p. 4.

11 Dorothy Gwendoline Howard 'Buddy' Elmes, b. 27 April 1914 (Armadale, Melbourne), d. 16 February 1942 (Radji Beach, Bangka Island, Indonesia).

12 Virtual War Memorial Australia, vwma.org.au

13 On 2 March 1942, 'Elmes, Dorothy Gwendoline Howard', vwma.org.au.

14 Ernest Lloyd (1917–1994).

15 Hal Richardson, 'The Japanese Leopard with Unchanging Spots', *The Sun* (Sydney), 8 September 1946, p. 4.

16 Vivian Bullwinkel interview, *Vivian Bullwinkel An Australian Heroine*, Waterbyrd Filmz, 2007.

17 'The Japanese Leopard with Unchanging Spots', *The Sun* (Sydney), 8 September 1946, p. 4.

18 *Ibid.*

19 Manners, *Bullwinkel*, p. 79.

20 Ernest Charles Watson, b. October 1874 (Clapham Common, UK), d. 16 February 1942 (Radji Beach, Bangka Island, Indonesia).

21 McDougall, *By Eastern Windows*, p. 181.

22 *Ibid.*, p. 187.

23 *Ibid.*

24 Vivian Bullwinkel's testimony, Australian War Crimes Board of Inquiry, Melbourne, 29 October 1945, p. 2, AWM 54, 1010/4/24, Part 2.

25 Ellen Fanning, 'A War Crime has been Censored: Truth Revealed About a WWII Massacre on Bangka Island', abc.net.au, 2 June 2023.

26 'Mother Perpetuates Memory of Heroic Army Nurse Shot by Japs', *The Courier-Mail* (Brisbane), 29 January 1946, p. 1.

27 The Last Post Ceremony commemorating the service of (WFX11175) Sister Alma May Beard, 13th Australian General Hospital, Royal Australian Army Nursing Service, Second World War, awm.gov.au

28 Manners, *Bullwinkel*, p. 81.

29 Richardson, 'The Japanese Leopard with Unchanging Spots', *The Sun* (Sydney), 8 September 1946, p. 4.

30   Shaw, *On Radji Beach*, ebook ed.,
     loc. 2983.
31   Vivian Bullwinkel interview, *Vivian
     Bullwinkel An Australian Heroine*,
     Waterbyrd Filmz, 2007.

Chapter Fifteen
1   *Ibid.*
2   Crisp, 'Thoughts of a Brave Lady', *Army
     Magazine*, 1 December 1992, p. 30.
3   *Ibid.*
4   *Ibid.*
5   McDougall, *By Eastern Windows*, p. 184.
6   Most likely Stoker Ernest Lloyd.
7   'HMS Vyner Brooke',
     muntokpeacemuseum.org.
8   *Ibid.*
9   Probably magistrate Ernest Watson or
     stockbroker Tom Betteridge.
10   Richardson, 'The Japanese Leopard with
     Unchanging Spots', *The Sun* (Sydney),
     8 September 1946, p. 4.
11   'HMS Vyner Brooke',
     muntokpeacemuseum.org
12   McDougall, *By Eastern Windows*, p. 186.
13   *Ibid.*, p. 187.
14   *Ibid.*
15   'The Japanese Leopard with
     Unchanging Spots', *The Sun* (Sydney),
     8 September 1946, p. 4.
16   Vivian Gordon Bowden CBE (28 May
     1884 – 17 February 1942).
17   Manners, *Bullwinkel*, p. 84.

Chapter Sixteen
1   *Ibid.*
2   *Ibid.*, p. 85.
3   1939 England and Wales Register,
     Yorkshire East Riding, Kingston-Upon-
     Hull, National Archives, London.
4   'Darwin Bombed Heavily in Two Day
     Raids', *The Courier-Mail* (Brisbane),
     20 February 1942, p. 1.
5   'When Bombs Rained from the Sky',
     Northern Territory News, 18 February 2017.
6   Vivian Bullwinkel interview, *Vivian
     Bullwinkel An Australian Heroine*,
     Waterbyrd Filmz, 2007.
7   Manners, *Bullwinkel*, p. 89.
8   *Ibid.*
9   Petty Officer Hajime Toyoshima,
     b. 29 March 1920 (Kagawa Prefecture,
     Japan), d. 5 August 1944 (Cowra, NSW).

10   Matthias Ulungura (1921–1980).
11   Manners, *Bullwinkel*, p. 90.
12   *Ibid.*
13   *Ibid.*, p. 92.

Chapter Seventeen
1   *Ibid.*, p. 93.
2   Eva Bullwinkel to Vivian, February
     1942, AWN, PR01216, Series 2.
3   Vivian Bullwinkel diary, AWM,
     PR01216, Series 1, 1/1/1.
4   *Ibid.*
5   Sister Vivian Bullwinkel's testimony,
     Australian War Crimes Board of Inquiry,
     Melbourne, 29 October 1945, p. 1,
     AWM 54, 1010/4/24, Part 2.
6   Manners, *Bullwinkel*, p. 97.
7   *Ibid.*, p. 98.
8   *Ibid.*, p. 99.
9   *Ibid.*
10   *Ibid.*, p. 103.

Chapter Eighteen
1   Jeffrey, *White Coolies*, p. 25.
2   Vivian Bullwinkel interview, 1993,
     Vivian Bullwinkel: An Australian Heroine,
     Waterbyrd Filmz, 2007.
3   *Ibid.*
4   Manners, *Bullwinkle*, p. 104.
5   Jeffrey, *White Coolies*, p. 25.
6   Barbara Angell, *A Woman's War:
     The Exceptional Life of Wilma Oram*,
     New Holland, 2011, p. 79, 103.
7   Jeffrey, *White Coolies*.
8   Manners, *Bullwinkle*, p. 110.
9   *Ibid.*
10   'S.A. Nurses' Moving Story', *The Advertiser*
     (Adelaide), 18 September 1945, p. 5.
11   Shaw, *On Radji Beach,* ebook ed.,
     loc. 3251.
12   Jeffrey, *White Coolies*.
13   *Ibid.*
14   *Ibid.*
15   *Ibid.*
16   *Ibid.*
17   Manners, *Bullwinkle*, p. 115.
18   Simons, *While History Passed*, p. 40.
19   Manners, *Bullwinkle*, p. 117.
20   Simons, *While History Passed*, p. 36.

Chapter Nineteen
1   Jess Gregory MacAuley (nee Doyle),
     b. 27 November 1911 (Sydney), d. 1993
     (Wellington, New Zealand).

2   Veronica Ann Turner (nee Clancy), manuscript, AWM, MSS1086.
3   Jeffrey, *White Coolies*.
4   Manners, *Bullwinkel*, p. 118.
5   Jessie Blanch (Mrs Jessie Eaton-Lee) interview transcript with Barb Angell, 6 May 1998, p. 3, from angellpro.com.au
6   *Ibid.*
7   Simons, *While History Passed*, p. 36.
8   Jeffrey, *White Coolies*, p. 31.
9   Manners, *Bullwinkel*, p. 119.
10   Simons, *While History Passed*, p. 37.
11   *Ibid.*
12   Manners, *Bullwinkel*, p. 120.
13   Simons, *While History Passed*, p. 37.
14   *Ibid.*
15   Eileen Mary Ita Short, b. 15 January 1904 (Maryborough, Qld), d. 25 April 1975 (Toowoomba, Qld).
16   Manners, *Bullwinkel*, p. 121.
17   *Ibid.*
18   Sarah Fulford, *Training, Ethos, Camaraderie and Endurance of World War Two Australian POW Nurses*, Department of Social Sciences and Security Studies, Curtin University, espace.curtin.edu.au, p. 92.
19   Jeffrey, *White Coolies*, p. 33.
20   Simons, *While History Passed*, p. 38.
21   *Ibid.*, p. 50.
22   Susannah de Vries, *Heroic Australian Women in War*, HarperCollins, 2004, p. 549.
23   Simons, *While History Passed*, p. 39.
24   *Ibid.*
25   Jeffrey, *White Coolies*.
26   Private Papers of Lieutenant AJ Mann RNVR, Imperial War Museum, London, Documents 23736.
27   'Struggle to Safety,' *The Age* (Melbourne), 19 March 1942, p. 3.
28   On 26 March 1942 at the Muntok prison hospital, Bangka Island, Indonesia.

Chapter Twenty
1   Simons, *While History Passed*, p. 40.
2   Jeffrey, *White Coolies*.
3   *Ibid.*
4   *Ibid.*
5   Recollections of Florence Elizabeth Syer (nee Trotter), pows-of-japan.net
6   Jessie Blanch interview with Barb Angell, 6 May 1998, p. 2. angellpro.com.au

7   Ada Corbett (Mickey) Syer, b. 15 November 1910 (Melbourne, Vic.), d. 4 April 1991 (Narrabeen, NSW).
8   Pat Darling, *Portrait of a Nurse*, Don Wall, 2001, p. 35.
9   Simons, *While History Passed*, p. 63.
10   Winstanley, Recollections of Florence Elizabeth Syer (nee Trotter), pows-of-japan.net
11   Jean Ashton, *Jean's diary: a POW diary, 1942–1945*, Jill Ashton, 2003, p. 7.
12   Simons, *While History Passed*, p. 44.
13   Margaret Dryburgh, b. 24 February 1890 (Sunderland, UK), d. 21 April 1945 (Bangka Island, Indonesia).
14   'The Vocal Orchestra (1943–44)', singingtosurvive.com
15   Christian Sarah Mary Oxley, b. 7 June 1912 (Charters Towers, Qld), d. 16 April 1994 (Southport, Qld).
16   Winstanley, Recollections of Florence Elizabeth Syer (nee Trotter), pows-of-japan.net
17   Jeffrey, *White Coolies*.
18   Simons, *While History Passed*, p. 78.
19   Angell, *A Woman's War*, p. 136.
20   Jessie Blanch interview with Barb Angell, 6 May 1998, p. 7. angellpro.com.au.
21   Simons, *While History Passed*, p. 45.
22   Jeffrey, *White Coolies*.
23   Lillian Violet Kenneison (nee Whatmore), b. 1895 (Ceylon), d. 22 July 1956 (Chermside, Qld).
24   Edith 'Edie' Cynthia Rose Leembruggen (nee Kenneison), b. 26 November 1927 (Batu Caves, Kuala Lumpur, Malaya), d. 2 October 2008 (Perth, WA).
25   Edie Leembruggen interview, *Vivian Bullwinkel An Australian Heroine*, Waterbyrd Filmz, 2007.
26   *Ibid.*
27   Ernest James Kenneison MBE, b. 9 May 1877 (Horsell, UK), d. 13 February 1942 (Bangka Strait, Indonesia).
28   Natalie Lynch, '"Little Bet You Helped Save My Life": An unlikely friendship formed in the horrors of war', awm.gov.au
29   *Ibid.*
30   Manners, *Bullwinkel*, p. 134.

Chapter Twenty-one

1   Jeffrey, *White Coolies*, p. 125.
2   Angell, *A Woman's War*, 136.
3   Cevia Warman died on 9 March 1942.
4   Manners, *Bullwinkel*, p. 130.
5   Janet Darling (Pat, nee Gunther), transcript of interview, 2nd May 2003, australiansatwarfilmarchive.unsw.edu.au/archive/5.
6   Betty Jeffrey, *White Coolies*, p. 69.
7   Jean Ashton, *Jean's Diary: A POW Diary 1942–1945,* Published by Jill Ashton, 2003, p. 37.
8   'Australia, with Mr. Curtin, Looks to America', *The Daily Mirror* (Sydney), 29 December 1941, p. 2.
9   Ian Townsend, *Line of Fire,* Fourth Estate, 2017.
10   Manners, *Bullwinkel*, p. 131.
11   Manners, *Bullwinkel*, p. 133.
12   Simons, *While History Passed*, p. 62.
13   *Ibid.*, p. 48.
14   *Ibid.*, p. 89.
15   'The Vocal Orchestra (1943–44)', singingtosurvive.com
16   Manners, *Bullwinkel*, p. 137.
17   *Ibid.*
18   Shaw, *On Radji Beach*, ebook ed., loc. 3548.
19   Manners, *Bullwinkel*, p. 165.
20   Darling, *Portrait of a Nurse*, p. 62.
21   Jessie Blanch interview with Barb Angell, 6 May 1998, angellpro.com.au.
22   *Ibid.*
23   *Ibid.*
24   Simons, *While History Passed*, p. 62.
25   Vivian Bullwinkel interview, 1993, *Vivian Bullwinkel: An Australian Heroine*, Waterbyrd Filmz, 2007.
26   Jeffrey, *White Coolies*.
27   Margaret Constance Norah Chambers (nee Hope), b. 26 April 1905 (Singapore), d. 1989 (Jersey, UK).
28   'Former Local Man Injured on Service', *Barrier Miner* (Broken Hill), 2 November 1942, p. 1.
29   Bullwinkel, John William: Service Number 407780, NAA: A9301, 407780, p. 14.
30   aircrewremembered.com
31   Simons, *While History Passed*, p. 62.
32   Angell, *A Woman's War,* p. 116.
33   Manners, *Bullwinkel*, p. 139.

Chapter Twenty-two

1   *Ibid.*, p. 140.
2   Turner, Veronica Ann (nee Clancy) manuscript, AWM MSS 1086.
3   Manners, *Bullwinkel*, p. 140.
4   Recollections of Florence Elizabeth Syer (nee Trotter), pows-of-japan.net
5   *Ibid.*
6   *Ibid.*
7   Manners, *Bullwinkel*, p. 141.
8   *Ibid.*, p. 142.
9   *Ibid.*
10   Angell, *A Woman's War,* p. 132.
11   Miller famously said pressure in sport, even at the highest level, was nothing. Real pressure, he said, was being a mile up in the air 'with a Messerschmitt on your arse'.
12   Sergeant Basil Eastwood.
13   Sub-Lieutenant Uichi Komai was killed in action soon afterwards in the Philippines.
14   Ellen Savage (1912–1985).
15   The *Centaur's* wreckage was finally discovered in 2009 off the southern tip of Moreton Island. It lies 2059 metres under the surface.
16   'Burma–Thailand Railway', nma.gov.au
17   Manners, *Bullwinkel*, p. 145.
18   Simons, *While History Passed*, p. 64.
19   *Ibid.*
20   *Ibid.*
21   Recollections of Florence Elizabeth Syer (nee Trotter), pows-of-japan.net
22   Simons, *While History Passed*, p. 64.
23   Manners, *Bullwinkel*, p. 151.
24   'The Vocal Orchestra', singingto survive.com
25   Recollections of Florence Elizabeth Syer (nee Trotter), pows-of-japan.net
26   'The Vocal Orchestra', singingto survive.com
27   *Ibid.*
28   Manners, *Bullwinkel*, p. 151.
29   *Ibid.*
30   Recollections of Florence Elizabeth Syer (nee Trotter), pows-of-japan.net.
31   Simons, *While History Passed*, p. 70.

Chapter Twenty-three

1   Manners, *Bullwinkel*, p. 152.
2   Simons, *While History Passed*, p. 72.
3   Recollections of Florence Elizabeth Syer (nee Trotter), pows-of-japan.net.

4   Simons, *While History Passed*, p. 77.
5   Manners, *Bullwinkel*, p. 148.
6   *Ibid.*
7   Vivian Bullwinkel interview, 1993, *Vivian Bullwinkel: An Australian Heroine*, Waterbyrd Filmz, 2007.
8   Simons, *While History Passed*, p. 75.
9   Recollections of Florence Elizabeth Syer (nee Trotter), pows-of-japan.net
10 Manners, *Bullwinkel*, p. 149.
11 Angell, *A Woman's War*, p. 140.
12 *Ibid.*, p. 137.
13 Manners, *Bullwinkel*, p. 152.
14 Simons, *While History Passed*, p. 76.
15 'Cowra breakout', awm.gov.au
16 Sister Nesta James's testimony, Australian War Crimes Board of Inquiry, AWM, PR01216, Series 8/1/4.
17 Sister Vivian Bullwinkel's testimony, Australian War Crimes Board of Inquiry, Melbourne, 29 October 1945, p. 9, AWM54 1010/4/24B.
18 Papers of Vivian Bullwinkel, AWM, PR01216, Series 1: 1/2/9.
19 Recollections of Florence Elizabeth Syer (nee Trotter), pows-of-japan.net
20 Simons, *While History Passed*, p. 81.
21 *Ibid*, p. 84.
22 Recollections of Florence Elizabeth Syer (nee Trotter), pows-of-japan.net
23 *Ibid.*
24 *Ibid.*
25 'Wilhelmina Rosalie Raymont', muntokpeacemuseum.org
26 Catherine Kenny, *Captives: Australian Army Nurses in Japanese Prison Camps*, University of Queensland Press, 1986, p. 95.
27 Manners, *Bullwinkel*, p. 159.
28 Kenny, *Captives*, p. 95.
29 Darling, *Portrait of a Nurse*, p. 73.
30 Simons, *While History Passed*, p. 86.
31 Betty Jeffrey diary, 8 February 1945, AWM, PR01780.

Chapter Twenty-four
1   Kenny, *Captives*, p. 95.
2   Simons, *While History Passed*, p. 85.
3   *Ibid.*, p. 75.
4   Irene 'Rene' Ada Singleton, b. 21 June 1908 (Melbourne, Vic.), d. 20 February 1945 (Sumatra, Indonesia).
5   Simons, *While History Passed*, p. 89.

6   Betty Jeffrey diary, 20 March 1945, AWM, PR01780.
7   Simons, *While History Passed*, p. 89.
8   Darling, *Portrait of a Nurse*.
9   Simons, *While History Passed*, p. 95.
10 *Ibid.*
11 *Ibid.*, p. 97.
12 Manners, *Bullwinkel*, p. 162.
13 *Ibid.*
14 Kenny, *Captives*, p. 92.
15 Simons, *While History Passed*, p. 101.
16 *Ibid*, p. 104.
17 Kenny, *Captives*, p. 98.
18 Simons, *While History Passed*, p. 107.
19 Manners, *Bullwinkel*, p. 164.
20 Simons, *While History Passed*, p. 89.
21 Betty Kenneison interview, *Vivian Bullwinkel: An Australian Heroine*, Waterbyrd Filmz, 2007.
22 Manners, *Bullwinkel*, p. 164.
23 Betty Kenneison interview, *Vivian Bullwinkel: An Australian Heroine*, Waterbyrd Filmz, 2007.
24 *Ibid.*
25 Manners, *Bullwinkel*, p. 166.
26 Kenny, *Captives*, p. 95.
27 Rubina Dorothy Freeman, b. 17 June 1913 (Randwick, NSW), d. 8 August 1945 (Sumatra, Indonesia).
28 Simons, *While History Passed*, p. 89.
29 Manners, *Bullwinkel*, p. 166.
30 Simons, *While History Passed*, p. 109.
31 Kenny, *Captives*, p. 97.
32 Simons, *While History Passed*, p. 111; Kenny, *Captives*, p. 97.

Chapter Twenty-five
1   Simons, *While History Passed*, p. 112.
2   Kenny, *Captives*, p. 97
3   Recollections of Florence Elizabeth Syer (nee Trotter), pows-of-japan.net
4   Eva Bullwinkel to Viv, 21 August 1945, AWM, PR01216, Series 2, 2/4/98.
5   'Australian Welcome to P.O.W. Nurses', *The Age* (Melbourne), 25 October 1945, p. 3.
6   Simons, *While History Passed*, p. 113.
7   Coral Craig, 'From Prison to Piccadilly', *Woman's Day and Home*, 22 January 1951, p. 9.
8   Albert Plesman Jnr, b. 19 October 1922 (The Hague, Netherlands), d. 27 February 2015 (Rome, Italy).

9   Gideon Francois Jacobs, *Prelude to the Monsoon*, Purnell & Sons, 1966, p. 64.
10 *Ibid.*, p. 136.
11 Manners, *Bullwinkel*, p. 173.
12 Haydon Wallace Lennard, b 4 July 1909 (Annandale, NSW), d. 22 April 1987 (Fairlight, NSW).
13 Manners, *Bullwinkel*, p. 176.
14 Angell, *A Woman's War*, p. 188.
15 *Ibid.*
16 Kenny, *Captives*, p. 145.
17 'Nurses "Like Skeletons"', *The Daily Telegraph* (Sydney), 18 September 1945, p. 3.
18 Kenny, *Captives*, p. 145. Joyce recovered and for many years was chief radiographer at the Royal Brisbane Hospital.
19 Statham, Vivian (nee Bullwinkel), Service Number: VFX61330, NAA: A14472, VFX61330, p. 45.
20 Manners, *Bullwinkel*, p. 177.
21 Kenny, *Captives*, p. 144.
22 'Nurses "Like Skeletons"', *The Daily Telegraph* (Sydney), 18 September 1945, p. 3.
23 *Ibid.*
24 'Sister Was Left for Dead on Beach', *The Sydney Morning Herald*, 18 September 1945, p. 3.
25 Annie Moriah Sage (1895–1969).
26 Kenny, *Captives*, p. 146.
27 *Ibid.*, p. 147, quoting Beryl Maddock (nee Chandler), *Flight Sister,* unpublished book, p. 177.
28 Report of Dr Harry M Windsor, Major, 2/14th AGH, 19 September 1945. NAA MP742/1 Item 336/1/1289, Medical Report 'A', p. 27, AWM, 11/2/14.
29 Manners, *Bullwinkel*, p. 177.

Chapter Twenty-six
1   'Nurses "Like Skeletons"', *The Daily Telegraph* (Sydney), 18 September 1945, p. 3.
2   Captain Mavis Hannah interviewed by Dr Amy McGrath, 13 July 1981, Tape No TRC 1087/1, National Library of Australia.
3   'Sister Was Left for Dead on Beach', *The Sydney Morning Herald*, 18 September 1945, p. 3.

4   Eva Bullwinkel to Viv, 18 August 1945, AWM, PR01216, Series 2: 2/4/99.
5   'Nurses "Like Skeletons"', *The Daily Telegraph* (Sydney), 18 September 1945, p. 3.
6   Statham, Vivian (nee Bullwinkel), Service Number: VFX61330, NAA: A14472, VFX61330, p. 43.
7   *Ibid.*, p. 44.
8   *Ibid.*, p. 45.
9   *Ibid.*
10 Manners, *Bullwinkel*, p. 179.
11 Statham, Vivian (nee Bullwinkel), Service Number: VFX61330, NAA: A14472, VFX61330, p. 47.
12 Commander, 2 Australian POW Reception Group to Adjutant-General, October 1945, point 5, MP 742, 336/1/1289, Australian Archives, Melbourne.
13 'Nurses Will Leave Singapore this Week', *News* (Adelaide), 2 October 1945, p. 1.
14 *Ibid.*
15 Manners, *Bullwinkel*, p. 184.
16 'Shipping', *The West Australian* (Perth), 13 October 1945, p. 9.
17 Manners, *Bullwinkel*, p. 185.
18 'Nurses Return', *The West Australian* (Perth), 19 October 1945, p. 8.
19 'How Nurses Died at Banka', *Daily Mirror* (Sydney), *ibid.*, p. 9.?
20 'Sister Bullwinkel Reaches Fremantle', *Barrier Miner* (Broken Hill), *ibid.*, p. 8.
21 'How Nurses Died at Banka', *Daily Mirror* (Sydney), *ibid.*, p. 9.
22 'Warm Welcome for P.O.W. Nurses', *The Herald* (Melbourne), *ibid.*, p. 5.
23 'Nurses Return', *The West Australian* (Perth), *ibid*, p. 8.
24 Manners, *Bullwinkel*, p. 185.
25 'Australian Welcome to P.O.W. Nurses', *The Age* (Melbourne), 25 October 1945, p. 3.
26 Manners, *Bullwinkel*, p. 186.
27 Sister Vivian Bullwinkel's testimony, Australian War Crimes Board of Inquiry, Melbourne, 29 October 1945, AWM54 1010/4/24B.

Chapter Twenty-seven
1   'Injured Nurse Saved Sailor', *News* (Adelaide), 6 November 1945, p. 3.

2   Barbara Helen Crowhurst (nee Shegog), b. 11 August 1890, d. 29 May 1950 (Adelaide, SA).

3   Vivienne Helen Crowhurst, b. 20 June 1931 (Adelaide, SA), d. 23 December 2010 (Strathalbyn, SA).

4   'Big Citizens Welcome to Sister Bullwinkel', *Barrier Miner* (Broken Hill), 14 January 1946, p. 3.

5   'Round of Functions for Sister V. Bullwinkel,' *Barrier Miner* (Broken Hill), 19 January 1946, p. 6.

6   'V.C. Proposal', *News* (Adelaide), 21 November 1945, p. 2.

7   'Japanese Sadism to P.O.W.s', *The Sydney Morning Herald*, 11 April 1946, p. 1.

8   *Ibid.*

9   'Sedatives Given to Japs Before Execution', *The Canberra Times*, 21 March 1946, p. 1.

10 Statham, Vivian (nee Bullwinkel), Service Number: VFX61330, NAA: A14472, VFX61330, p. 43.

11 *Ibid.*

12 Captain Mavis Hannah Interviewed by Dr Amy McGrath, 13 July 1981, Tape No. TRC 1087/1, National Library of Australia.

13 'Net Closing on Jap Murderers of Nurses', *The Herald* (Melbourne), 29 August 1946, p. 3.

14 *Ibid.*

15 Vivian Bullwinkel, address to the Hollywood RGH 40th anniversary, 16 February 1987, AWM, PR01216, 2020.545.1, Wallet 4.

16 *Ibid.*

17 Vivian Bullwinkel interview, 1993, *Vivian Bullwinkel: An Australian Heroine*, Waterbyrd Filmz, 2007.

18 Manners, *Bullwinkel*, p. 190.

19 Vivian Bullwinkel, address to the Hollywood RGH 40th anniversary, 16 February 1987, AWM, PR01216, 2020.545.1, Wallet 4.

20 'Sandakan Death March', *Cairns Post*, 21 December 1946, p. 1.

21 Manners, *Bullwinkel*, p. 192.

22 On 12 July 1948.

23 National Archives of Australia, 3004097.

24 'S.A. Nurse in New Honors List', *News* (Adelaide), 6 March 1947, p. 1.

25 'Banka Island Massacre', *The West Australian* (Perth), 31 May 1947, p. 15.

26 Vivian Bullwinkel speech after receiving Florence Nightingale Medal, 23 July 1947, AWM, PR01216, Series 4.

27 Manners, *Bullwinkel*, p. 202.

28 'About the ANMC', australiannursesmemorialcentre.org.au

29 'War Nurses Appeal for Memorial Centre', *The Riverine Herald* (Echuca), 3 January 1948, p. 7.

30 Vivian Bullwinkel, address to the Hollywood RGH 40th anniversary, 16 February 1987, AWM, PR01216, 2020.545.1, Wallet 4.

31 About the ANMC', australiannursesmemorialcentre.org.au

32 Chloe Horrabin, 'Nursing War Hero Vivian Bullwinkel's Legacy Burns Brightly', *Australian Nursing and Midwifery Journal*, 21 April 2023, anmj.org.au

33 Young, Allan [sic] Livingston, Service Number: VX47581, NAA: B883, VX47581, p. 1.

34 David Young, Interview with the author.

35 'Tokyo War Crimes Trial', nationalww2museum.org

36 'Million Mile Manhunt for Japanese War Criminals', *The Sun* (Sydney), 5 June 1950, p. 11.

37 'The Japanese', muntokpeacemuseum.org

38 'They Machine Gunned Us in the Water', *The Sunday Mail*, 20 January 2002.

39 'Nurse Speaks Out Against Japs Admission', *Sporting Globe* (Melbourne), 16 November 1949, p. 10.

Chapter Twenty-eight

1   'Bradman Receives Accolade', *The Mercury* (Hobart), 16 March 1949, p. 8.

2   Heroines in Legacy Ceremony', *The Sun* (Sydney), 17 August 1949, p. 16.

3   'Matron Paschke Memorial to be Unveiled on Sunday Week', *The Horsham Times,* 22 April 1949, p. 1.

4   'High Tribute Paid to Heroic Nursing Sister', *Barrier Daily Truth* (Broken Hill), 10 October 1949, p. 3.

5   'Ex-Army Nurses on Way to U.K.', *News* (Adelaide), 29 September 1950, p. 2.

6   Coral Craig, 'From Prison to Piccadilly', *Woman's Day and Home*, 22 January 1951, p. 9.

7   'The Good Queen', *The Age* (Melbourne), 26 March 1953, p. 5.

8   'Queen Mary Knew of Nurses Heroism', 10 April 1952, p. 4.

9   *Ibid.*

10   'The Good Queen', *The Age* (Melbourne), 26 March 1953, p. 5.

11   'Australian Heroine Abroad', *The Advertiser* (Adelaide), 17 March 1953, p. 2.

12   'London Cheers Aust. Nurses', *Brisbane Telegraph*, 6 July 1953, p. 6.

13   'Liner's Gesture to Nurse', *The Advertiser* (Adelaide), 21 September 1953, p. 4.

14   'Family Notices', 16 February 1954, p. 20.

15   'Australian Military Forces', *Commonwealth of Australia Gazette*, 26 January 1956, p. 294.

16   *Ibid.*, 22 February 1962, p. 653.

17   'Singapore Memorial', *The Australian Women's Weekly*, 27 February 1957, p. 21.

18   John Sorrell, 'War Heroine Heads Staff of Hospital', *The Age*, 22 February 1961.

19   Manners, *Bullwinkel*, p. 209.

20   David Young, Interview with the author.

21   John Bullwinkel speech at the dedication of Vivian Bullwinkel statue, 2 August 2023.

22   Joan Holland interview, *Vivian Bullwinkel: An Australian Heroine*, Waterbyrd Filmz, 2007.

23   Margaret Wiseman interview, *ibid.*

24   Dr Olga Kanitsaki interview with the author.

25   On 15 October 1965, AWM, PR01216, 2020.545.1, Wallet 2.

26   Francis West Statham, b. 25 June 1916 (Toowoomba, Qld), d. 3 December 1999 (Perth, WA).

27   Pamela Statham-Drew, 'Statham, Francis West (Frank) (1916–1999)', *Australian Dictionary of Biography*, published online 2022.

28   Manners, *Bullwinkel*, p. 211.

29   *Ibid.*, p. 212.

Chapter Twenty-nine

1   Recollections of Phyllis Schumann, 'Rescue Flight Brings Vietnamese Orphans Out of Saigon', anzacportal. dva.gov.au

2   'Vietnam Waifs Fly In', *The Sun-Herald* (Sydney), 6 April 1975, p. 1, 3.

3   Recollections of Phyllis Schumann, 'Rescue Flight Brings Vietnamese Orphans Out of Saigon', anzacportal. dva.gov.au

4   Vivian Bullwinkel interview, 1993, *Vivian Bullwinkel: An Australian Heroine*, Waterbyrd Filmz, 2007.

5   Recollections of Phyllis Schumann, 'Rescue Flight Brings Vietnamese Orphans Out of Saigon', anzacportal. dva.gov.au

6   *Ibid.*

7   Val Seeger interview, *Vivian Bullwinkel: An Australian Heroine,* Waterbyrd Filmz, 2007.

8   Recollections of Phyllis Schumann, 'Rescue Flight Brings Vietnamese Orphans Out of Saigon', anzacportal. dva.gov.au

9   Vivian Bullwinkel interview, 1993, *Vivian Bullwinkel: An Australian Heroine,* Waterbyrd Filmz, 2007.

10   Ian W. Shaw, *Operation Babylift*, Hachette, 2019, p. 224.

11   *The Age* (Melbourne), 19 April 1975.

12   Vivian Bullwinkel interview, 1993, *Vivian Bullwinkel: An Australian Heroine,* Waterbyrd Filmz, 2007.

13   Vivian Bullwinkel, address to the Hollywood RGH 40th Anniversary, 16 February 1987, AWM, PR01216, 2020.545.1, Wallet 4.

14   *Ibid.*

15   *Ibid.*

16   Margaret Wiseman interview, *Vivian Bullwinkel: An Australian Heroine.*

17   Joan Holland interview, *ibid.*

Chapter Thirty

1   Natalie Lynch, 'Little Bet You Helped Save My Life', awm.gov.au

2   Pamela Statham-Drew, 'Statham, Francis West (Frank) (1916–1999)', *Australian Dictionary of Biography*, published online 2022.

3   Vivian Bullwinkel, Address to the Graduates of No. 144 Pilots Course, Point Cook, Victoria, 1988, AWM 2020.545.1, Wallet 4.

4   Manners, *Bullwinkel*, p. 222.

5   Vivian Bullwinkel interview, 1993, *Vivian Bullwinkel: An Australian Heroine,* Waterbyrd Filmz, 2007.

6   Manners, *Bullwinkel*, p. 224.
7   'Nurses Dedicate Island Memorial',
    Army, 8 April 1993, p. 6.
8   'Bangka Island', anzacday.org.au
9   'Bangka Island', anzacday.org.au
10 Norman Abjorensen, 'Murdered Nurses
    Were Probably Raped by Japanese
    Officers Says Academic', *The Canberra
    Times*, 22 September 1993, p. 3.
11 *Ibid.*
12 Ralph Armstrong, *A Short Cruise on
    the Vyner Brooke*, George Mann, 2003,
    pp. 53-54.
13 Author interview with Vivian
    Bullwinkel's nephew John Bullwinkel.
14 'Memorial Salutes Dedicated Service
    of Uniformed Angels', *Army*, 6 March
    1997, p. 4.
15 Eric Germann to Vivian Bullwinkel,
    15 December 1998, John Bullwinkel
    collection.
16 *Ibid.*
17 'Eric Harrison Germann',
    muntokpeacemuseum.org.
18 Eric Germann to Vivian Bullwinkel,
    15 December 1998, John Bullwinkel
    collection.
19 Tom Moody, 'Bangka Island massacre
    survivor Ernest Lloyd was one of three
    survivors of a horrific war crime',
    southwalesargus.co.uk, 27 May 2019.
20 Edie Leembruggen interview, *Vivian
    Bullwinkel: An Australian Heroine*,
    Waterbyrd Filmz, 2007.
21 Peter Cosgrove interview, *ibid.*

Epilogue
1   John Bullwinkel speech at the
    dedication of Vivian Bullwinkel statue,
    2 August 2023.
2   Niki Burnside and James Vyver,
    'Australian War Memorial Criticised
    for Not Funding Statue of Lieutenant
    Colonel Vivian Bullwinkel', abc.net.au,
    2 August 2023.
3   Claire Hunter, 'Guess You Will Be
    Thinking I've Gone Up in Smoke',
    awm.gov.au, 20 June 2018.
4   Tess Lawrence, 'Vivian Bullwinkel, the
    Bangka Island Massacre and the Guilt of
    the Survivor', independentaustralia.net,
    19 February 2017.
5   *Ibid.*
6   Ellen Fanning, 'A War Crime Has Been
    Censored', abc.net.au, 2 June 2023.
7   Interview with the author.
8   *Ibid.*
9   *Ibid.*
10 Gary Nunn, 'Bangka Island: The WW2
    Massacre and a "Truth Too Awful to
    Speak"', bbc.com, 18 April 2019.
11 Professor Kylie Ward speech at the
    dedication of Vivian Bullwinkel statue,
    2 August 2023.

In memory of

Olive Paschke, Vima Bates, Ellenor Calnan, Mary Clarke, Millie Dorsch, Caroline Ennis, Kit Kinsella, Gladys McDonald, Lavinia Russell, Marjorie Schuman, Merle Trenerry, and Mona Wilton, who were lost at sea off Bangka Island

and of

Lainie Balfour-Ogilvy, Alma Beard, Ada Bridge, Flo Casson, Mary Cuthbertson, Irene Drummond, 'Buddy' Elmes, Lorna Fairweather, Peggy Farmaner, Clarice Halligan, Nancy Harris, Minnie Hodgson, Ellen Keats, Janet 'Jenny' Kerr, Ellie McGlade, Kathleen Neuss, Flo Salmon, Jean Stewart, Mona Tait, Rosetta Wight, and Bessie Wilmott, who were murdered on Radji Beach

Pearl Mittelheuser, Win Davis, Blanche Hempsted, Gladys Hughes, Mina Raymont, Rene Singleton, Shirley Gardam and Dot Freeman, who died as Prisoners of War

Vivian Bullwinkel (Statham), Jean Ashton, Pat Blake (Dixon), Jessie Blanch (Eaton-Lee), Veronica Clancy (Turner), Cecilia Delforce (McPhee), Jess Doyle (MacAuley), Jenny Greer (Pemberton), Pat Gunther (Darling), Mavis Hannah (Allgrove), Iole Harper (Burkitt), Nesta James (Noy), Betty Jeffrey, Vi McElnea, Sylvia Muir (McGregor), Wilma Oram (Young), Chris Oxley, Eileen Short, Jessie Simons (Hookway), Val Smith, Mickey Syer (Corbitt), Flo Trotter (Syer), Joyce Tweddell, and Beryl Woodbridge, who made it home.

RIP